D0874360

THE WASHINGTON MANUAL™

Infectious Diseases   Subspecialty Consult

SECOND EDITION

Editors

Nigar Kirmani, MD

Professor of Medicine
Division of Infectious Diseases
Department of Internal Medicine
Washington University School of Medicine
St. Louis, Missouri

Keith F. Woeltje, MD, PhD

Professor of Medicine
Division of Infectious Diseases
Department of Internal Medicine
Washington University School of Medicine
St. Louis, Missouri

Hilary M. Babcock, MD

Assistant Professor of Medicine
Division of Infectious Diseases
Department of Internal Medicine
Washington University School of Medicine
St. Louis, Missouri

Series Editors

Thomas M. De Fer, MD

Professor of Medicine
Washington University School of Medicine
St. Louis, Missouri

Katherine E. Henderson, MD

Assistant Professor of Clinical Medicine
Department of Medicine
Washington University School of Medicine
Barnes-Jewish Hospital
St. Louis, Missouri

PRAIRIE STATE COLLEGE
LIBRARY

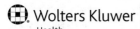 Wolters Kluwer | Lippincott Williams & Wilkins
Health
Philadelphia • Baltimore • New York • London
Buenos Aires • Hong Kong • Sydney • Tokyo

Senior Acquisitions Editor: Sonya Seigafuse
Senior Product Manager: Kerry Barrett
Vendor Manager: Alicia Jackson
Senior Marketing Manager: Kimberly Schonberger
Senior Manufacturing Manager: Benjamin Rivera
Editorial Coordinator: Katie Sharp
Design Coordinator: Stephen Druding
Production Service: Integra Software Services Pvt. Ltd.

© **2013 by Department of Medicine, Washington University School of Medicine**

Printed in China

All rights reserved. This book is protected by copyright. No part of this book may be reproduced in any form by any means, including photocopying, or utilized by any information storage and retrieval system without written permission from the copyright owner, except for brief quotations embodied in critical articles and reviews. Materials appearing in this book prepared by individuals as part of their official duties as U.S. government employees are not covered by the above-mentioned copyright.

Library of Congress Cataloging-in-Publication Data

The Washington manual infectious diseases subspecialty consult. —2nd ed. / editors, Nigar Kirmani, Keith F. Woeltje, Hilary M. Babcock.
  p. ; cm. — (Washington manual subspecialty consult series)
  Infectious diseases subspecialty consult
  Includes bibliographical references and index.
  ISBN 978-1-4511-1364-8 — ISBN 1-4511-1364-1
  I. Kirmani, Nigar. II. Woeltje, Keith F. III. Babcock, Hilary. IV. Washington University (Saint Louis, Mo.). School of Medicine. V. Title: Infectious diseases subspecialty consult. VI. Series: Washington manual subspecialty consult series.
  [DNLM: 1. Communicable Diseases—Handbooks. 2. Diagnosis, Differential—Handbooks. 3. Patient Care Planning—Handbooks. WC 39]

616.9—dc23

2012025731

The Washington Manual™ is an intent-to-use mark belonging to Washington University in St. Louis to which international legal protection applies. The mark is used in this publication by LWW under license from Washington University.

Care has been taken to confirm the accuracy of the information presented and to describe generally accepted practices. However, the authors, editors, and publisher are not responsible for errors or omissions or for any consequences from application of the information in this book and make no warranty, expressed or implied, with respect to the currency, completeness, or accuracy of the contents of the publication. Application of the information in a particular situation remains the professional responsibility of the practitioner.

The authors, editors, and publisher have exerted every effort to ensure that drug selection and dosage set forth in this text are in accordance with current recommendations and practice at the time of publication. However, in view of ongoing research, changes in government regulations, and the constant flow of information relating to drug therapy and drug reactions, the reader is urged to check the package insert for each drug for any change in indications and dosage and for added warnings and precautions. This is particularly important when the recommended agent is a new or infrequently employed drug.

Some drugs and medical devices presented in the publication have Food and Drug Administration (FDA) clearance for limited use in restricted research settings. It is the responsibility of the health care provider to ascertain the FDA status of each drug or device planned for use in their clinical practice.

To purchase additional copies of this book, call our customer service department at (800) 638-3030 or fax orders to (301) 223-2320. International customers should call (301) 223-2300.

Visit Lippincott Williams & Wilkins on the Internet: at LWW.com. Lippincott Williams & Wilkins customer service representatives are available from 8:30 am to 6 pm, EST.

10 9 8 7 6 5 4 3 2 1

CCS1012

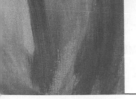

Contributing Authors

Hilary M. Babcock, MD
Assistant Professor of Medicine
Division of Infectious Diseases
Department of Internal Medicine
Washington University School of Medicine
St. Louis, Missouri

Thomas C. Bailey, MD
Professor of Medicine
Division of Infectious Diseases
Department of Internal Medicine
Washington University School of Medicine
St. Louis, Missouri

Erik R. Dubberke, MD
Assistant Professor of Medicine
Division of Infectious Diseases
Department of Internal Medicine
Washington University School of Medicine
St. Louis, Missouri

Michael J. Durkin, MD
Instructor in Medicine
Division of Infectious Diseases
Department of Internal Medicine
Washington University School of Medicine
St. Louis, Missouri

Jessica R. Grubb, MD
Assistant Professor of Medicine
Division of Infectious Diseases
Department of Internal Medicine
Washington University School of Medicine
St. Louis, Missouri

José E. Hagan, MD
Clinical Fellow
Division of Infectious Diseases
Department of Internal Medicine
Washington University School of Medicine
St. Louis, Missouri

Zhuolin Han, MD
Clinical Fellow
Division of Infectious Diseases
Department of Internal Medicine
Washington University School of Medicine
St. Louis, Missouri

Jeffrey P. Henderson, MD
Assistant Professor of Medicine
Division of Infectious Diseases
Department of Internal Medicine
Washington University School of Medicine
St. Louis, Missouri

Hitoshi Honda, MD
Clinical Fellow
Division of Infectious Diseases
Department of Internal Medicine
Washington University School of Medicine
St. Louis, Missouri

Cynthia Johnson, MD
Clinical Fellow
Division of Infectious Diseases
Department of Internal Medicine
Washington University School of Medicine
St. Louis, Missouri

Amelia M. Kasper, MD
Resident
Division of Infectious Diseases
Department of Internal Medicine
Washington University School of Medicine
St. Louis, Missouri

Nigar Kirmani, MD
Professor of Medicine
Division of Infectious Diseases
Department of Internal Medicine
Washington University School of Medicine
St. Louis, Missouri

Robyn S. Klein, MD
Associate Professor of Medicine
Division of Infectious Diseases
Department of Internal Medicine
Washington University School of Medicine
St. Louis, Missouri

F. Matthew Kuhlmann, MD
Instructor of Medicine
Division of Infectious Diseases
Department of Internal Medicine
Washington University School of Medicine
St. Louis, Missouri

Michael A. Lane, MD
Assistant Professor of Medicine
Division of Infectious Diseases
Department of Internal Medicine
Washington University School of Medicine
St. Louis, Missouri

Steven J. Lawrence, MD
Assistant Professor of Medicine
Division of Infectious Diseases
Department of Internal Medicine
Washington University School of Medicine
St. Louis, Missouri

Susana Lazarte, MD
Clinical Fellow
Division of Infectious Diseases
Department of Internal Medicine
Washington University School of Medicine
St. Louis, Missouri

Stephen Y. Liang, MD
Clinical Fellow
Division of Infectious Diseases
Department of Internal Medicine
Washington University School of Medicine
St. Louis, Missouri

Luis A. Marcos, MD
Clinical Fellow
Division of Infectious Diseases
Department of Internal Medicine
Washington University School of Medicine
St. Louis, Missouri

Jonas Marschall, MD
Assistant Professor of Medicine
Division of Infectious Diseases
Department of Internal Medicine
Washington University School of Medicine
St. Louis, Missouri

Jay R. McDonald, MD
Assistant Professor of Medicine
Division of Infectious Diseases
Department of Internal Medicine
Washington University School of Medicine
St. Louis, Missouri

Diana Nurutdinova, MD
Instructor in Medicine
Division of Infectious Diseases
Department of Internal Medicine
Washington University School of Medicine
St. Louis, Missouri

Rachel Presti, MD
Assistant Professor of Medicine
Division of Infectious Diseases
Department of Internal Medicine
Washington University School of Medicine
St. Louis, Missouri

Hilary Reno, MD
Instructor in Medicine
Division of Infectious Diseases
Department of Internal Medicine
Washington University School of Medicine
St. Louis, Missouri

David J. Riddle, MD
Instructor in Medicine
Division of Infectious Diseases
Department of Internal Medicine
Washington University School of Medicine
St. Louis, Missouri

David J. Ritchie, PharmD
Clinical Pharmacist, Infectious Diseases
Barnes-Jewish Hospital
Professor of Pharmacy Practice
St. Louis College of Pharmacy
St. Louis, Missouri

Carlos Santos, MD
Assistant Professor of Medicine
Division of Infectious Diseases
Department of Internal Medicine
Washington University School of Medicine
St. Louis, Missouri

Molly F. Sarikonda, MD
Clinical Fellow
Division of Infectious Diseases
Department of Internal Medicine
Washington University School of Medicine
St. Louis, Missouri

Toshibumi Taniguchi, MD
Clinical Fellow
Division of Infectious Diseases
Department of Internal Medicine
Washington University School of Medicine
St. Louis, Missouri

Brent W. Wieland, MD
Clinical Fellow
Division of Infectious Diseases
Department of Internal Medicine
Washington University School of Medicine
St. Louis, Missouri

Keith F. Woeltje, MD, PhD
Professor of Medicine
Division of Infectious Diseases
Department of Internal Medicine
Washington University School of Medicine
St. Louis, Missouri

Chairman's Note

I t is a pleasure to present the new edition of *The Washington Manual™ Subspecialty Consult Series: Infectious Diseases Subspecialty Consult.* This pocket-size book continues to be a primary reference for medical students, interns, residents, and other practitioners who need ready access to practical clinical information to diagnose and treat patients with a wide variety of disorders. Medical knowledge continues to increase at an astounding rate, which creates a challenge for physicians to keep up with the biomedical discoveries, genetic and genomic information, and novel therapeutics that can positively impact patient outcomes. The *Washington Manual Subspecialty Series* addresses this challenge by concisely and practically providing current scientific information for clinicians to aid them in the diagnosis, investigation, and treatment of common medical conditions.

I want to personally thank the authors, who include house officers, fellows, and attendings at Washington University School of Medicine and Barnes-Jewish Hospital. Their commitment to patient care and education is unsurpassed, and their efforts and skill in compiling this manual are evident in the quality of the final product. In particular, I would like to acknowledge our editors, Drs. Nigar Kirmani, Keith Woeltje, and Hilary Babcock, and the series editors, Drs. Tom De Fer and Katherine Henderson, who have worked tirelessly to produce another outstanding edition of this manual. I would also like to thank Dr. Melvin Blanchard, Chief of the Division of Medical Education in the Department of Medicine at Washington University School of Medicine, for his advice and guidance. I believe this Subspecialty Manual will meet its desired goal of providing practical knowledge that can be directly applied at the bedside and in outpatient settings to improve patient care.

Victoria J. Fraser, MD
Dr. J. William Campbell Professor
Interim Chairman of Medicine
Codirector of the Infectious Disease Division
Washington University School of Medicine

Preface

We are delighted to introduce the long-awaited second edition of *The Washington Manual™ Infectious Diseases Subspecialty Consult*. The chapters have been contributed primarily by faculty and fellows from the Infectious Diseases Division in the Department of Internal Medicine at the Washington University School of Medicine in St. Louis.

Infectious disease is an exciting field in constant evolution. Even since the release of the first edition of this manual, there have been new diseases, new diagnostic methods, and new treatment challenges with the development of multiple-drug–resistant organisms. There continues to be a need for specialists in this field. Infectious disease specialists treat patients of all ages, deal with all organ systems, and collaborate with nearly all other medical specialties and subspecialties. In infectious disease, no case is exactly the same, so there is no "cookbook" approach to these problems. This makes each case intriguing, and even the most mundane cases have appeal. It is our hope that this manual stimulates interest in infectious disease among its readers and inspires them to pursue a career in this specialty.

This manual complements the *Washington Manual of Medical Therapeutics* by providing more in-depth coverage of infectious diseases. We have focused on providing easy-to-follow guidance for the diagnosis and treatment of infectious diseases likely to be seen by medical house officers and hospitalists. Diseases are organized primarily by organ system to facilitate generating a useful differential diagnosis based on a patient's presentation. By providing practical guidance for common problems, the manual serves not as a comprehensive textbook, but rather as a go-to reference that can be kept handy on the wards.

It should be noted that the dosing information in the text assumes normal renal function unless otherwise indicated. Dosing information for impaired renal function is available in Chapter 20: Antimicrobial Agents.

We would like to offer special thanks to Katie Sharp for her extensive assistance in keeping the project organized and moving forward. This book wouldn't have been possible without her. We would also like to thank Dr. Tom De Fer in the Department of Medicine for his editorial guidance. And finally we'd like to recognize Dr. Victoria Fraser, the J. William Campbell Professor in the Department of Medicine. She is an outstanding clinician, researcher, and administrator. Initially as a faculty member, then as cochief of the Infectious Diseases Division, and now as Chair of Medicine, her mentorship has been invaluable. Thanks for everything, Vicky, even if it is exhausting trying to keep up with you.

N.K.
K.F.W.
H.M.B.

Contents

Approach to the Infectious Disease Consultation

F. Matthew Kuhlmann and Hilary M. Babcock

GENERAL PRINCIPLES

- The greatest challenge in the infectious disease consultation is the breadth of the subspecialty. Disease manifestations involve all specialties and organ systems. Infectious disease consultation requires thorough evaluation, organized thought processes, and an ability to appropriately consider rare but significant diagnoses.
- **Four general categories of infectious disease consults**
  - **Diagnostic dilemmas** are by far the most challenging consultation; they are classified as consults where a diagnosis remains elusive. Types of consults include evaluations for fever of unknown origin and other seemingly mysterious illnesses. Thorough evaluation and history describing details of the patient's potential exposures is critical.
  - **Therapeutic management** involves management of a specific infection as it relates to the overall care of the patient, such as an infected knee implant.
  - **Antibiotic management** ensures appropriate choice, dose, and duration of antibiotics for a given infection.
  - **Occupational health and infection prevention** ensure the health of employees, patients, and visitors within health care facilities.
- **The ten commandments for effective consultation**
  Established in 1983 by Goldman and others and modified by Salerno in 2007, the following rules provide a framework for effective patient care and communication with requesting physicians.[1,2] Knowing the specific expectations of the requesting physician allows you to address the concerns leading to the consultation. Always remember that a physician requests a service from the consultant much like a consumer buys products from a vendor.
  - **Determine your customer**. Are you providing *management* for a surgeon or *guidance* for an internist? What specific question should be answered?
  - **Establish urgency**. How quickly should the patient be seen? Several potential infectious diseases, such as necrotizing fasciitis or cerebral malaria, require emergent consultation to initiate proper therapy.
  - **Look for yourself**. Although one does not need to repeat every excruciating detail in written consultation, each important detail should be reconfirmed.
  - **Be as brief as appropriate**. Write concise assessments that adequately explain your rationale.
  - **Be specific and humble**. Write clear plans. Provide help in executing the plans when requested. Such help may include order writing or obtaining additional information from hospitals or health departments.
  - **Provide contingency plans**. Determine likely problems and provide guidance for their remediation. Provide around-the-clock contact information in order to assist in addressing such problems when they arise.
  - **Determine the appropriate level of management**. How much should you intervene regarding order writing and dictating patient care? This should be negotiated with the requesting physician during initial discussions.

○ **Teach with tact and pragmatism**. Provide educational materials or discussions appropriate to the given situation.

○ **Talk is essential**. Always call the requesting physician with your recommendations.

○ **Follow up daily**. Daily written notes should be provided until problems are no longer active as determined by yourself and the requesting physician. Provide appropriate long-term follow-up care.

- **"Curbside" consultation**

Frequently, requesting physicians ask for opinions based on limited conversation. Such consultations, called "curbside consultations," are considered a courtesy and promote collegiality. When providing curbside consultation, one should always speak in general terms and avoid providing absolute recommendations. Frequently, important historical details are unintentionally omitted, limiting the ability to provide accurate advice. Generalized guidelines for providing curbside consultation are provided below.

○ **Appropriate for curbside consultation**
  - Dose or duration of antibiotics for simple infections
  - Choice of antibiotics for simple infections

○ **Inappropriate for curbside consultation**
  - Complex patient problems
  - Uncertainty regarding question asked by the requesting physician
  - Infections due to highly resistant organisms, rare organisms, or bloodstream infections

- **Patient concerns**

Many patients may feel that additional questioning by a consultant is redundant or insulting. Frequently, a thorough review of the written record followed by empathetic consultations will provide improved rapport with the patient. The following suggestions may be beneficial in alleviating patient fear:

○ Advise patients that you are visiting them on the request of their primary physician and that you will work closely with that physician to provide the best care possible.

○ Consider telling the patient that you have reviewed his/her history and have additional specific questions that you would like to ask before providing an opinion on his/her care.

○ Ask the patient to confirm your brief understanding of his/her history and to supplement information with important details. After the initial conversation, specific or open-ended questions regarding the history of the patient's illness can be asked.

○ Do not provide information that directly contradicts the clinical care of the primary provider. Reasons for following a specific care plan may not be readily apparent at the time of the patient encounter and should be clarified with the requesting physician prior to instituting changes.

STRUCTURE OF CONSULT NOTES

Consult notes are written in a fashion similar to the admission history and physical. Details relating to specific sections follow.

- **History of present illness (HPI)**. The admission HPI provides the structure for the consultation HPI. Provide a thorough review of the patient's current illness (onset, severity, duration, location, etc.) and hospital course. Specific details of positive findings or pertinent negative findings from the review of systems, past medical/surgical history, family history, and social history should be included.

- **Review of systems**. A thorough review of systems should be obtained. Patients may forget to include significant history in their initial encounters. Such details may provide additional information leading to a diagnosis.
- **Past medical and surgical history**
  - Specific details should be summarized in the HPI, with additional information supplemented in the body of the consultation note.
  - Review detailed histories of immunosuppression due to illness or medications.
  - Details of surgeries and surgical findings related to infections should be summarized.
  - Pertinent vaccination history can be summarized.
- **Medications**
  - Review histories of any antimicrobial therapy that has been administered in the past several months. Note doses, durations, and any available drug levels.
  - Any immunosuppressive medications should be noted.
  - Note drugs that frequently interact with antimicrobials, especially warfarin.
- **Allergies**. Note not only the drugs, especially antibiotics, but also the type of reaction (rash vs. anaphylaxis, etc.).
- **Social history**. This section could be alternatively named *exposure history*, as many behaviors place patients at risk for specific infections. General topics to review include the following:
  - *Living environment.* In what geographical region does the patient reside? Does the patient live in a stable home or is he/she homeless? Does the patient live in an urban or rural environment?
  - *Work history.* Different jobs involve exposures to various infectious or toxic agents.
  - *Animals.* Specific zoonoses can be diagnosed based on the exposures to certain domestic or wild animals.
  - *Travel history.* The patient may have traveled to areas that harbor specific infections, even within their native country. Any travel history over a patient's lifetime may be considered important.
  - *Sexual history.* The number of partners places a patient at risk for sexually transmitted infections, and the nature of such interactions may be important, leading to additional diagnoses, e.g., oropharyngeal gonococcal infections.
- **Physical exam**. A detailed exam can provide additional clues to the cause of a patient's illness or complications from a patient's medical interventions. Rashes are highly indicative of specific infections or toxicities from antibiotics. Thorough dermatological, oral, ocular, and lymph node exams are especially important. Detailed descriptions of infected lesions remain essential.
- **Data**
  - One should review all serological, radiological, and pathological studies and consider reviewing the data with the microbiologist, radiologist, or pathologist.
  - Trends in routine chemistries should be described, as they are much more informative than one isolated time point. Note the differential on complete blood counts as neutropenia and lymphopenia are not evident from the total blood cell count. For patients receiving long-term antibiotics, recent liver function testing should be noted.
  - Note specific details of microbiological culture data, both positive and negative cultures.
    - Site of collection (e.g., peripheral vs. central line, right arm vs. left arm, specific drains)
    - Time of collection

- Full susceptibility profiles
- All identified microorganisms
  - Especially note any prior serological data such as viral, fungal, or bacterial antibody titers.
- **Assessment.** Summarize the case and describe the rationale for your recommendations as noted in the ten commandments for effective consultation; communicate your assessment directly to the requesting physician.
- **Plan.** Outline your recommendations in an easy-to-read format, supplement with details only if they are not provided in your assessment.

REFERENCES

1. Goldman L, Lee T, Rudd P. Ten commandments for effective consultations. *Arch Intern Med.* 1983;143:1753-1755.
2. Salerno SM, Hurst FP, Halvorson S, Mercado DL. Principles of effective consultation: an update for the 21st-century consultant. *Arch Intern Med.* 2007;167:271-275.

The Acute Febrile Patient and Sepsis

Stephen Y. Liang and Jay R. McDonald

APPROACH TO THE ACUTE FEBRILE PATIENT

GENERAL PRINCIPLES

Definition

- Fever has classically been defined as a body temperature of ≥38.0°C (100.4°F). Recent evidence suggests that the upper limit of normal oral temperature may be 37.2°C (98.9°F) in the early morning and 37.7°C (99.9°F) overall in healthy adults, though significant variability exists between individuals.[1]
- Febrile response in the elderly patient is frequently blunted, leading some to define fever in this population as a persistent oral temperature ≥37.2°C (98.9°F), rectal temperature ≥37.5°C (99.5°F), or a rise in temperature of ≥1.3°C (2.3°F) above baseline.[2]
- Oral temperatures are generally 0.4°C (0.7°F) lower than rectal temperatures. Axillary and tympanic temperatures may be unreliable.

Etiology

- Infectious causes of fever lasting less than 2 weeks are legion and may range from self-limited viral to serious bacterial infections. Differential diagnosis hinges heavily upon the history and physical examination. Fevers of unknown origin lasting more than 3 weeks are discussed in Chapter 3.
- Noninfectious causes of fever may include neoplastic, rheumatologic, endocrine, thromboembolic, and medication-related disorders.
- While hyperpyrexia (>41.5°C or 106.7°F) may be encountered with severe infection, it is more common with central nervous system hemorrhage.
- **Hyperthermia** is a distinct entity apart from fever and may result from environmental factors, endocrine disorders (hyperthyroidism), and certain medications (e.g., anesthetics, neuroleptic agents, recreational drugs).

Pathophysiology

- Thermoregulation is mediated by the hypothalamus.
- Exogenous pyrogens (e.g., microbes, toxins) induce host macrophages and other phagocytic cells, triggering the release of endogenous cytokines (e.g., interleukin [IL]-1, IL-6, tumor necrosis factor [TNF]-α, interferons).
- These endogenous pyrogens modulate an inflammatory acute phase response and promote prostaglandin E2 (PGE2) synthesis. It is thought that PGE2 acts upon the hypothalamus, precipitating a rise in body temperature.

DIAGNOSIS

Clinical Presentation

History
- **Clarify the patient's definition of "fever,"** whether it is subjective, tactile, or measured, and if so, by what route. Characterize the magnitude, duration, and consistency of the fever.
- **Establish a time line of all symptoms** in relation to the start of the fever. While the cause may be obvious in many cases, a thorough review of systems may uncover additional symptomatology characteristic of specific infections (e.g., myalgias, rashes, lymphadenopathy). Look for temporal relationships between fever and medical interventions (e.g., surgeries, catheters, mechanical ventilation, antibiotics, prolonged hospitalizations).
- **Ascertain the immune status of the patient.** Neoplasm, chemotherapy, immunosuppressive therapy (to prevent transplant rejection or treat rheumatologic disorders), corticosteroid use, human immunodeficiency virus (HIV) infection, and primary immunodeficiency disease (e.g., humoral immune or severe combined immunodeficiencies) all influence the spectrum of infections possible.
- Obtain a complete past medical history, surgical history (including all prosthetics, foreign materials, and implantable devices), and medication list (prescription, over-the-counter, alternative). Use of antipyretics should be noted. When available, a vaccination record should be reviewed, particularly in asplenic and immunocompromised patients.
- A social history should identify environmental, occupational, recreational, sexual, dietary, animal, and travel exposures as well as sick contacts.
- Family members can frequently provide additional insight into the patient's illness and exposure history.

Physical Examination
A thorough and methodical approach to the physical examination helps ensure that subtle findings are not missed (see Table 2-1).

Febrile Syndromes
- When used in conjunction with the history and physical, common febrile syndromes help guide the differential diagnosis by suggesting organ-specific disease processes.
- Fever and headache is concerning for meningitis, while fever with focal neurological deficits or seizure may suggest encephalitis, cerebral abscess, subdural empyema, or epidural abscess.
- Fever and chest pain mandates a search for pneumonia, but may also be seen with pericarditis, esophagitis, and mediastinitis.
- Depending on the location and history, fever and abdominal pain may raise the suspicion of cholecystitis, appendicitis, intra-abdominal abscess, peritonitis, diverticulitis, colitis, or a host of other pathologies.
- Other febrile syndromes (e.g., rash [Table 2-2], lymphadenopathy [Table 2-3], jaundice, and splenomegaly) may be indicative of an underlying systemic infection (Table 2-4).

TABLE 2-1	PHYSICAL EXAMINATION FINDINGS AND CLINICAL SYNDROMES TO CONSIDER IN THE PATIENT WITH FEVER
Location	**Findings and associations**
Eyes	Retinitis and other lesions (e.g., Roth spots), uveitis, hypopyon, conjunctival suffusion/hemorrhage, conjunctivitis, visual field deficits
Ears	Otitis media/externa, mastoiditis
Face, nose, throat	Sinus tenderness, pharyngitis (erythema, exudate), mucosal lesions, thrush, periodontitis, peritonsillar abscess, muffled voice (epiglottitis)
Neck	Neck stiffness (meningitis, retropharyngeal abscess), tenderness along the sternocleidomastoid muscle (internal jugular septic thrombophlebitis), thyromegaly
Heart	Murmurs (endocarditis), rubs, distant sounds
Lungs	Crackles, rhonchi, wheezes, dullness to percussion
Abdomen	Focal tenderness, peritoneal signs, hepatomegaly, splenomegaly, ascites
Genitourinary/ rectum	Male: urethritis, prostatitis, orchitis, epididymitis
	Female: cervicitis, adnexal mass/tenderness, foreign body (e.g., tampon)
	Rectum: perirectal fluctuance (abscess), ulcers, Fournier gangrene
Back	Pressure sores, decubitus ulcers, costovertebral angle tenderness
Extremities	Stigmata of endocarditis (Osler nodes, Janeway lesions, splinter hemorrhages), clubbing, palmar/plantar rashes, track marks
Neuro	Altered mental status, focal neurologic deficits, ataxia
Skin	Cellulitis, cutaneous abscess, sinus tracts, crepitus, necrotizing soft tissue infection, rash (petechiae, purpura, macules, papules, vesicles, ulcers, eschars)
Musculoskeletal	Effusion, septic arthritis, spinous process tenderness
Lymph	Any lymphadenopathy, lymph node fluctuance or drainage
Devices	Pacemaker/defibrillator, tunneled intravenous catheter, implantable port, orthopedic hardware

Diagnostic Testing

Laboratories
- **Initial testing**
  - ○ Laboratory evaluation of fever should be driven by the nature and severity of the patient's symptoms. In the inpatient setting, the following tests are a reasonable starting point to screen for abnormalities:
    - ▪ Complete blood count with differential (leukocytosis, neutrophilia, bandemia, neutropenia, anemia, thrombocytopenia)
    - ▪ Metabolic panel (hyponatremia, acidosis, impaired renal function)

TABLE 2-2	DIFFERENTIAL DIAGNOSIS OF INFECTIONS CAUSING FEVER AND RASH	
Rash	**Potential causes**	
Petechiae/purpura	Meningococcemia	RMSF
	Gonococcemia	Relapsing fever
	Subacute bacterial endocarditis	Rat bite fever
	Enterovirus	Hepatitis B (acute)
	EBV	Viral hemorrhagic fevers
	Rubella	
Macules/papules	Lyme disease	Typhoid fever (rose spots)
	Meningococcemia	Syphilis (secondary)
	Gonococcemia	RMSF and other *Rickettsia*
	Mycoplasma	Typhus (epidemic, murine, and scrub)
	Adenovirus	Parvovirus B19
	Enterovirus	Hepatitis B
	EBV	Rubeola
	HHV-6	Rubella
	Coxsackievirus	HIV
		Dengue
Nodules	Ecthyma gangrenosum (*Pseudomonas* sepsis)	Disseminated fungal infection (candidiasis, histoplasmosis, blastomycosis, coccidioidomycosis, sporotrichosis)
	Disseminated atypical mycobacterial infection	
Erythema nodosum	*Streptococcus* spp.	Mycobacteria
	Yersinia spp.	Histoplasmosis
	Mycoplasma pneumoniae	Coccidioidomycosis
	Chlamydia spp.	
Vesicles	Enterovirus	VZV
	Echovirus	Coxsackievirus (hand-foot-mouth)
	HSV	Poxviruses
Pustules	*Pseudomonas aeruginosa*	Gonococcemia
	Staphylococcus spp.	
Bullae	*Streptococcus* spp. (group A)	*Pseudomonas aeruginosa*
	Staphylococcus spp.	*Vibrio vulnificus*

Ulcers	Anthrax	Melioidosis
	Chancroid	Mycobacteria
	Glanders	Plague
	Granuloma inguinale	Syphilis
	Leprosy	Tularemia
	Lymphogranuloma venereum	Dracunculiasis
	All invasive fungal infections	Amebiasis
	HSV	Leishmania
Eschars	*Rickettsia* spp.	Tularemia
	Anthrax	Plague
	Poxvirus	Disseminated aspergillosis
		Blastomycosis
	Leishmaniasis	Mucormycosis
Lesions involving the palms and soles	Meningococcemia	RMSF and other *Rickettsia* spp.
	Subacute bacterial endocarditis	Ehrlichiosis
		Rat bite fever
	Syphilis (secondary)	VZV
	Enterovirus	
Oral lesions	HSV	Enterovirus
	VZV	Syphilis (secondary)
		Histoplasmosis (ulcer)

CMV, cytomegalovirus; EBV, Epstein-Barr virus; HSV, herpes simplex virus; HHV, human herpes virus; HIV, human immunodeficiency virus; RMSF, Rocky Mountain spotted fever; VZV, varicella zoster virus.

- Liver tests (transaminitis, cholestasis)
- Coagulation studies (disseminated intravascular coagulation)
- Urinalysis (urinary tract infection, active urinary sediment)
- HIV screening is strongly recommended, particularly in high-prevalence areas.
- **Cultures should be obtained prior to antimicrobials whenever possible.** However, collection of cultures should not delay antimicrobial administration in an unstable patient.
  - Blood cultures (preferably a minimum of 2 to 3) should be obtained from a febrile patient within the first 24 hours of presentation when endocarditis, bacteremia, or catheter-associated bloodstream infection is suspected. Each culture should consist of 20 to 30 mL of blood drawn from a single site at a single time point. In the case of catheter-associated bloodstream infection, at least one culture should be obtained through the infected catheter. Specialized blood culture media may be required to effectively isolate fungi, mycobacteria, viruses, and rare organisms (e.g., *Brucella* spp.).
  - Urine cultures should be obtained if a urinary tract infection is suspected.

TABLE 2-3	DIFFERENTIAL DIAGNOSIS OF INFECTIONS CAUSING FEVER AND LYMPHADENOPATHY	
Distribution	**Potential causes**	
Generalized	Cat scratch disease	Brucellosis
	Syphilis (secondary)	Mycobacteria
	Typhoid fever	Leptospirosis
	CMV	Rubella
	EBV	Rubeola
	HIV	Dengue
	Histoplasmosis	Toxoplasmosis
	Blastomycosis	Visceral leishmaniasis
	Coccidioidomycosis	
Cervical	Streptococci (group A)	Mycobacteria
	Diphtheria	EBV
	Numerous other viruses	
Regional	Streptococci	Mycobacteria
	Staphylococci	Tularemia
	Cat scratch disease	Plague
	Syphilis (secondary, epitrochlear)	Typhus
	HSV	Sporotrichosis
	Toxoplasmosis	Filariasis
	Trypanosomiasis	
Inguinal	Syphilis (primary)	Lymphogranuloma venereum
	Chancroid	Granuloma inguinale
	HSV	

CMV, cytomegalovirus; EBV, Epstein-Barr virus; HSV, herpes simplex virus; HIV, human immunodeficiency virus.

- Sputum and bronchoalveolar lavage cultures may be obtained to guide antibiotic therapy of pneumonia, particularly in intensive care unit (ICU) and severely immunocompromised patients where fungal and mycobacterial infections are also suspected.
  - Stool cultures, parasite examination, and tests for *Clostridium difficile* infection should be considered in a febrile patient with diarrhea.
  ○ If osteomyelitis is suspected, an erythrocyte sedimentation rate and C-reactive protein may be helpful if highly elevated.
- **Subsequent testing**
  ○ In cases where meningitis or encephalitis is suspected, lumbar puncture should be performed before the initiation of antibiotics if possible. Cerebrospinal fluid should be sent for cell count, glucose, protein, culture, Gram stain, culture, and other specialized tests based on clinical suspicion.

TABLE 2-4	DIFFERENTIAL DIAGNOSIS OF INFECTIOUS CAUSES OF SELECTED FEBRILE SYNDROMES	
Syndrome	**Potential causes**	
Fever and jaundice	Sepsis	Q fever
	Cholangitis	Leptospirosis
	Hepatic abscesses	
	CMV	Viral hepatitis
	EBV	Rift Valley fever
	HIV	Viral hemorrhagic fevers
	Malaria	Fascioliasis
	Hepatic flukes	
Fever and splenomegaly	Endocarditis	Brucellosis
	Typhoid fever	Rickettsiosis
	Miliary tuberculosis	
	EBV	CMV
	Malaria	Echinococcosis
	Visceral leishmaniasis	Trypanosomiasis
	Schistosomiasis	
Fever without localizing symptoms	Tuberculosis	Brucellosis
	Endocarditis	Q fever
	Mycotic aneurysm	Rat bite fever
	Intra-abdominal abscess	Leptospirosis
	Osteomyelitis	Rickettsiosis
	Typhoid fever	Ehrlichiosis
	Cat scratch disease	Whipple disease
	CMV	HIV
	Coccidioidomycosis	Toxoplasmosis
	Histoplasmosis	Malaria

CMV, cytomegalovirus; EBV, Epstein-Barr virus; HIV, human immunodeficiency virus.

○ As a general rule, all fluid collections suspected of being infected (e.g., pleural fluid, ascites, abscess) should be sampled and sent for cell count, culture, and other appropriate analytic studies.

○ Superinfected chronic wounds (e.g., decubitus or diabetic foot ulcers) should be debrided first and then cultured from the base of the wound. Superficial cultures are contaminated with skin flora that may or may not be responsible for the infection.

○ Intravascular catheters strongly suspected as sources of infection should be removed after blood cultures are obtained through the lumen and the catheter tip should be sent for culture.

○ Throat and nasopharyngeal cultures may help identify viral and streptococcal upper respiratory infections. Testing for influenza, particularly in immunocompromised and elderly patients, should be considered if the season is appropriate or an epidemic is underway.

○ Disease-specific serologies and other specialized laboratory tests (e.g., polymerase chain reaction [PCR]) may be indicated in the appropriate clinical context.

Imaging
- Chest radiography should be obtained if pulmonary complaints exist.
- Computed tomography (CT), magnetic resonance imaging, ultrasound, and nuclear studies may be indicated based on presenting symptoms and clinical suspicion. Consultation with a radiologist regarding the best modality for visualizing pathology (e.g., abscess, osteomyelitis, cerebral disease) can be helpful in avoiding excessive imaging.
- Echocardiography should be pursued if endocarditis is suspected based on the presence of a new heart murmur and other clinical criteria.

Diagnostic Procedures
- Tissue biopsy for pathology, culture, and other specialized testing may be needed to establish diagnoses of osteomyelitis, disorders associated with lymphadenopathy (e.g., cat scratch disease, toxoplasmosis), and disseminated infections (e.g., tuberculosis, atypical mycobacteria, histoplasmosis).
- When possible, appropriate cultures should be obtained during any surgical intervention to treat an infectious complication (e.g., endocarditis, pacemaker lead infection, graft or hardware infection).

TREATMENT

Antimicrobial Therapy
- In the outpatient setting, most fevers in healthy adults are associated with transient, self-limited viral infections and are frequently overtreated with antimicrobials.
- An emphasis should be placed on establishing an infectious etiology for the fever to guide appropriate antimicrobial coverage.
- Situations warranting empiric antimicrobial therapy before a definitive diagnosis can be made include the following:
  ○ Acute clinical deterioration (e.g., respiratory distress, altered mental status, hemodynamic instability, sepsis)
  ○ Immunocompromised state (e.g., HIV, neoplasm, transplant, immunosuppressive therapy)
  ○ Elderly patients (in whom atypical and muted presentations of serious infection are common)
- Choice of empiric antimicrobial should be based upon the type of infection suspected (e.g., pneumonia, meningitis, cellulitis), common microorganisms implicated, concern for multidrug resistance among those organisms, and local antimicrobial susceptibility patterns.

Antipyretic Therapy
- Antipyretics can be given for symptom relief but they do not alter outcomes. In patients with cardiovascular or pulmonary disease, antipyretics may reduce some of the metabolic demands of fever.
- Nonsteroidal antiinflammatory drugs including acetaminophen, ibuprofen, and aspirin inhibit the synthesis of inflammatory prostaglandins through the cyclooxygenase pathway and trigger other antipyretic pathways, reducing hypothalamus-mediated fever.
- Corticosteroids also have antipyretic properties but generally are not indicated for fever control alone.

- External cooling methods including cooling blankets, fans, and water sponging effect heat loss through conduction, convection, and evaporation, respectively. Rebound hyperthermia may result if antipyretic medications are not used and shivering is not controlled.

SPECIAL CONSIDERATIONS

Fever in the Intensive Care Unit

- New, unexplained fevers complicate a significant number of ICU admissions and prolonged hospitalizations.[3,4] The causes can be wide ranging, underscoring the complexity of these patients (Table 2-5).

TABLE 2-5	DIFFERENTIAL DIAGNOSIS OF A NEW FEVER IN THE INTENSIVE CARE UNIT	

Infectious	Intravascular catheter–related infection:
	  Cellulitis/abscess
	  Tunnel infection
	  Bloodstream infection
	  Suppurative phlebitis
	Pneumonia:
	  Hospital acquired
	  Ventilator associated
		Urinary tract infection
		Clostridium difficile infection
		Surgical site infection
		Sinusitis
		Otitis media
		Parotitis
		Transfusion-related infection
		Retained foreign body (e.g., tampon)

Noninfectious	Drug fever
	  Antimicrobials
	  Anticonvulsants
	  Antihistamines
	  Antihypertensives
	  Antiarrhythmics
	Neuroleptic malignant syndrome
	  Antipsychotics (haloperidol)
	Serotonin syndrome
	  Selective serotonin reuptake inhibitors
	Malignant hyperthermia
	  Succinylcholine
	  Halothane
	Withdrawal syndromes
	  Alcohol
	  Opiates
	  Barbiturates
	  Benzodiazepines
		Acalculous cholecystitis
		Acute myocardial infarction
		Adrenal insufficiency
		Cerebrovascular accident
		Gout
		Hyperthyroidism (thyroid storm)
		Intracranial hemorrhage
		Mesenteric ischemia/infarction
		Pancreatitis
		Thromboembolic diseases (deep vein thrombosis/pulmonary embolus)
		Transfusion reactions
		Tumor lysis syndrome

- In reviewing the medical history of the ICU patient, a strong emphasis should be placed on understanding not only the patient's initial clinical presentation and primary diagnosis but also the sequence of medical interventions (e.g., new medications, procedures, surgeries, health care–associated devices, respiratory support) that have taken place since admission.
- Nursing observations regarding patient hemodynamics, oxygen requirements, tracheal secretions, catheter sites, skin breakdown, wounds, diarrhea, and other clinically relevant conditions can lend valuable insight into the patient's hospital course.
- **Health care–associated infections** are responsible for a sizable portion of these fevers.
  - **Intravascular catheter–associated bloodstream infection**.[5] Infection rates differ by type (uncuffed > tunneled > peripheral), location (femoral vein > internal jugular vein > subclavian vein), duration, frequency of manipulation, and method of placement (use of sterile precautions).
    - At least one blood culture should be obtained through the infected catheter and one culture from a peripheral site by venipuncture.
    - The intravascular catheter in question should be promptly removed and the catheter tip sent for culture if sepsis, embolic disease, or tunnel infection is suspected.
    - Peripheral intravenous catheters should be changed every 72 hours regardless of fever.
  - **Ventilator-associated pneumonia**. Infection occurring more than 48 hours after endotracheal intubation and mechanical ventilation.
    - Chest radiography or CT with evolving infiltrates coupled with clinical cues (increased purulent tracheal secretions and/or oxygen requirement) help secure the diagnosis.
    - Bronchoscopy to obtain accurate lower respiratory tract cultures and Gram stains should be considered.
    - Blood cultures and diagnostic thoracentesis of associated pleural effusions may also be helpful in identifying a causative organism.
  - **Urinary tract infection**.[6] Risk factors include having an indwelling urethral catheter, suprapubic catheter, ureteral stent, or nephrostomy.
    - Urinalysis and urine culture should be obtained from the sampling port of the catheter and never the drainage bag.
    - Infected catheters should be removed promptly if possible.
  - ***C. difficile* infection**.[7] Spectrum of disease may range from diarrhea to ileus and toxic megacolon. Leukemoid reactions with extremely high white blood cell counts are occasionally seen.
    - Send a stool specimen for *C. difficile* toxin by enzyme immunoassay or PCR and for fecal leukocytes.
    - Consider empiric therapy with metronidazole or oral vancomycin if illness is severe.
  - **Sinusitis**. Nasotracheal/nasogastric intubations, nasal packing, and maxillofacial trauma may prevent drainage of the facial sinuses (especially maxillary) leading to bacterial overgrowth.
    - CT of the facial sinuses should be performed. Sinus puncture and aspiration under sterile conditions is diagnostic.
    - Empiric antibiotic therapy and removal of the nasotracheal or nasogastric tube are indicated in most cases.
  - **Surgical site infection**. See discussion on postoperative fever.

- o **Wound infection**. Prolonged or chronic debilitation increases the risk of pressure sores and decubitus ulcers, which are prone to infection.
  - Examine the back, sacrum, and other dependent areas thoroughly for wounds.
  - Document the number, size, and depth of any wounds and any signs of super-infection or necrosis.
- o **Transfusion-related infection**. However rare, bacterial infection may be trans-mitted through blood product transfusion. Cytomegalovirus (CMV) transmitted by donor leukocytes present in the blood product can precipitate a mononucleo-sis-like syndrome in healthy adults or disseminated disease in the immunocom-promised (particularly if the recipient is CMV seronegative).
  - Identify the timing of all blood product transfusions in relation to onset of fever. If a bacterial infection is suspected, obtain a recipient blood culture from a site opposite that of the transfusion and culture the donor blood product.
  - Administer leukocyte-reduced blood components to immunocompromised patients to prevent CMV disease.
- **Noninfectious causes** of a new, unexplained fever in the ICU include the following:
  - o **Drug fever**. Antimicrobials (e.g., sulfonamides, penicillins, cephalosporins, vanco-mycin, nitrofurantoin), anticonvulsants (e.g., phenytoin, carbamazepine, barbitu-rates), H1- and H2-blocking antihistamines, antihypertensives (e.g., hydralazine, methyldopa), and antiarrhythmics (e.g., quinidine, procainamide) are common offenders. Relative bradycardia, rash, leukocytosis, and eosinophilia may or may not be present.
    - Establish a time line of start and stop dates for all suspect medications (particu-larly antimicrobials).
    - The time between discontinuation of the offending agent and resolution of fever can be variable and up to a week.
  - o **Thromboembolic disease**. Deep vein thrombosis and pulmonary embolus occa-sionally present with isolated fever.
  - o **Endocrine disease**. Adrenal insufficiency and thyroid storm may present with fever, tachycardia, and hypotension that can be easily mistaken for sepsis.
  - o **Transfusion reactions**
    - **Febrile nonhemolytic transfusion reactions are common** (1 in 100 units) and occur when recipient antibodies react against antigens on donor leukocytes and platelets, triggering cytokine release anywhere from 30 minutes to several hours after a transfusion.
    - Acute hemolytic transfusion reactions result from ABO mismatch and occur when preformed recipient antibodies rapidly destroy donor erythrocytes leading to fever, flank pain, and hemoglobinuria. This is considered a medical emergency.
- Recent guidelines suggest that a body temperature of ≥38.3°C (100.9°F) or <36°C (96.8°F) is a reasonable threshold for initiating an evaluation for infection in the ICU patient. Remember that critically ill patients with serious infection may be normothermic or hypothermic in the context of extensive burns, open abdominal wounds, continuous renal replacement therapy, extracorporeal membrane oxygen-ation, or a host of medical illnesses (e.g., congestive heart failure, end-stage liver or renal disease, myxedema coma). Evaluation for infection should be guided ulti-mately by clinical suspicion.
- If infection is suspected, empiric antimicrobial therapy should be initiated imme-diately after appropriate cultures have been obtained. The risk of infection with multidrug-resistant pathogens should be taken into account along with local antimicrobial susceptibility patterns.

Postoperative Fever

- **Fever within the first 72 hours after surgery** is common and generally self-limited. Cytokine release from surgical trauma is thought to play a part.
  - ○ **Wound infections are uncommon during the first three postoperative days**. When an early infection is evident, myonecrosis secondary to *Clostridium* species and group A streptococci must be considered and may require antibiotics and emergent surgical debridement. Toxic shock syndrome may accompany serious infection with group A streptococci or *Staphylococcus aureus.*
  - ○ Noninfectious causes of fever may include thromboembolism, hematoma, transfusion reactions, and adrenal insufficiency. Malignant hyperthermia may manifest as muscle rigidity, tachycardia, and hyperthermia up to 10 hours after induction of general anesthesia.
- **Fever more than 72 hours after surgery** is significant and more likely to be associated with infection.
  - ○ Wound infections, intra-abdominal infections, abscesses, infected hematomas, and the sequelae of anastomotic leaks are typically seen around the fourth or fifth day after surgery.
  - ○ Health care–associated infections including pneumonia, urinary tract infection (in the setting of urinary catheterization), intravenous catheter–related infections (cellulitis, thrombophlebitis, bloodstream infection), and *C. difficile* infection related to antibiotic exposure are also more common.
  - ○ Acalculous cholecystitis, pancreatitis, and thromboembolism are noninfectious etiologies that must also be considered.
- Postoperative fever may also result from surgical site inflammation, seroma, or hematoma without infection.
- Classic teaching maintains that the differential diagnosis of postoperative fever should focus on the **"five Ws": wind** (pneumonia), **water** (urinary tract infection), **wound**, **walking** (thromboembolism), and **"wonder" drugs** (medication reaction). Opinions differ on whether atelectasis causes fever.
- History gathering should focus on understanding the preoperative presentation (including existing infection), surgical procedure (duration, complexity, blood products, perioperative prophylactic antibiotics, complications including intra-operative contamination; Table 2-6), and postoperative course (cough, diarrhea, pain, and changes in character or volume of surgical drain output or wound drainage). Hardware and foreign material inserted during the surgery should be documented. The possibility of drug fever should be examined through a chronology of all medications (e.g., antibiotics, anesthetics) received during and after surgery.
- Chest radiography, urinalysis, and urine culture are suggested for the evaluation of fever presenting more than 72 hours after surgery and for any febrile postoperative patient who has had a urinary catheter in place for ≥72 hours. Hemodynamic instability with concern for bacteremia or pending sepsis should prompt blood cultures.
- All surgical wounds should be examined daily for erythema, induration, and purulent discharge. Surgical and percutaneous drain reservoirs and their exit sites should likewise be inspected for evidence of infection.
- All infected surgical wounds should be cultured and in many cases opened to facilitate drainage.
- **Superficial wound cultures are seldom helpful in the absence of a clinically apparent infection**.
- If an abscess or deep infection is suspected, be aggressive about obtaining further imaging and surgical evaluation to determine whether operative or radiology-guided drainage is necessary. All fluid collections requiring drainage should be sent for culture.

TABLE 2-6	COMMON CAUSES OF POSTOPERATIVE FEVER ASSOCIATED WITH SPECIFIC TYPES OF SURGERY	
Neurosurgery	Meningitis	Posterior fossa syndrome
	Deep vein thrombosis	Hypothalamic dysfunction
	Intracranial hemorrhage	
Cardiothoracic surgery	Pneumonia	Mediastinitis
	Endocarditis	Sternal wound infection
Abdominal surgery	Abscess	Peritonitis
	Infected hematoma/seroma	Pancreatitis
	Anastomotic leak (e.g., bowel, biliary)	Splenoportal thrombosis
Obstetrical or gynecologic surgery	Urinary tract infection	Pelvic thrombophlebitis
	Pelvic abscess	Toxic shock syndrome (vaginal packing)
	Postpartum endometritis	
Urologic surgery	Urinary tract infection	Deep infection (prostate, perinephric)
Orthopedic surgery	Prosthetic infection	Deep vein thrombosis
	Infected hematoma	Fat embolism
Vascular surgery	Graft infection	Blue toe syndrome (atherothrombotic embolism)
	Postimplantation syndrome	

- Be vigilant of intravenous catheter–associated infections, *C. difficile* infection, and noninfectious causes of fever already discussed with fever in the ICU patient.
- Empiric antimicrobial therapy is generally unnecessary for fever presenting within the first 72 hours of surgery, unless infection is clinically evident or uncovered on laboratory evaluation or imaging. Continuation of perioperative prophylactic antibiotics for early postoperative fever does not prevent infection and likely selects for resistant organisms.

Fever in the Immunocompromised Patient

- Immunocompromised patients are at heightened risk not only for community-acquired infections but also for an extensive range of opportunistic infections.
- Atypical and nonspecific clinical presentations abound. Muted inflammatory responses arising from neutropenia, corticosteroids, and other forms of immuno-suppressive therapy may conceal serious infections.
- The medical history should assess the severity of the patient's immunocompromised state and risk factors for primary infection or reactivation of latent disease (Table 2-7).
- The etiology of fever in the immunocompromised patient varies depending upon the underlying disease and its subsequent therapy. Markers of immune status and approximately derived windows of susceptibility to infection help inform the differential diagnosis.
- In addition to the opportunistic infections discussed below, it is important to keep in mind that immunocompromised patients are also at risk for common community-acquired infections (e.g., bacterial pneumonia, influenza) as well as health care–associated

TABLE 2-7	KEY ASPECTS OF THE MEDICAL HISTORY IN EVALUATING THE IMMUNOCOMPROMISED PATIENT WITH FEVER
All immunocompromised patients	• Any history of tuberculosis • Chronic infections (e.g., hepatitis B and C) • Disseminated infections (e.g., mycobacteria, endemic mycoses) • Opportunistic infections (e.g., *Pneumocystis jiroveci, Cryptococcus neoformans, Toxoplasma gondii, Mycobacterium avium complex*) • Chemoprophylaxis against opportunistic infections (dose, duration) • Baseline serologies (e.g., CMV, *T. gondii*) • Known colonization with multidrug-resistant organisms • Presence of long-term intravascular access (tunneled catheters vs. implantable ports) • Sick contacts • Environmental exposures
HIV infection	• CD4+ cell count and HIV viral load • Antiretroviral therapy (date started, adherence) • Recent unprotected sex • Presence of immune reconstitution inflammatory syndrome
Chemotherapy-related neutropenia	• Type and location of neoplasm (solid organ vs. hematologic) • Chemotherapy (dose, duration, number of days since last cycle) • Other therapies (e.g., surgery, radiation) and any associated complications • Relapse vs. remission of disease
Solid organ transplantation	• Date and type of organ transplant • Immediate and delayed surgical complications associated with transplant • Immunosuppressive regimens (dose, duration, serum levels) • Presence of graft rejection • Donor and recipient CMV serology
Hematopoietic stem cell transplantation	• Date and type of transplant (allogeneic vs. autologous) • Immunosuppressive regimen (dose, duration) • Presence of GVHD • Donor CMV serology (if allogeneic transplant)

CMV, cytomegalovirus; HIV, human immunodeficiency virus; GVHD, graft versus host disease.

TABLE 2-8	DIFFERENTIAL DIAGNOSIS OF INFECTIOUS CAUSES OF FEVER IN A PATIENT WITH HIV
Meningitis/encephalitis/ other CNS disorders	Any CD4+: *Streptococcus pneumoniae, Neisseria meningitidis, Listeria monocytogenes,* HSV
	CD4+ <100: *Cryptococcus neoformans, Toxoplasma gondii* (encephalitis, cerebral abscess)
	CD4+ <50: CMV and VZV (encephalitis), EBV-associated lymphoma,[a] JC polyomavirus (progressive multifocal leukoencephalopathy)[a]
Pneumonia	Any CD4+: *S. pneumoniae, Haemophilus influenzae, Mycoplasma pneumoniae, Legionella pneumophila, Staphylococcus aureus, Mycobacterium tuberculosis*
	CD4+ <200: *Pneumocystis jiroveci,* endemic fungi
	CD4+ <100: *C. neoformans, T. gondii*
	CD4+ <50: *Mycobacterium avium complex, Aspergillus* spp., CMV, VZV
Esophagitis	CD4 <200: *Candida albicans,* CMV, HSV
Diarrhea	Any CD4+: *Salmonella, Shigella, Campylobacter, Escherichia coli, L. monocytogenes, Clostridium difficile;* rotavirus, norovirus, *Giardia lamblia*[a]
	CD4+ <100: CMV (colitis), *Cryptosporidium,*[a] *Microsporidia,*[a] *Cyclospora,*[a] *Isospora*[a]
Rash	Any CD4+: *Staphylococcus* and *Streptococcus* spp. (cellulitis, abscess); VZV (herpes zoster)
Disseminated infection	CD4+ <100 (generally): *Mycobacterium avium complex, Mycobacterium tuberculosis, Histoplasma capsulatum, Coccidioides immitis, Bartonella henselae, Penicillium marneffei, Cryptococcus neoformans*

HIV, human immunodeficiency virus; CNS, central nervous system; CMV, cytomegalovirus; HSV, herpes simplex virus; VZV, varicella zoster virus; EBV, Epstein-Barr virus.

[a]For completeness, several important opportunistic infections not typically associated with fever are included as well.

infections (e.g., intravascular catheter–associated bloodstream infection, *C. difficile* infection), given their frequent contact with the hospital environment and exposure to antimicrobials either as chemoprophylaxis or to treat active infection.

- ○ **Human immunodeficiency virus**
  - The CD4+ lymphocyte cell count is a reasonably accurate gauge of susceptibility to opportunistic infections in the HIV patient (Table 2-8).
  - Patients recently started on antiretroviral therapy may present with immune reconstitution inflammatory syndrome, an inflammatory immune response against pathogens that may have previously been clinically silent (e.g., mycobacteria, *Pneumocystis jiroveci,* endemic fungi, CMV).

- Noninfectious causes of fever particular to HIV include neoplasm (non–Hodgkin lymphoma and occasionally visceral Kaposi sarcoma), drug fever (e.g., trimethoprim–sulfamethoxazole, dapsone), hypersensitivity reaction (abacavir, nevirapine, efavirenz), and Castleman disease (angiofollicular lymph node hyperplasia).

○ **Chemotherapy-related neutropenia**
  - **Neutropenic fever.**[8] Absolute neutrophil count of <500 cells/mm^3 or <1,000 cells/mm^3 with an anticipated decline below 500 cells/mm^3 over the next 48 hours coupled with the presence of a single temperature of ≥38.3°C (100.9°F) or a persistent temperature of ≥38.0°C (100.4°F) for more than an hour.
  - Mucosal barriers compromised by chemotherapy may allow translocation of intestinal flora into the bloodstream, leading to bacteremia (*Enterococcus*, gram-negative bacteria) and candidemia. Hepatosplenic candidiasis, seen mostly in patients with acute leukemia, may present with fever, abdominal pain, and elevated alkaline phosphatase. Mucositis predisposes to bacteremia with oral flora (*Streptococcus viridans*, anaerobes). Cutaneous breakdown can lead to cellulitis, abscess, and bacteremia with gram-positive and gram-negative organisms alike.
  - Neutropenic enterocolitis (typhlitis) manifesting as a necrotizing cecal infection can extend to the terminal ileum and ascending colon, leading to bowel perforation.
  - Invasive mold infections (*Aspergillus*, *Fusarium*, *Zygomycetes*) presenting as pneumonia, sinusitis, central nervous system infection, or skin infections are also encountered.
  - **Solid organ transplantation**
  - Infections occurring shortly after organ transplant are largely related to surgical complications (e.g., anastomotic leaks, wound dehiscence, infected fluid collections) and prolonged hospitalization.
  - As immunosuppressive therapy to prevent acute rejection takes effect, opportunistic infections (e.g., mycobacteria, *Aspergillus*, *P. jiroveci*, herpesviruses) become more common by 1 month after transplant. CMV donor–recipient mismatch leading to primary CMV infection carries the highest risk of invasive disease (pneumonitis, hepatitis, colitis).
  - As the risk of acute graft rejection declines over time, the need for immunosuppression stabilizes and decreases. At 6 months posttransplant, community-acquired infections are more likely than opportunistic ones. Patients still on significant doses of immunosuppressive therapy remain prone to the latter.

○ **Hematopoietic stem cell transplantation**
  - The preengraftment phase comprises the first 3 weeks after conditioning chemotherapy and allogeneic stem cell transplant. Bone marrow suppression is profound and patients are at high risk for all of the infections associated with chemotherapy-related neutropenia.
  - Bone marrow recovery marks the beginning of the **immediate postengraftment phase** typically lasting from 3 weeks to 3 months after allogeneic stem cell transplant. Invasive fungal and viral infections (e.g., CMV) as well as other opportunistic infections (e.g., *P. jiroveci*) are possible depending on antimicrobial prophylaxis strategies. Acute graft versus host disease (GVHD) may necessitate additional immunosuppressive therapy.
  - Six months after transplant, the recipient enters the **late postengraftment phase**. If a recipient has not developed GVHD by this point, immune function may be largely restored within 1 to 2 years. However, recipients with chronic GVHD on immunosuppression remain prone to a wide array of opportunistic infections.

○ A more comprehensive discussion of infections seen in each of these immunocompromised states and their management shall be undertaken in later chapters.

- Empiric broad-spectrum antimicrobial therapy is almost universally indicated in the initial management of fever in the immunocompromised patient pending a thorough investigation for infection.

Fever in the Returned Traveler

- Fever is a common complaint among returned travelers seeking medical care.[9]
- The differential diagnosis of fever in the returned traveler can be broad and elusive. Geographic-specific infections not routinely encountered in daily practice may present alongside globally distributed infections (e.g., influenza) and illnesses not necessarily specific to travel (e.g., pneumonia).
- A thorough travel history should include the following:
  - Departure and return dates
  - Itinerary (e.g., all geographic locations visited, length of stay at each site, urban vs. rural setting, nature of the accommodations, modes of transportation)
  - Purpose of travel (tourism, work, visiting family or friends)
  - Activities (e.g., freshwater swimming, caving, hunting, agriculture, missionary work, health care)
  - Sick contacts (including fellow travelers)
  - Sexual contacts
  - Animal contacts (e.g., domestic animals, rodents, exotic wildlife, insects, ticks)
  - Type of food consumed (e.g., undercooked food, unpasteurized dairy products)
  - Source of water
  - Childhood and pretravel immunizations
  - Chemoprophylaxis (start and start dates, adherence)
- Knowledge of geographic-specific infections and their usual incubation periods (Table 2-9) can help in narrowing the list of suspect pathogens. Published by the Centers for Disease Control and Prevention (www.cdc.gov), the Yellow Book can be an invaluable travel medicine asset. Likewise, ProMED-mail (www.promedmail.org), a global electronic reporting system sponsored by the International Society for Infectious Diseases, can provide timely information about outbreaks of emerging infectious diseases around the world
- **Malaria is the most common cause of fever in the returned traveler** and should always be considered highest on the differential if travel has occurred in an endemic area. Serial thick and thin blood smears should be obtained to evaluate for parasitemia.
- **Enteric fever** (*Salmonella typhi* or *Salmonella paratyphi*) acquired through fecal–oral spread may present as fever, abdominal discomfort, and constipation. Diarrhea may or may not be present early in the infection. **Dengue fever**, **rickettsioses**, and **leptospirosis** are also commonly encountered in tropical regions. Poor sanitation, inadequate hand hygiene, and food or waterborne exposures increase the risk of acquiring **viral hepatitis** and **infectious diarrheas** (bacterial, viral, or parasitic). Emerging infections including Chikungunya fever should also be considered based on location of travel.
- Upper respiratory tract infections, bacterial pneumonia, urinary tract infections, and viral syndromes (including mononucleosis secondary to CMV or Epstein-Barr virus) that may occur irrespective of geography traveled are likewise common.
- Noninfectious causes of fever related to travel may include medications (e.g., chemoprophylaxis or antibiotic therapy prescribed during travel) and thromboembolism related to prolonged venous stasis during transit.
- Empiric antimicrobial therapy may be necessary in the clinically deteriorating patient with suspected malaria, rickettsiosis, leptospirosis, or other infection before a definitive diagnosis can be made.

TABLE 2-9	INCUBATION PERIODS OF SELECTED CAUSES OF FEVER IN THE RETURNED TRAVELER		
	<10 days	**10–21 days**	**>21 days**
	Bacterial enteritis	Typhoid and paratyphoid	Tuberculosis
	Bacterial pneumonia	Rickettsiosis (flea-borne, louse-borne, and scrub typhus, Q fever)	Rickettsiosis (Q fever)
	Meningococcemia		Syphilis (secondary)
	Typhoid and paratyphoid		
	Rickettsiosis (RMSF, African tick bite fever, Mediterranean spotted fever, scrub typhus, Q fever)	Brucella	Brucella
		Leptospirosis	Bartonellosis (chronic)
	Relapsing fever		
	Leptospirosis		
	Respiratory viruses (e.g., Chikungunya, influenza, SARS)	Acute HIV	Acute HIV
		CMV	CMV
		Flaviviruses	EBV
	Arboviruses (dengue, Japanese encephalitis, yellow fever)	Viral hemorrhagic fevers	Viral hepatitis
	Viral hemorrhagic fevers	Rabies	Rabies
		Measles	
		Histoplasmosis	
		Coccidioidomycosis	
	Malaria	Malaria	Malaria (especially *Plasmodium vivax* or in the context of ineffective chemoprophylaxis)
	Amebic dysentery	Babesiosis	
	Fascioliasis	Giardia	
	African trypanosomiasis (acute)	Toxoplasmosis	Babesiosis
		Amebic dysentery	Amebic liver disease
		African trypanosomiasis (acute)	Schistosomiasis
			Leishmaniasis
			Filariasis
			African trypanosomiasis (chronic)

CMV, cytomegalovirus; EBV, Epstein-Barr virus; HIV, human immunodeficiency virus; RMSF, Rocky Mountain spotted fever; SARS, severe acute respiratory syndrome.

Adapted from Freedman DO. Infections in returning travelers. In: Mandell GL, Bennett JE, Dolin R, eds. *Mandell, Douglas, and Bennett's Principles and Practice of Infectious Diseases.* 7th ed. Philadelphia, PA: Elsevier; 2009:4019-4028.

SEPSIS

GENERAL PRINCIPLES

Definitions

- Sepsis is positioned along a continuum of increasingly maladaptive host inflammatory responses to an infecting organism, spanning from systemic inflammatory response syndrome (SIRS) to septic shock and multiple organ dysfunction syndrome (Table 2-10).
- SIRS may occur with any process associated with inflammation (e.g., infection, pancreatitis, trauma/burn, surgery, thromboembolism, autoimmune disease, and vasculitis).
- Sepsis and septic shock stem from infection.

Pathophysiology

- The host response to infection is normally comprised of a localized inflammatory process mediated by phagocytic cells with little host tissue damage or physiological derangement. Pattern recognition receptors on these immune cells, including toll-like receptors, selectively bind to damage-associated molecular patterns on invading pathogens, triggering a balance of proinflammatory and antiinflammatory reactions, thereby eliminating the infection. In sepsis, this balance is unseated, leading to a predominantly proinflammatory, antiinflammatory, or mixed picture.
- The systemic proinflammatory state of sepsis, severe sepsis, and septic shock is orchestrated by cytokine (e.g., IL-1, TNF-α) and noncytokine (e.g., nitric oxide) mediators, resulting in endothelial damage, microvascular dysfunction, impaired tissue oxygenation, and organ injury. The antiinflammatory state is marked by immunosuppression and anergy.

Etiology

- Major causes of sepsis include respiratory, bloodstream, intra-abdominal, and urinary tract infections. Gram-positive and gram-negative bacteria comprise the majority of the causative organisms implicated in sepsis (Table 2-11). Fungal sepsis (mainly with *Candida* spp.) has also become increasingly common, particularly among immunocompromised patients and patients receiving parenteral feeding.
- Fulminant sepsis can accompany bacteremia with *Neisseria meningitidis*, *S. aureus*, *Yersinia pestis*, *Bacillus anthracis*, and *Capnocytophaga canimorsus* among a handful of other organisms. Asplenic patients are at particular risk for fulminant sepsis with encapsulated organisms (*Streptococcus pneumoniae*, *Haemophilus influenzae*, and *N. meningitidis*).

DIAGNOSIS

- Blood cultures (minimum of two to three sets) should be obtained from separate sites preferably before antibiotics have been administered. In the case of catheter-associated bloodstream infection, at least one blood culture should be obtained through the infected catheter.
- Appropriate imaging to identify or confirm sites of infection should be sought as the patient's clinical and hemodynamic status permits.
- Additional diagnostic testing (e.g., lumbar puncture, abscess drainage) should be driven by the type of infection suspected.

TABLE 2-10	SEPSIS AND THE SPECTRUM OF HOST INFLAMMATORY RESPONSE TO INFECTION
SIRS	Requires two or more of the following: • Fever (temperature >38.3°C [100.9°F]) • Hypothermia (temperature <36°C [96.8°F]) • Tachycardia (heart rate >90 beats/min) • Tachypnea (respiratory rate >20 breaths/min or hyperventilation [$Paco_2$ <32 mm Hg]) • White blood cell count >12,000 cells/mm^3, <4,000 cells/mm^3, or >10% bands
Sepsis	SIRS + documented infection

Severe sepsis	Sepsis + sepsis-induced organ dysfunction or tissue hypoperfusion as evidenced by any of the following:
	• Sepsis-induced hypotension
	  ○ Systolic blood pressure <90 mm Hg
	  ○ Mean arterial pressure <70 mm Hg
	  ○ Systolic blood pressure decrease >40 mm Hg or <2 standard deviations below normal for age without an alternative etiology
	• Urinary output <0.5 mL/kg for >2 h, despite adequate fluid resuscitation
	• Lactate >2 mmol/L
	• Creatinine >2 mg/dL
	• Acute lung injury with Pao_2/Fio_2 <250 in the absence of pneumonia
	• Acute lung injury with Pao_2/Fio_2 <200 in the presence of pneumonia
	• Platelet count <100,000 cells/mm^3
	• Coagulopathy (INR >1.5)
	• Disseminated intravascular coagulopathy

Septic shock	Severe sepsis + sepsis-induced hypotension unresponsive to fluid resuscitation
Refractory septic shock	Septic shock unresponsive to vasopressors
MODS	Altered organ function involving ≥2 organ systems

SIRS, systemic inflammatory response syndrome; MODS, multiple organ dysfunction syndrome; INR, international normalized ratio.

TREATMENT

Antimicrobial Therapy

• Early empiric antimicrobial therapy reduces mortality and improves patient outcomes in sepsis.[10,11]

TABLE 2-11	BACTERIAL PATHOGENS FREQUENTLY ASSOCIATED WITH SEPSIS	
Meningitis	*Streptococcus pneumoniae* *Listeria monocytogenes*	*H. influenzae* *Neisseria meningitidis*
Pneumonia	*S. pneumoniae* *Haemophilus influenzae* *Staphylococcus aureus*	*Klebsiella pneumoniae* *Pseudomonas aeruginosa*
Biliary tract infection	*Enterococcus* spp. *Escherichia coli*	*K. pneumoniae*
Intra-abdominal infection	*E. coli* *Bacteroides fragilis*	*Enterococcus* spp. (rare)
Urinary tract infection	*E. coli* *Klebsiella* spp. *Enterobacter* spp.	*Proteus* spp. *P. aeruginosa* *Enterococcus* spp.
Soft tissue and skin infection	*Staph. aureus* Group A streptococci	*Clostridium perfringens*
Intravascular catheter infection	*Staph. aureus* *Enterococcus faecalis*	*P. aeruginosa*

Adapted from Munford RS, Suffredini AF. Sepsis. In: Mandell GL, Bennett JE, Dolin R, eds. *Mandell, Douglas, and Bennett's Principles and Practice of Infectious Diseases.* 7th ed. Philadelphia, PA: Elsevier; 2009:987-1010.

- An empiric regimen should target anticipated pathogens and penetrate suspected sites of infection. As always, the risk of multidrug-resistant infection and local antimicrobial susceptibility patterns should be considered.
- Broad-spectrum empiric antimicrobial therapy should cover both gram-positive and gram-negative bacteria.
  - If *Pseudomonas* **is not suspected**, a combination of vancomycin with one of the following is generally acceptable:
    - Third- or fourth-generation cephalosporin (e.g., ceftriaxone, cefotaxime)
    - β-lactam/β-lactamase inhibitor (e.g., ampicillin-sulbactam, piperacillin-tazobactam, ticarcillin-clavulanate)
    - Carbapenem (e.g., meropenem, imipenem)
  - If *Pseudomonas* **is a concern**, a combination of vancomycin with one or two of the following is recommended:
    - Antipseudomonal cephalosporin (e.g., cefepime, ceftazidime)
    - Antipseudomonal β-lactam/β-lactamase inhibitor (e.g., piperacillin-tazobactam, ticarcillin-clavulanate)
    - Antipseudomonal carbapenem (e.g., meropenem, imipenem)
    - Aminoglycoside (e.g., gentamicin, amikacin; although frequently added for synergy, this practice is not well supported by evidence)
    - Fluoroquinolone with antipseudomonal activity (e.g., ciprofloxacin)
    - Monobactam (e.g., aztreonam)

○ For patients with documented colonization or previous infection with a multidrug-resistant organism or who have had prolonged or repeated hospitalizations or exposures to a health care setting, empiric therapy should include appropriate coverage:
  ■ Methicillin-resistant *S. aureus*: vancomycin
  ■ Vancomycin-resistant enterococcus: linezolid, daptomycin
  ■ Extended-spectrum β-lactamase producing gram-negative bacteria: carbapenem

- In clinical situations where fungemia is strongly suspected, empiric coverage with an echinocandin or amphotericin B may be warranted until blood cultures have been finalized.
- **Once a pathogen has been isolated in culture and antibiotic susceptibilities determined, empiric antimicrobial therapy should be de-escalated and narrowed accordingly**.
- Duration of therapy should be individualized and guided by the patient's clinical improvement and type of infection (e.g., pneumonia, bloodstream infection).

Source Control

- In addition to antimicrobial therapy, physical interventions are frequently necessary to eradicate primary infectious foci and prevent spread.[12]
- **All abscesses and infected fluid collections** (e.g., empyema) **should be drained**. Complicated intra-abdominal infections (e.g., abscess, cholangitis, necrotizing pancreatitis, peritonitis secondary to organ perforation) may require laparotomy or percutaneous drainage. Necrotizing soft tissue infections mandate emergent surgical debridement.
- **Infected intravascular catheters, urinary catheters, and prosthetic devices should be removed promptly**.
- Endocarditis may necessitate valve replacement.

Other Therapies

- Supportive care of sepsis in the ICU focuses on aggressive volume resuscitation and hemodynamic stabilization to restore perfusion and limit organ dysfunction. Intravenous fluids, vasopressors, and red blood cell transfusions are administered to normalize physiologic parameters including mean arterial pressure, central venous pressure, central venous oxygenation saturation, and urine output.
- Mechanical ventilation may be necessary in the face of pending respiratory compromise in many cases.
- Adjunctive therapies including intensive glycemic control, intravenous glucocorticoids, and recombinant human activated protein C remain controversial, each in their own right. Most agree that glycemic control in critical illness contributes to improved outcomes but differ on what blood glucose range is optimal.

OUTCOME/PROGNOSIS

Even with appropriate and timely medical care, the overall mortality for sepsis remains as high as 40% in critically ill patients. The role of the infectious disease specialist in guiding appropriate antimicrobial therapy and advocating for source control in the patient with sepsis can be crucial in determining clinical outcomes.

REFERENCES

1. Mackowiak PA, Wasserman SS, Levine MM. A critical appraisal of 98.6°F, the upper limit of the normal body temperature, and other legacies of Carl Reinhold August Wunderlich. *JAMA* 1992;268:1578-1580.
2. Norman DC. Fever in the elderly. *Clin Infect Dis* 2000;31:148-151.
3. Dimopoulos G, Falagas ME. Approach to the febrile patient in the ICU. *Infect Dis Clin N Am* 2009;23:471-484.
4. O'Grady NP, Barie PS, Bartlett JG *et al.* Guidelines for evaluation of new fever in critically ill adult patients: 2008 update from the American College of Critical Care Medicine and the Infectious Diseases Society of America. *Crit Care Med* 2008;36:1330-1349.
5. Mermel LA, Allon M, Bouza E *et al.* Clinical practice guidelines for the diagnosis and management of intravascular catheter-related infection: 2009 update by the Infectious Diseases Society of America. *Clin Infect Dis* 2009;49:1-45.
6. Hooton TM, Bradley SF, Cardenas DD *et al.* Diagnosis, prevention, and treatment of catheter-associated urinary tract infection in adults: 2009 international clinical practice guidelines from the Infectious Diseases Society of America. *Clin Infect Dis* 2010;50:625-663.
7. Cohen SH, Gerding DN, Johnson S *et al.* Clinical practice guidelines for *Clostridium difficile* infection in adults: 2010 update by the Society for Healthcare Epidemiology of American (SHEA) and the Infectious Diseases Society of America (IDSA). *Infect Control Hosp Epidemiol* 2010;31:431-455.
8. Freifeld AG, Bow EJ, Sepkowitz KA *et al.* Clinical practice guideline for the use of antimicrobial agents in neutropenic patients with cancer: 2010 update by the Infectious Diseases Society of America. *Clin Infect Dis* 2011;52:e56-93.
9. Wilson ME, Weld LH, Boggild A et al. Fever in returned travelers: results from the GeoSentinel Surveillance Network. *Clin Infect Dis* 2007;44:1560-1568.
10. Dellinger RP, Levy MM, Carlet JM et al. Surviving Sepsis Campaign: International guidelines for management of severe sepsis and septic shock: 2008. *Crit Care Med* 2008;36:296-327.
11. Kumar A. Optimizing antimicrobial therapy in sepsis and septic shock *Crit Care Clin* 2009;25.733-751.
12. Marshall JC, al Naqbi. Principles of source control in the management of sepsis. *Crit Care Clin* 2009;25:753-768.

Fever of Unknown Origin

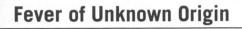

3

Stephen Y. Liang and Nigar Kirmani

GENERAL PRINCIPLES

Definition

Classic fever of unknown origin (FUO) is defined as an illness lasting >3 weeks with temperatures >38.3°C (101°F) on multiple occasions and no established etiology after 3 days of inpatient hospitalization or three outpatient visits, despite appropriate investigations.

Etiology

Infections account for a third of all cases of FUO in the United States, followed by neoplasm (20% to 30%), connective tissue disorders (10% to 20%), and miscellaneous disorders (15% to 20%). A definitive cause may not be found in up to 15% of cases.

Infectious Diseases

- The differential diagnosis of infectious causes of FUO can be extensive (Table 3-1).
- In many instances, FUO may constitute an atypical presentation of a common disease rather than a typical presentation of a rare disease.
- Causes of FUO vary significantly by geography. Infections acquired in endemic regions through travel or residence may present to care as FUO in nonendemic areas.

Bacterial Infections

- **Tuberculosis** remains an important cause of FUO. In particular, disseminated (miliary) and certain forms of extrapulmonary tuberculosis (e.g., renal, mesenteric lymphadenitis) may present initially with vague and protean manifestations.
- **Subacute bacterial endocarditis** with *Streptococcus viridans* and **culture-negative endocarditis** with less virulent organisms (e.g., *Coxiella burnetii*, *Bartonella* spp., *Brucella*, HACEK [*Haemophilus parainfluenzae*, *Aggregatibacter* spp., *Cardiobacterium hominis*, *Eikenella corrodens*, *Kingella kingae*] group organisms) may manifest insidiously as FUO in the context of a new heart murmur with or without peripheral stigmata. Blood cultures can be negative if patients have received antibiotics.
- **Occult abscesses** in the abdomen or pelvis may arise in the context of recent surgery, infection (e.g., cholecystitis, cholangitis, appendicitis, diverticulitis, urinary tract infection), diabetes mellitus, or immunosuppression. Septic emboli from endocarditis commonly lead to splenic abscesses. Dental abscesses can also be a rare cause of FUO.
- **Occult osteomyelitis** may present as FUO accompanied by musculoskeletal complaints. Vertebral osteomyelitis should be suspected in elderly patients with a history of fever and recurrent urinary tract infections.
- **Typhoid fever** (*Salmonella typhi*), acquired through travel and ingestion of contaminated food or water, may present with persistent fever, abdominal pain, relative bradycardia, hepatosplenomegaly, rose spots, and leukopenia.

TABLE 3-1	CAUSES OF CLASSIC FEVER OF UNKNOWN ORIGIN	
Etiology	**Common**	**Uncommon**
Infectious diseases	*Bacteria* Abscess Subacute bacterial endocarditis Culture-negative endocarditis Osteomyelitis Tuberculosis Typhoid fever Cat scratch disease	*Bacteria* Chronic sinusitis Brucellosis Q fever Rat bite fever Leptospirosis Relapsing fever Ehrlichiosis Scrub and murine typhus Melioidosis Lymphogranuloma venereum Whipple disease
	Virus Epstein-Barr virus Cytomegalovirus Human immunodeficiency virus	*Virus* Parvovirus B19 Chikungunya fever *Fungus* Coccidioidomycosis Histoplasmosis *Parasite* Malaria Babesiosis Toxoplasmosis Trichinosis Visceral leishmaniasis
Neoplastic disorders	Lymphoma Leukemia Myelodysplastic syndrome Renal cell carcinoma Hepatocellular carcinoma Liver metastases Pancreatic carcinoma	Atrial myxoma Central nervous system tumors Multiple myeloma Hemophagocytic lymphohistiocytosis Colon carcinoma
Rheumatic disorders	Temporal arteritis Polymyalgia rheumatica Adult-onset Still disease	Wegener granulomatosis Takayasu arteritis Behçet disease Cryoglobulinemic vasculitis

	Polyarteritis nodosa	Kikuchi-Fujimoto disease
	Systemic lupus erythematosus	Polyarticular gout/pseudogout
	Rheumatoid arthritis	
Miscellaneous disorders	Drug fever	Thromboembolic disease
	Hematoma	Periodic fever syndromes
	Alcoholic hepatitis	Sweet syndrome
	Crohn disease	Schnitzler syndrome (with hives)
	Sarcoidosis	
	Subacute thyroiditis	Hypothalamic dysfunction
		Hyperthyroidism
		Pheochromocytoma
		Adrenal insufficiency
		Factitious fever

Adapted from Cunha BA. Fever of unknown origin: clinical overview of classic and current concepts. *Infect Dis Clin N Am.* 2007;21:867-915.

- **Cat scratch disease** (*Bartonella henselae*) should be suspected in the patient with fever, lymphadenopathy, and recent history of a cat bite or scratch.
- **Q fever** (*Coxiella burnetii*) may manifest as a flu-like illness after close contact with cattle, sheep, and goats or the consumption of contaminated dairy products.
- **Brucellosis** is marked by undulant fevers, sweating, and migratory arthralgias. It has been associated with the consumption of unpasteurized milk or goat cheese.

Viral Infections
- **Epstein-Barr virus** and **cytomegalovirus (CMV)** may present as fever, fatigue, lymphadenopathy, and transaminitis. Leukopenia and atypical lymphocytes seen on peripheral smear may aid in diagnosis.
- **Human immunodeficiency virus (HIV)**/acquired immune deficiency syndrome (**AIDS**) and associated opportunistic infections (e.g., mycobacteria, CMV) and neoplasms can manifest as FUO in the absence of antiretroviral therapy and adequate antibiotic prophylaxis.

Fungal Infections
- Endemic mycoses including **histoplasmosis** and **coccidioidomycosis** should be considered in patients reporting travel to or residence in geographic locations traditionally associated with these fungi.
- Disseminated histoplasmosis and tuberculosis bear many similarities.

Parasitic Infections
- **Toxoplasmosis** in immunocompetent patients may present with fever, lymphadenopathy, and myalgias in the setting of ingestion of raw or partially cooked meat or exposure to cat litter. A peripheral smear may reveal atypical lymphocytes.
- **Visceral leishmaniasis** (kala-azar) involving the liver, spleen, and bone marrow can manifest with FUO accompanied by weight loss, malaise, hepatosplenomegaly, anemia, and elevated liver function tests after travel to an endemic region.

Neoplasm

- **Lymphoma**, especially non-Hodgkin lymphoma, remains the most common neoplastic etiology of FUO. Fever, night sweats, weight loss, and lymphadenopathy warrant further evaluation with imaging and lymph node biopsy.
- **Leukemias** and **myelodysplastic syndromes** may be identified on peripheral smear but ultimately require a bone marrow biopsy for diagnosis.
- **Renal cell carcinoma** may present with fever and hematuria. **Hepatocellular carcinoma** and **metastatic liver cancer** also frequently present as FUO.
- **Atrial myxoma** should be considered in the patient with fever, weight loss, a heart murmur, and negative blood cultures.

Connective Tissue Disorders

- In young and middle-aged adults, **adult-onset Still disease** ("juvenile rheumatoid arthritis") is marked by fever >39°C (102.2°F), arthritis, and an evanescent salmon-pink rash. Lymphadenopathy and splenomegaly coupled with leukocytosis and elevated erythrocyte sedimentation rate (ESR), C-reactive protein (CRP), ferritin (>1,000 ng/mL), and liver enzymes may suggest the diagnosis.
- In the patient over age 50, **temporal arteritis** may present with a constellation of fever, headache, jaw claudication, and abrupt vision loss. Tenderness to palpation or diminished pulsation over the temporal artery coupled with an ESR >50 mm/h mandates temporal artery biopsy.
- **Polymyalgia rheumatica** presents with bilateral aching and morning stiffness of the neck, torso, shoulders, and hip girdle with ESR > 40 mm/h.

Miscellaneous Disorders

- **Drug fever** may arise from any number of medications. Antimicrobials (e.g., sulfonamides, penicillins, cephalosporins, vancomycin, nitrofurantoin), anticonvulsants (e.g., phenytoin, carbamazepine, barbiturates), H1 and H2 blocking antihistamines, antihypertensives (e.g., hydralazine, methyldopa), and antiarrhythmic drugs (e.g., quinidine, procainamide) are common causes. Rash and eosinophilia may or may not be present.
- **Factitious fever** is a psychiatric illness. Manipulation of thermometers may lead to spurious readings, while self-administration of nonsterile injections can cause intentional infections.
- **Periodic fever syndromes** (e.g., familial Mediterranean fever, tumor necrosis factor 1–associated periodic syndrome, hyperimmunoglobulinemia D syndrome) are autoinflammatory and hereditary in nature.
- **Sarcoidosis** manifesting with fever, night sweats, weight loss, fatigue, cough, and lymphadenopathy can be mistaken for other granulomatous diseases, notably tuberculosis and histoplasmosis.
- **Alcoholic hepatitis** may be characterized by low-grade fevers, jaundice, hepatosplenomegaly, and abnormal liver function tests with an aspartate aminotransferase: alanine aminotransferase ratio of 2:1.
- **Crohn disease** frequently presents with fever, weight loss, abdominal pain, and diarrhea with or without gastrointestinal bleeding.
- Endocrine disorders including **hyperthyroidism**, **pheochromocytoma**, and **adrenal insufficiency** may occasionally surface as FUO.
- Unexplained fever may be the only presenting feature of a **deep vein thrombosis** or **pulmonary embolus**.

DIAGNOSIS

Clinical Presentation

A comprehensive history and physical examination focuses the diagnostic evaluation of FUO and spares the patient unnecessary tests and procedures.

History
- Establish a time line of any and all symptoms.
- Characterize all prior infections, malignancies, and their subsequent medical management. All surgeries, postsurgical complications, foreign materials, and prosthetic devices should be identified.
- Review all current prescription and over-the-counter medications.
- Obtain a complete social history including environmental, occupational, recreational, sexual, dietary, animal, and travel exposures.
- A family history should identify inherited malignancies and inflammatory disorders, as well as any common symptomatology or prior infections between family members.

Physical Examination
- **Verify the presence of fever.** Comparison of temperatures taken from multiple sites (oral, rectal, voided urine) can aid in clarifying a factitious fever.
- Most fevers peak in the late afternoon or early afternoon. Abnormal fever patterns may be helpful in selected cases provided that antipyretic medications or body cooling devices have not altered their periodicity.
  - Morning fever spikes: typhoid fever, tuberculosis, polyarteritis nodosa.
  - Double quotidian fevers (two temperature spikes within 24 hours): disseminated (miliary) tuberculosis, visceral leishmaniasis, or adult-onset Still disease.
  - Relative bradycardia: malaria, typhoid fever, drug fever, central nervous system disorder. Beware of confounding medications (e.g., β-blockers, calcium channel blockers).
- Inspect the eyes (including fundi). Palpate the sinuses and temporal arteries. Examine the oropharynx for ulcers, thrush, and evidence of dental infection. Look for thyromegaly.
- A new heart murmur may suggest bacterial endocarditis, marantic endocarditis (e.g., systemic lupus erythematosus), or atrial myxoma.
- Hepatomegaly, splenomegaly, and any abnormal abdominal masses should be noted. Genitourinary and rectal examination should be performed to look for ulcerative lesions and signs of perirectal abscess.
- Thoroughly examine the skin, joints, and all major lymph nodes.
- Repeat physical examination may be necessary to identify subtle and evolving findings as the FUO progresses with time.

Diagnostic Testing

Laboratories
- Basic laboratory evaluation should include a complete blood count with differential, liver function panel, urinalysis, and nonspecific inflammatory markers including an ESR, CRP, and ferritin level. Highly elevated ESR (>100 mm/h) can be suggestive of abscess, osteomyelitis, or endocarditis. Highly elevated ferritin levels favor noninfectious etiologies of FUO.

- **At least three blood cultures should be obtained, while the patient is off antibiotics, preferably during febrile episodes and several hours apart.**
- All patients should be screened for HIV infection and syphilis.
- Purified protein derivative (PPD) skin test is recommended. While a positive PPD may suggest infection, **a negative result cannot exclude it.**
- Additional laboratory tests may include antinuclear antibodies, rheumatoid factor, and serum protein electrophoresis if a rheumatologic diagnosis is being considered.
- Infection-specific serologies and other definitive diagnostic assays should be ordered based on the prevalence and degree of clinical suspicion for that disease in order to minimize the risk of false-positive results.

Imaging
- Obtain a screening chest radiogram if pulmonary complaints exist.
- Computed tomography (CT) of the abdomen and pelvis may be helpful in identifying occult abscesses, hematoma, or lymphadenopathy.
- Echocardiography should be reserved for patients with a heart murmur where endocarditis or other valvular abnormality is suspected.
- Nuclear medicine studies (e.g., gallium scintigraphy, indium white blood cell scanning, fluorodeoxyglucose positron emission tomography/CT) may be helpful in localizing occult infection, inflammation, or malignancy.

Diagnostic Procedures
- Tissue biopsy is frequently required to establish the etiology of FUO.
- All biopsied tissues should be sent for appropriate culture (e.g., bacterial, mycobacterial, fungal) and sensitivity in addition to pathology.
- **Liver biopsy** is useful in establishing the cause of granulomatous hepatitis, which may be seen in disseminated tuberculosis, histoplasmosis, or sarcoidosis.
- **Lymph node biopsy** is crucial in diagnosing lymphoma and can also aid with the identification of disseminated granulomatous infections, toxoplasmosis, and cat scratch disease.
- **Bone marrow biopsy** is necessary to confirm leukemia and myelodysplastic syndrome. It should be strongly considered with infections associated with bone marrow involvement (e.g., disseminated tuberculosis and histoplasmosis).
- **Exploratory laparotomy** is rarely indicated given modern imaging and guided biopsy techniques. However, in some circumstances (e.g., peritoneal tuberculosis), laparotomy may be necessary in order to obtain appropriate biopsy specimens and establish diagnosis.

TREATMENT

Antimicrobial Therapy
- In the absence of clinical deterioration or a severely immunocompromised state (neutropenic fever, solid organ or hematopoietic stem cell transplant, advanced AIDS, asplenia), empiric antibiotics are rarely indicated in the initial management

of fever without a clear source. In many cases, they may delay diagnosis and optimal antimicrobial therapy through partial treatment of infection (e.g., tuberculosis).

- Most infections associated with classic FUO are indolent and subacute. Emphasis should be placed on establishing a definitive diagnosis.
- Disseminated tuberculosis is one of the few exceptions where antimicrobial therapy is reasonable if the suspicion is high. Adequate cultures should be obtained prior to therapy to confirm diagnosis.
- Culture-negative endocarditis likewise warrants empiric therapy once adequate blood cultures have been obtained.

Other Interventions

- Withdrawal of offending medications frequently leads to resolution of a drug fever within 72 hours.
- Timely corticosteroid therapy and other immunosuppression are important in rheumatic disorders, particularly temporal arteritis.
- Chemotherapy, radiation, and surgery may be necessary depending on the type of neoplastic disorder identified.

PROGNOSIS

- Prognosis is dictated by timely diagnosis of life-threatening infections, malignancies, and other miscellaneous disorders.
- The longer the duration of FUO without progressive clinical deterioration, the less likely the FUO is infectious in nature.
- If no clear etiology of FUO has been found despite a thorough evaluation for infections, neoplasm, connective tissue disorders, and miscellaneous causes, patient mortality is generally low and prognosis is considered good. Spontaneous resolution of FUO is not uncommon. Long-term follow-up is indicated to monitor for recurrence of fever.

SPECIAL CONSIDERATIONS

In addition to the classic form, FUO has also been described in the context of several patient populations at heightened risk for infectious complications.

Health Care–Associated Fever of Unknown Origin

- Defined as fever >38.3°C (101°F) on several occasions in a hospitalized patient without an initial infection on admission and having no established cause after at least 3 days of investigation and 48 hours of culture incubation.
- Common etiologies include catheter-related infection, sinusitis, postoperative complications, *Clostridium difficile* infection, thromboembolic disease (deep vein thrombosis/pulmonary embolism), and drug fever (Table 3-2). Health care–associated and aspiration pneumonia must also be considered in the nonintubated patient.

TABLE 3-2	CAUSES OF HEALTH CARE–ASSOCIATED FEVER OF UNKNOWN ORIGIN
Risk factor	**Complication**
Central venous catheter	Insertion site infection
	Catheter-related bloodstream infection
	Suppurative thrombophlebitis
	Endocarditis
Arterial catheter	Insertion site infection
	Catheter-related bloodstream infection
Nasogastric, nasoendotracheal, endotracheal tube	Sinusitis
Urinary catheter	Urinary tract infection
Mechanical ventilation	Ventilator-associated pneumonia
Surgery	Surgical site infection
Recent antibiotic exposure	*Clostridium difficile* infection

Immunodeficiency and Fever of Unknown Origin

- Defined as fever >38.3°C (101°F) on several occasions in a patient with an absolute neutrophil count <500 cells/mm^3 (or anticipated decline below this level within the next 48 hours) with no established cause after at least 3 days of investigation and 48 hours of culture incubation.
- Opportunistic infections, invasive fungal infections, health care–associated infections, and drug fever are most frequently implicated (Table 3-3).

TABLE 3-3	CAUSES OF IMMUNE-DEFICIENT FEVER OF UNKNOWN ORIGIN
Bacteria	*Staphylococcus aureus*
	Coagulase-negative staphylococcus
	Streptococcus spp.
	Enterococcus spp.
	Pseudomonas aeruginosa
	Escherichia coli
	Enterobacteriaceae
	Klebsiella spp.
	Nocardia spp.
	Clostridium difficile
Virus	Human herpesviruses (HSV, CMV, EBV, VZV, HHV-6)
	Respiratory viruses (RSV, parainfluenza, influenza, rhinovirus, human metapneumovirus)

Fungi	*Candida* sp.
	Cryptococcus neoformans
	Aspergillus spp.
	Fusarium spp.
	Zygomycetes
	Histoplasma capsulatum
	Blastomyces dermatitidis
	Coccidioides immitis
	Pneumocystis jiroveci

CMV, cytomegalovirus; EBV, Epstein-Barr virus; HHV, human herpesvirus; HSV, herpes simplex virus; RSV, respiratory syncytial virus; VZV, varicella zoster virus.

- Repeated and prolonged hospitalization places immune-deficient patients at high risk of colonization and infection with multidrug-resistant organisms.
- Empiric antimicrobial therapy should be instituted promptly based on suspicion for serious bacterial or fungal infection.

HIV-Associated Fever of Unknown Origin

- Defined as fever >38.3°C (101°F) on several occasions in a patient with HIV infection, lasting more than 3 weeks with no established cause after 3 days of inpatient hospitalization and 48 hours of culture incubation.
- In patients with low CD4+ cell counts, opportunistic infections including infection with *Mycobacterium avium-intracellulare*, CMV, *Pneumocystis jiroveci*, *Cryptococcus neoformans*, and *Toxoplasma gondii* are frequently encountered, particularly in the absence of prophylactic antimicrobials. Tuberculosis, *Bartonella* infection, and endemic mycoses (histoplasmosis, coccidioidomycosis) remain important causes of FUO.
- Immune reconstitution inflammatory syndrome after the initiation of antiretroviral therapy can present as FUO with reactivation or worsening of preexisting opportunistic infections.
- Neoplastic disorders (lymphoma) and drug fever related to antiretroviral and prophylactic antimicrobial therapy are also common causes of FUO (Table 3-4).

TABLE 3-4	**CAUSES OF HIV-ASSOCIATED FEVER OF UNKNOWN ORIGIN**
Infectious disorders	*Mycobacterium tuberculosis*
	Mycobacterium avium-intracellulare
	Bartonella spp.
	CMV
	Pneumocystis jiroveci
	Cryptococcus neoformans
	Aspergillus spp.
	Histoplasma capsulatum
	Coccidioides immitis

(continued)

TABLE 3-4	(CONTINUED)
	Toxoplasma gondii
	Leishmania
	IRIS-associated opportunistic infection
Neoplastic disorders	Lymphoma (non-Hodgkin, central nervous system, B cell)
	Kaposi sarcoma
	Castleman disease
Rheumatic disorders	Systemic lupus erythematosus
Miscellaneous disorders	Drug fever

CMV, cytomegalovirus; HIV, human immunodeficiency virus; IRIS, immune reconstitution inflammatory syndrome.

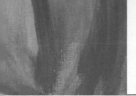

Bacteremia and Infections of the Cardiovascular Systems

4

Brent W. Wieland and Rachel Presti

BACTEREMIA AND FUNGEMIA

GENERAL PRINCIPLES

- Bacteremia is common in hospitalized patients and the incidence is increasing. This is likely due to the increasing use of central venous catheters (CVCs) and implantable cardiac devices and the increased severity of illness in hospitalized patients.
- Fungemia is the presence of fungi in the blood. Many of the principles of bacteremia and fungemia are the same. For general principles, the term *bacteremia* will refer to both entities unless specified.

Definition

- Bacteremia is defined as the presence of bacteria in the bloodstream. Bacteremia is not an uncommon event even in healthy, asymptomatic people. Transient bacteremia can be provoked by eating, brushing teeth, or minor scrapes and cuts. These transient episodes of bacteremia are usually eliminated by the host immune system. Clinical disease occurs when bacteremia overcomes the host's immune defense.
- There are many potential causes of bacteremia. Primary bacteremia is due to an intravascular source of infection, such as the heart and a blood vessel. Primary bacteremia can also occur when normal barriers to the bloodstream are disrupted, as with a vascular catheter, or due to trauma. Secondary bacteremia occurs when a bacterial infection of a noncardiovascular tissue is introduced into the vascular supply. Urinary tract infections, respiratory infections, infections of the gastrointestinal tract, and skin and soft tissue infections can all result in invasion of organisms into the bloodstream. Spontaneous secondary bacteremia may occur in immunosuppressed individuals due to translocation of gut bacteria into the bloodstream.

Epidemiology

- Clinically significant bacteremia occurs most commonly in hospitalized patients. Due to more frequent use of home intravenous (IV) catheters for hemodialysis and administration of chemotherapy, antibiotics, or parenteral nutrition, as well as more frequent implantation of cardiovascular devices, bacteremia is also becoming a problem in the outpatient setting.
- Bacteremia should be considered in any patient with fever who has implanted vascular devices or implanted cardiac devices, neutropenic patients, or in patients with evidence of bacterial infection at distant sites. It is critically important in these patient populations to obtain blood cultures prior to the institution of antibiotics in order to diagnose and identify the cause of bacteremia.

Etiology

- Many gram-negative, gram-positive, aerobic, or anaerobic bacteria can cause bacteremia. The source of infection can give clues to the possible organism involved. Clinical consideration should be given to the probable source of the infection.
  - Urinary tract infections are most commonly caused by aerobic gram-negative bacteria from the genus Enterobacteriaceae. *Escherichia coli* accounts for >50% of bacteremias associated with infections of the urinary tract.
  - Bacteremias with a respiratory source are commonly caused by *Streptococcus pneumoniae*, *Klebsiella pneumoniae*, and *Pseudomonas aeruginosa*.
  - If skin or soft tissue infection is the source, the most common organisms include normal gram-positive skin flora such as *Streptococcus* and *Staphylococcus* spp.
  - If an abdominal source is suspected, infection is likely from *E. coli* or other Enterobacteriaceae, *Bacteroides* spp., other anaerobes, or mixed organisms.
- Neutropenic patients are particularly at risk for infection with gram-negative organisms such as *P. aeruginosa*.
- Patients with prolonged hospitalization are at risk for bacteremia with resistant organisms such as *P. aeruginosa*, *Acinetobacter baumannii*, and methicillin-resistant *Staphylococcus aureus* (MRSA).
- Patients on antibiotics are also at risk for bacteremia caused by resistant organisms as well as fungi.
- Patients with *Staph. aureus* bacteremia as well as bacteremia from highly resistant organisms have a much higher mortality. Strong consideration should be given to consultation of an infectious disease specialist in these situations.[1]

DIAGNOSIS

- Upon suspicion of bloodstream infection, patients should be evaluated for the causative organism, the source of infection, and the severity of illness.
- Blood cultures should be obtained from two to three separate venipuncture sites, as well as from any indwelling vascular catheter, over 15 to 30 minutes. **If possible, cultures should be obtained prior to starting antibiotics**.
- The source should also be determined. Common causes include CVCs (which will be addressed in detail in a later section), the genitourinary tract, the respiratory tract, and the gastrointestinal tract. Additional workup, such as urinalysis, chest radiography, and abdominal imaging, should be determined based on clinical suspicion.
- Determining the causative organism as well as the source of bacteremia is of paramount importance, as this will determine the choice of treatment and the duration of therapy.

TREATMENT

- **Definitive treatment should be tailored to the results of culture and sensitivity testing**. Treatment should be initiated with parenteral antibiotics. In rare cases, route may be switched to oral antibiotics once the organism, susceptibilities, and source of infection are known.
- Duration of treatment will be based on the source of infection and the severity of illness.
- Empiric therapy should be based on the most likely causative organisms.

○ If the source of bacteremia is thought to be **skin or soft tissues**, the selected agent should be geared toward gram-positive organisms including streptococci and staphylococci. If there is a high local incidence of MRSA, vancomycin should be included in the initial empiric treatment. Otherwise, treatment may be initiated with nafcillin, oxacillin, clindamycin, or cephalosporins.

○ If the source is thought to be the urinary tract, treatment should be geared toward gram-negative organisms including *E. coli*. Empiric treatment could include a fluoroquinolone or a third-generation cephalosporin.

○ If the source is thought to be the **abdomen**, treatment should be effective against gram-negative and anaerobic organisms, specifically *E. coli* and *Bacteroides* spp. Empiric treatment could include a carbapenem, a β-lactam combined with a β-lactamase inhibitor, or a third- or fourth-generation cephalosporin combined with metronidazole.

○ In **neutropenic patients**, the initial antibiotic should be geared toward gram-negative organisms. The agent should have coverage against *P. aeruginosa*. Empiric treatment should be with an antipseudomonal cephalosporin, carbapenem, ciprofloxacin, or piperacillin/tazobactam. Neutropenic patients with hypotension, mucositis, evidence of a skin or catheter site infection, known MRSA colonization, or clinical deterioration should also be empirically covered with an agent effective against MRSA: vancomycin, linezolid, and daptomycin.

○ Patients who have been **hospitalized or in a health care setting** should initially be treated with broad-spectrum antibiotics with coverage against resistant organisms such as *P. aeruginosa* and MRSA. Treatment options are similar to options for neutropenic patients.

○ **Critically ill patients** should also be covered with broad-spectrum antibiotics until the causative organism is known. Consideration should also be given to antifungal coverage in critically ill patients.

• **Fungemia** is the presence of fungi in the blood. The most common fungi found in the bloodstream are *Candida* spp. Empiric antifungal choice should depend on the severity of illness and the prevalence of non-albicans *Candida* spp. in the hospital population. Most *Candida albicans* are sensitive to fluconazole. *Candida glabrata* and *Candida krusei* are commonly resistant to fluconazole. Echinocandins are preferred for infections due to *C. glabrata* and *C. krusei*. *Candida parapsilosis* is less sensitive to the echinocandins, and fluconazole is the preferred agent.

CATHETER-RELATED BACTEREMIA AND FUNGEMIA

GENERAL PRINCIPLES

• This section is specifically devoted to the treatment of catheter-related blood stream infections (CRBSIs). Many of the same principles of diagnosis and treatment are the same as in the previous section. This section will focus on the differences from other sources of bacteremia.

• The use of CVCs is a necessary component of health care delivery in hospitalized patient, and their use outside of hospitals is increasingly frequent.

• Infectious complications are becoming more common as the use of CVCs increases. Infections can range from insertion site skin and soft tissue infections, bacteremia, endocarditis, septic thrombophlebitis, and metastatic infections such as pulmonary abscesses, osteomyelitis, and intracranial abscesses.

Epidemiology

- The risk of developing a CRBSI is dependent upon several factors, including the type of catheter used, the location of the catheter, the setting (i.e., inpatient or outpatient; intensive care unit [ICU] or general wards), the duration of catheter placement, frequency of catheter manipulation, and patient-dependent factors and comorbidities such as diabetes and obesity.
- Peripheral IV catheters are associated with a low risk of bacteremia; however, inflammation or phlebitis is not uncommon when left in place for a prolonged duration.
- **Temporary, nontunneled CVCs and pulmonary artery catheters have the highest risk of infection**. The risk of infection with CVCs is dependent upon the site used. The subclavian vein is the preferred location with the lowest infection risk, followed by internal jugular vein. **Femoral venous catheters have the highest rates of infection and should be avoided whenever possible**. Catheters placed emergently are at higher risk for infection and should be replaced once a patient is stabilized.
- Tunneled CVCs have a lower risk of infection than nontunneled catheters. Peripherally inserted central venous catheters (PICC) also have lower rates of infection than nontunneled CVCs.
- Totally implanted venous catheters (ports) have the lowest overall risk of infection. Placement and removal of implanted venous catheters requires a surgical procedure.
- Overall, nontunneled CVCs account for about 90% of all CRBSIs.

Etiology

- The most common organisms identified in CRBSIs are gram-positive skin organisms. Coagulase-negative staphylococci are the most common organisms, followed by gram-negative organisms, *Staph. aureus*, enterococci, and *Candida*. Among gram-negative organisms, the most common organisms are Enterobacteriaceae (*E. coli*, *Klebsiella* spp., and *Enterobacter* spp.) and *P. aeruginosa*.
- CRBSI with *Staph. aureus* has the highest mortality with a rate of 8.2%.[2] Coagulase-negative staphylococcal CRBSI has the lowest associated mortality.
- Prolonged hospitalization, ICU admission, and prior antibiotic exposure increase the risk of more resistant organisms. Infection with *Candida* spp. should be considered in patients on broad-spectrum antibiotics and those receiving lipid-rich formulations, such as parenteral nutrition and propofol. Colonization of urinary catheters and endotracheal or tracheostomy tubes with *Candida* can predispose patients to fungemia.
- Bacteria usually enter the blood by migrating from the skin at the site of line insertion. Less commonly, the catheter may be hematogenously seeded by bacteria or fungi that entered the blood at a distant site.

Prevention

- **Most CRBSIs are preventable**. A multifaceted approach should be taken in attempts to prevent catheter infections.[3–5]
- Insertion of the catheter should be **performed under aseptic conditions** with proper hand hygiene, sterile gloves, cap, mask, gown, and full body drape. Skin cleansing should be performed using 2% chlorhexidine solution. The preferred site for insertion of a nontunneled CVC is the subclavian vein followed by the internal jugular vein.

- **The femoral vein should only be used for CVC insertion when there are no other options or in emergency situations**. When a femoral CVC is placed, it should be removed as soon as alternative venous access can be established.
- When the CVC is expected to be needed for a prolonged period of time, tunneled catheters, PICC, and totally implanted catheters should be utilized when feasible.
- CVCs should be **removed as soon as central venous access is no longer needed**. Routine catheter exchange and exchange of the catheter over a wire are not generally recommended.

DIAGNOSIS

- The most common presentation of a CRBSI is a **new fever in a patient with an intravascular catheter**. Any patient with a new fever and an intravascular device should be evaluated with vital signs and physical examination.
- The catheter should be evaluated for obvious signs of infection such as erythema or purulent drainage, although these signs are not commonly present.
- The patient should also be evaluated for alternative sources of fever.
- The diagnosis of a CRBSI is achieved by obtaining **a minimum of two cultures, with at least one via peripheral venipuncture**. The diagnosis is made if one or more cultures are positive with a pathogen associated with CRBSI in the absence of another source of blood stream infection (i.e., pneumonia and urinary tract infection).
- If a common skin contaminant (diphtheroids, *Bacillus* spp., coagulase-negative *Staphylococcus*, and *Propionibacterium* spp.) is grown in culture, it should be confirmed by growth in two or more cultures drawn on separate occasions.
- As always, cultures should be drawn prior to the administration of antibiotics whenever possible.

TREATMENT

- Antibiotic management of patients with a confirmed CRBSI should be **tailored to the identified pathogen. Empiric antibiotic coverage should target the most likely causative organisms**. The first-line agent for empiric treatment is **vancomycin**. In critically ill patients or patients with other comorbid conditions, the addition of gram-negative coverage or an antifungal agent should be considered.
- **Catheter removal is a key component** in the management of CRBSI. In general, all intravascular catheters should be removed if there is evidence of an insertion site infection (e.g., purulent drainage, erythema, induration, and pain at the site of insertion). Clinically, unstable patients in whom CRBSI is suspected should have the catheter removed as soon as possible.
- Nontunneled, nonimplanted CVCs should be removed in almost all circumstances when CRBSI is suspected. If CRBSI is suspected, the patient should be evaluated for alternative sites for venous access. If the patient has ongoing needs for central venous access, the existing catheter should be removed once alternative access is achieved. If the patient no longer has a need for central venous access, the existing catheter should be removed and a peripheral catheter placed.
- If a patient has persistent fevers without a clear source, consideration should be given to CVC removal or exchange even in the absence of positive blood cultures or evidence of an insertion site infection.

- In rare cases, when a patient is stable, and an uncomplicated CRBSI is due to coagulase-negative *Staphylococcus*, the physician may choose to retain the catheter if alternative access is problematic. If the catheter is retained, treatment should be with 10 to 14 days of effective parenteral antibiotics, sometimes accompanied by antibiotic lock therapy.[6, 7]
- If salvage of a long-term CVC is desired and the patient has an uncomplicated infection with an organism other than *Staph. aureus* or *Candida* spp., consideration may be given to using antibiotic lock therapy. **There is no consensus on the protocol of antibiotic lock therapy** and it may differ between institutions. This should usually be done in consultation with an infectious disease specialist and in conjunction with the local pharmacy.
- Infection of a long-term CVC (e.g., tunneled catheter or totally implanted catheter) presents a unique challenge when it comes to catheter removal. The choice to remove or retain the catheter is dependent upon the causative organism, the indication for the long-term catheter, and the presence or absence of an alternative site for vascular access.
- Complicated infection of a long-term CVC is defined as the presence of abscess or tunnel infection or the presence of endocarditis or metastatic focus of infection. Long-term CVCs should be removed in all cases of complicated CRBSIs.
- The following are details in the treatment of uncomplicated long-term CVC infection due to specific organisms:
  - ○ ***Staph. aureus***. Long-term CVC should be removed followed by 4 to 6 weeks of effective parenteral antibiotics. Shorter courses can only be considered if the patient is not diabetic or immunocompromised, the catheter is removed, blood cultures are negative and fevers have resolved at 72 hours and there is no evidence of endocarditis on transesophageal echocardiogram, and there is no evidence of suppurative thrombophlebitis, or other metastatic infection. Due to the high morbidity and mortality, *Staph. aureus* blood stream infections are best managed in consultation with an infectious disease specialist.[1] Some guidelines suggest that all patients with *Staph. aureus* bacteremia should be evaluated with an echocardiogram; however, this remains controversial.
  - ○ **Gram-negative bacilli**. If possible, remove the long-term CVC followed by 7 to 14 days of effective parenteral antibiotics. If vascular access is difficult and infection is uncomplicated, it is reasonable to attempt to treat through the infection with 10 to 14 days of effective parenteral antibiotics, and antibiotic lock therapy should be considered in conjunction with pharmacy. If there is persistent bacteremia or no clinical improvement, the catheter should be removed followed by 7 to 14 days of effective antibiotics.
  - ○ ***Candida*** **spp**. Long-term CVC should be removed as soon as possible followed by 14 days of appropriate antifungal therapy.
  - ○ ***Enterococcus*** **spp**. Long-term CVC may be retained if infection is uncomplicated. Treat with 10 to 14 days of effective parenteral antibiotics. Antibiotic lock therapy can be considered in conjunction with pharmacy. If there is persistent bacteremia, or no clinical improvement, the catheter should be removed followed by 7 to 14 days of effective antibiotics.
  - ○ **Coagulase-negative *Staphylococcus***. Long-term CVC may be retained if infection is uncomplicated. Treat with 10 to 14 days of effective parenteral antibiotics. Antibiotic lock therapy can be considered in conjunction with pharmacy. If there is persistent bacteremia or no clinical improvement, the catheter should be removed followed by 7 to 14 days of effective antibiotics. The exception to this is infection with *Staphylococcus lugdunensis*, which should be treated more aggressively with catheter removal and further evaluation as for *Staph. aureus*.
- Figure 4-1 presents a summary of the management of CRBSIs.[2]

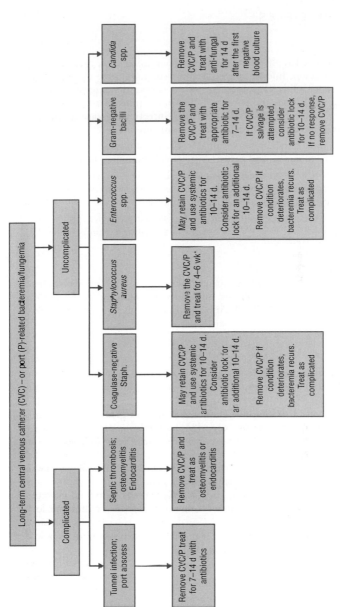

FIGURE 4-1 Management of central venous catheter-related bacteremia and fungemia.

*A shorter course of antibiotics may be considered (≥14 d) if catheter is removed, infection is uncomplicated, bacteremia and fevers resolve within 72 hours, and the patient is nondiabetic, nonneutropenic, nonimmunosuppressed, patient is without prosthetic intravascular device (e.g., graft and pacemaker), transesophageal echocardiogram is negative, and ultrasound is negative for septic thrombophlebitis.

Adapted from Mermel LA, Allon M, Bouza E, et al. Clinical practice guidelines for the diagnosis and management of intravascular catheter-related infection: 2009 Update by the Infectious Diseases Society of America. *Clin Infect Dis.* 2009;49:1-45.

NATIVE VALVE ENDOCARDITIS

GENERAL PRINCIPLES

Definition

- Endocarditis is defined as inflammation of the inner lining of the heart and heart valves, or endocardium. Infections are the most common cause of endocarditis (i.e., infective endocarditis [IE]). Infection of the endocardium, most commonly the heart valves, is a serious and potentially life-threatening disease. Presentation may be acute or subacute. **Consultation with an infectious disease specialist is recommended in most cases of suspected or confirmed IE**.

- Acute IE has the onset of symptoms within 3 to 10 days of presentation. The course of acute IE may be fulminant and patients may rapidly become critically ill.

- Subacute IE is more indolent and symptoms may be present for weeks or months. The frequent symptoms of subacute endocarditis are fever, fatigue, and weight loss and patients may have evidence of embolic phenomena.

- This section reviews native valve endocarditis, but similar principles apply to prosthetic valve endocarditis (PVE). PVE is covered in a separate section.

Epidemiology

Risk factors for the development of IE include prior endocarditis, valve replacement, valvular damage (e.g., age-related sclerosis, mitral valve prolapse, and history of rheumatic fever), and IV drug use (IVDU). Also any condition that increases the risk of bacteremia will increase the risk of endocarditis.

Etiology

- **The organisms most commonly associated with native valve endocarditis are *Staph. aureus*, *Streptococcus* spp. (classically *S. viridans*), and *Enterococcus* spp**.

- Less common causes of native valve endocarditis include gram-negative bacilli, HACEK organisms (*Haemophilus* spp. [*H. aphrophilus*, *H. parainfluenzae*, *H. paraphrophilus*], *Aggregatibacter actinomycetemcomitans*, *Cardiobacterium hominis*, *Eikenella corrodens*, and *Kingella kingae*), coagulase-negative staphylococci, fungi, *Bartonella* spp. (*B. henselae* or *B. quintana*), *Tropheryma whippelii*, *Legionella* spp., *Chlamydia* spp., *Abiotrophia* spp., (previously called nutritionally deficient streptococci), and *Coxiella burnetii*. When no pathogen is identified, but the diagnostic criteria are met, this is termed culture-negative endocarditis.

- Patient demographics may give a clue to the possible causative organism in IE.
  - Patients with poor dentition or following dental procedures are more commonly infected with viridans group streptococci.
  - Patients with indwelling venous catheters are at more risk for staphylococcal endocarditis.
  - IVDU may lead to pseudomonal or fungal endocarditis, although *Staphylococcus* spp. are still more common.

○ Nosocomial infection may be due to any number of gram-negative organisms or staphylococci including MRSA.

- **Culture-negative endocarditis** accounts for approximately 5% of cases of endocarditis, when strict diagnostic criteria are followed. **The most common reason for negative cultures is antibiotic administration prior to blood cultures being drawn**. True culture-negative endocarditis presents a unique challenge and may prompt additional diagnostics such as serology or polymerase chain reaction (PCR) testing for organisms such as *Bartonella, Coxiella, Legionella,* and *T. whippelii.* Bacterial 16S ribosomal RNA gene sequencing has shown promise in identifying the etiologic agent when the valve is removed and subjected to testing.

Pathophysiology

- The classic lesion of endocarditis is the valvular vegetation. Vegetations are made up of fibrin, platelets, microorganisms, and cells. The vegetation tends to form in areas of turbulent blood flow. This is most common when a valve is congenitally abnormal or damaged by some other factor. When microorganisms seed a damaged part of the endocardium, a vegetation forms creating a protective barrier.

- The most commonly involved area is the ventricular surface of the mitral valve, followed by the aortic valve; however, any area of the endocardium may be involved. There is a classic relationship between tricuspid valve endocarditis and IVDU.

Prevention

- The American Heart Association has published guidelines for antimicrobial prophylaxis to prevent IE (Table 4-1).[8]
- In 2007, these guidelines were significantly revised in recognition of the data showing that antimicrobial prophylaxis prevents an exceedingly small number of cases of IE and that the risk of antibiotic-associated adverse events exceeded the benefit for preventing IE.
- The updated guidelines were changed to only recommend antibiotic prophylaxis for the subset of patients at the greatest risk of developing IE.
- It is no longer recommended to give antibiotic prophylaxis for patients with bicuspid aortic valve, mitral valve prolapse with regurgitation, or hypertrophic cardiomyopathy.
- Antibiotic prophylaxis is not recommended prior to procedures with lower associated risk of bacteremia such as gastrointestinal procedures (including colonoscopy with biopsy), genitourinary procedures, respiratory procedures (unless incision or biopsy of the respiratory mucosa is planned), and vaginal or cesarian births.
- Antimicrobial prophylaxis can be considered in high-risk patients who are undergoing surgical procedures in which bacteremia is likely, such as incision and drainage of a skin abscess or gastrointestinal manipulation in the setting of an active colon infection, or genitourinary procedure in the setting of an active genitourinary infection.

TABLE 4-1   INFECTIVE ENDOCARDITIS PROPHYLAXIS

I. **Endocarditis prophylaxis is recommended only for the following cardiac conditions**: prosthetic valves; previous endocarditis; unrepaired congenital heart disease, including palliative shunts or conduits; repaired congenital heart disease with prosthetic material during the first 6 mo after procedure or with residual defects at or adjacent to the site of the prosthetic device; cardiac valvulopathy in transplant recipients.

II. Regimens for dental, oral, or respiratory tract procedures (including dental extractions, periodontal or endodontal procedures, professional teeth cleaning, bronchoscopy with biopsy, rigid bronchoscopy, surgery on respiratory mucosa, and tonsillectomy).

Clinical scenario	Drug and dosage
Standard prophylaxis	Amoxicillin 2 g PO 1 h before procedure
Unable to take PO	Ampicillin 2 g IM or IV or cefazolin or ceftriaxone 1 g IM or IV within 30 min before procedure
Penicillin-allergic patient	Clindamycin 600 mg PO, or cephalexin 2 g PO, or clarithromycin or azithromycin 500 mg PO 1 h before procedure
Penicillin-allergic and unable to take PO	Clindamycin 600 mg IV or cefazolin or ceftriaxone 1 g IV within 30 min before procedure

III. **Gastrointestinal and genitourinary procedures do not require routine use of prophylaxis**. High-risk patients infected or colonized with enterococci should receive amoxicillin, ampicillin, or vancomycin to eradicate the organism prior to urinary tract manipulation.

IV. Prophylaxis is recommended for procedures on infected skin, skin structures, or musculoskeletal tissue ONLY for patients with cardiac conditions outlined above. An antistaphylococcal penicillin or cephalosporin should be used.

—

Adapted from Wilson W, Taubert KA, Gewitz M, et al. Prevention of infective endocarditis: guidelines from the American Heart Association: a guideline from the American Heart Association Rheumatic Fever, Endocarditis, and Kawasaki Disease Committee, Council on Cardiovascular Disease in the Young, and the Council on Clinical Cardiology, Council on Cardiovascular Surgery and Anesthesia, and the Quality of Care and Outcomes Research Interdisciplinary Working Group. *Circulation.* 2007;116:1736-1754.

DIAGNOSIS

Clinical Presentation

History
- Patients with endocarditis may present with a wide spectrum of complaints.
- **The most common symptoms include fevers, weight loss, malaise, fatigue, night sweats, low back pain, arthralgias, and evidence of embolic phenomenon** (e.g., rash, hematuria, lung abscess, and stroke).

- Depending upon the extent of the valve damage, patients may also present with symptoms of left or right heart failure, shortness of breath, syncope, or arrhythmias.

Physical Examination
- Physical examination may reveal fever, findings consistent with heart failure or valve regurgitation, new murmur, splenomegaly, and evidence of embolic phenomenon.
- An abnormal neurologic examination may be present due to central nervous system (CNS) embolism or due to a ruptured mycotic aneurysm.
- Cutaneous findings may include petechiae, Osler nodes (painful subcutaneous nodules frequently on the pads of the fingers and toes), Janeway lesions (nonpainful hemorrhages found in the palms, soles, fingers, and toes), splinter hemorrhages (small linear hemorrhages underneath the fingernails or toenails), Roth spots (clear centered retinal hemorrhages), and subconjunctival hemorrhages.

Diagnostic Criteria
The most commonly used diagnostic criteria are the Duke criteria (Table 4-2).[9,10]

Diagnostic Testing
Laboratories
- **The key to the diagnosis of IE is obtaining adequate blood cultures**.
  - At least two to three blood cultures should be obtained by peripheral venipuncture, separated in time by at least 30 minutes each. Blood cultures should be obtained prior to the initiation of antibiotics.
  - If the patient is hemodynamically stable and not acutely ill, there is no urgent need to start antibiotics until the diagnosis is confirmed.
  - As long as antibiotics are not given prior to blood cultures being obtained, a microbiological diagnosis will frequently be made with blood cultures alone.
  - Due to advancements in laboratory techniques, organisms previously thought to be "slow-growing" or fastidious (i.e., HACEK organisms) are now usually identified in routine culture within 5 days.
- Serologic testing for unusual causes of endocarditis (e.g., *Coxiella* or *Bartonella* antibodies) is indicated only if cultures are negative or if the patient's travel or exposure history suggests an alternative diagnosis (i.e., chronic endocarditis with history of travel to Iraq, Afghanistan, or the Netherlands, or exposure to livestock for *Coxiella*; homelessness or cat exposure for *Bartonella*).
- Routine laboratory evaluation is frequently nonspecific. Some common abnormalities include leukocytosis, elevated inflammatory markers (erythrocyte sedimentation rate [ESR] and C-reactive protein [CRP]), anemia, proteinuria, and hematuria. Renal failure is not uncommon, due to immune complex deposition in the kidneys.

Electrocardiography
Electrocardiogram should be performed whenever endocarditis is considered. Findings may reveal a new conduction abnormality (bundle branch block, atrioventricular block, or fascicular block) in the setting of myocardial invasion or valvular abscess.

3 2783 00124 7637

PRAIRIE STATE COLLEGE
LIBRARY

TABLE 4-2	DUKE CRITERIA FOR THE DIAGNOSIS OF ENDOCARDITIS

Definite endocarditis requires two major criteria; one major criterion and three minor criteria; or five minor criteria

Possible endocarditis requires one major and one minor criterion; or three minor criteria

No endocarditis: when the criteria above are not met, there is no evidence to confirm the diagnosis of IE

Major criteria

- Positive blood culture suggestive of IE:
  - Typical organism isolated from at least two separate blood cultures: viridans streptococci, *Staphylococcus aureus*, HACEK organisms, *Streptococcus bovis*, or *Enterococcus* spp. in the absence of an alternative primary site of infection OR
  - Persistently positive blood cultures: at least two cultures drawn 12 h apart or three cultures with first and last drawn at least 1 h apart OR
  - One culture (or phase 1 IgG > 1:800) for *Coxiella burnetii*
- Evidence of endocardial involvement: echocardiogram showing oscillating intracardiac mass without alternative explanation; or abscess; or new partial dehiscence of prosthetic valve; or new valvular regurgitation

Minor criteria

- Predisposition to IE: prior IE, IVDU, prosthetic heart valve, or cardiac lesion causing turbulent blood flow
- Documented fever ≥38°C (100.4°F)
- Vascular phenomenon: arterial embolism, pulmonary infarct, mycotic aneurysm, intracranial or conjunctival hemorrhage, or Janeway lesions
- Immunologic phenomena: Osler nodes, Roth spots, glomerulonephritis, or positive rheumatoid factor
- Microbiologic findings not meeting major criteria

HACEK, *Haemophilus* spp. (*H. aphrophilus*, *H. parainfluenzae*, *H. paraphrophilus*), *Aggregatibacter actinomycetemcomitans*, *Cardiobacterium hominis*, *Eikenella corrodens*, and *Kingella kingae*; IE, infective endocarditis; IVDU, intravenous drug use.

Imaging

- **The second most important aspect of diagnosis is cardiac imaging. The gold standard in cardiac imaging is transesophageal echocardiography (TEE).** Transthoracic echocardiography (TTE) also plays a role in the diagnosis of IE. TEE is more sensitive than TTE (93% and 46%, respectively) but both tests are specific.[11] Both modalities can assess for cardiac dysfunction, but TEE usually provides more anatomical detail.
- Based on the clinical impression, a physician may choose to perform a TTE first. The choice of which test to order first depends on factors such as clinical suspicion and patient-specific demographics.[12]

- ○ If the index of suspicion for IE is intermediate or high, TEE should be the initial imaging modality. Also, if patient's body habitus or underlying lung disease may interfere with TTE, TEE should be performed as the initial study.
- ○ If the index of suspicion for IE is low, TTE is a reasonable initial test. If TTE is negative in this scenario, alternative diagnoses should be sought. If no alterative diagnosis has been made after a thorough evaluation, or the clinical suspicion of IE increases, then TEE may be performed as the definitive test. Also, if a patient is unstable or has another contraindication for TEE, or if TEE is not readily available, TTE can be the first test of choice.
- Chest radiography is nonspecific and may be normal, or it may show evidence of heart failure or of metastatic lung abscesses.

TREATMENT

Medications
- Adequate medical treatment of endocarditis is difficult and **requires long-term antibiotics**. Bacteria can persist in vegetations where they are isolated from host defenses or they may form biofilms, which are layers of a slime-like glycocalyx which protects the organisms from phagocytosis. Also, when organisms are in biofilms, they can enter dormant stages of reproduction making antibiotics less effective.
- **In general, high serum concentrations of antibiotics are needed** to diffuse into the vegetations, which are avascular and walled off with fibrin and other components. The recommendations are to give high doses of effective, parenteral, bactericidal antibiotics, sometimes in combination, for a prolonged period of time.
- Empiric antibiotics should be initiated in cases of suspected acute IE **after** blood cultures are obtained. In general, initial coverage should be broad and should cover *Staph. aureus*, including methicillin-resistant strains (MRSA). If the clinical scenario suggests gram-negative endocarditis, empiric antibiotics should include appropriate coverage, such as a third- or fourth-generation cephalosporin. Empiric gentamicin may be used as well, although its utility and safety in many scenarios are currently under question.
- When patients are clinically stable and there is a suspicion for subacute endocarditis, antibiotics need not be given empirically. Appropriate antibiotics should be initiated after culture results are known.
- Specific antibiotic treatment for IE is presented in Table 4-3.[13]
- For non-HACEK gram-negative organisms, antibiotics should be tailored to the susceptibility of the organism. Identity (ID) consultation is recommended.
- Fungal endocarditis should be treated initially with a lipid formulation of amphotericin B. The mortality of fungal endocarditis is high and early surgical evaluation is suggested.

Surgical Management
- IE can be treated with medical management alone in about 60% of cases. About 40% of cases require surgical intervention with either valve replacement or valve repair.
- The main indication for valve replacement surgery is symptomatic congestive heart failure due to valve dysfunction. Patients with symptomatic congestive heart failure as well as patients with acute or fulminate infections should be evaluated by a cardiac surgeon with experience in valvular surgery.

TABLE 4-3 TREATMENT OF NATIVE VALVE ENDOCARDITIS CAUSED BY SPECIFIC ORGANISMS

Organism	Antibiotic regimen	Duration	Notes
Viridians streptococci			
Penicillin MIC <0.12 µg/mL	• Penicillin G 12-18 MU IV q24h or ceftriaxone • Above **PLUS** gentamicin • Vancomycin if PCN allergic	• 4 or 2 wk total if in combination with gentamicin	
Penicillin MIC 0.12–0.5 µg/mL	• Penicillin G 4MU IV q4h or ceftriaxone **PLUS** gentamicin • Vancomycin if PCN allergic	• 4 wk total with 2 wk of gentamicin	
Penicillin MIC > 0.5 µg/mL	• Ampicillin–sulbactam **PLUS** gentamicin • Vancomycin **PLUS** gentamicin	• 4–6 wk	
Enterococcus species (same as prosthetic valve endocarditis)			
Penicillin-susceptible	• Ampicillin **PLUS** gentamicin • Vancomycin	• 4–6 wk	• Substitute streptomycin 7 mg/kg q12h for high-level gentamicin resistance
Penicillin-resistant	• β-Lactamase production: ampicillin–sulbactam **PLUS** gentamicin • Intrinsically resistant: vancomycin **PLUS** gentamicin	• 6 wk	
Vancomycin- and ampicillin-resistant	• Linezolid or daptomycin • Quinupristin/dalfopristin ± doxycycline	• ≥8 wk	• Consult infectious diseases specialist
Staphylococcus species			
Methicillin-sensitive *Staph. aureus* and coagulase-negative staphylococci	• Oxacillin/nafcillin • ±Gentamicin • Vancomycin if PCN allergic	• 8 wk	• Gentamicin use is controversial and should be used no more than 3–5 d • Vancomycin troughs should be followed with a goal of 15–20 µg/dL

Methicillin-resistant *Staph. aureus* and coagulase-negative staphylococci	• Vancomycin • Daptomycin is alternative, only approved for right-sided endocarditis		
HACEK organisms and culture-negative IE	• Ceftriaxone or ampicillin–sulbactam or ciprofloxacin	• 4 wk	• HACEK = *Haemophilus* spp., *Actinobacillus*, *Cardiobacterium*, *Eikenella*, and *Kingella*

IE, infective endocarditis; MIC, minimum inhibitory concentration; PCN, penicillin.

Dosing: Ceftriaxone 2 g IV q24h; gentamicin 1 mg/kg q8h; vancomycin 15 mg/kg IV q12h for normal renal function; ampicillin–sulbactam 3 g IV q6h; ampicillin 2 g IV q4h; oxacillin/nafcillin 2 g IV q4h; rifampin 300 mg PO q8h; cefazolin 2 g IV q8h; daptomycin 6 mg/kg/d; linezolid 600 mg IV q12h; ciprofloxacin 400 mg IV q12h.

Baseline and weekly audiometry recommended for patients receiving aminoglycosides >7 d.

Monitor aminoglycoside and vancomycin levels. Goal vancomycin trough levels are 15–20 µg/mL.

Adapted from Baddour LM, Wilson WR, Bayer AS, et al. Infective endocarditis: diagnosis, antimicrobial therapy, and management of complications: a statement for healthcare professionals from the Committee on Rheumatic Fever, Endocarditis, and Kawasaki Disease, Council on Cardiovascular Disease in the Young, and the Councils on Clinical Cardiology, Stroke, and Cardiovascular Surgery and Anesthesia, American Heart Association: endorsed by the Infectious Diseases Society of America. *Circulation*. 2005;111:e394-e434.

- Patients with fungal IE and *Pseudomonas* IE respond poorly to medical therapy alone. Cardiac surgical evaluation is suggested in these cases.
- Patients with a myocardial abscess, moderate or severe valvular regurgitation, and patients who do not clear blood cultures within 2 to 3 days of effective treatment should also be considered for surgery.

COMPLICATIONS

- **Mycotic aneurysms** are abnormal aneurysmal dilations of arteries caused by IE.
  - They are caused either by direct infection of the arterial wall, immune complex deposition in the blood vessel wall, or embolic occlusion of the vasa vasorum.
  - The incidence of mycotic aneurysms in IE is unknown.
  - Mycotic aneurysms are most commonly in the cerebral circulation but may also exist in other vascular distributions.
  - Usually, these are clinically silent until they rupture. Ruptured CNS mycotic aneurysms have approximately 80% mortality.[13] Routine screening is not indicated; however, if CNS symptoms develop, the clinician should have a low threshold to evaluate with neurological imaging and neurosurgical evaluation.
- Embolic events are common complications of endocarditis. Emboli most commonly travel to the cerebral, renal, splenic, pulmonary, coronary, and systemic circulation. This can result in abscess formation or ischemic damage to distant tissue.

- **Immunologic complication**s are also common in IE. IE stimulates the cellular and humoral immune system, which may result in hypergammaglobulinemia, splenomegaly, and the deposition of immune complexes in distant organs such as the kidneys. Rheumatoid factor and antinuclear antibodies may develop and may play a role in the pathogenesis of IE.
- **Renal dysfunction** in IE is not uncommon. This may occur due to several different processes including abscess formation, infarction, and glomerulonephritis.

PROSTHETIC VALVE ENDOCARDITIS

GENERAL PRINCIPLES

- This section is specifically devoted to endocarditis involving prosthetic valves. Many of the principles are the same as in native valve endocarditis; however, the etiologic agents and the treatment are different.
- PVE more frequently requires surgery in order to achieve a cure. Early surgical consultation with a cardiac surgeon is suggested in PVE.

Etiology

- PVE can be divided into early PVE and late PVE based on the time from valve placement to the time of infection. There is no consensus regarding the cutoff between early- and late-onset PVE. The etiologic agents responsible are differently distributed between early and late PVE.
- **The vast majority of early-onset PVE is caused by *Staph. aureus* and coagulase-negative staphylococci.**
- **Late-onset PVE is still predominantly caused by staphylococci; however, other organisms associated with native valve endocarditis begin to increase in frequency.**

Epidemiology

PVE accounts for up to a third of all cases of IE. IE is more common among patients with mechanical prosthetic valves rather than bioprosthetic valves.[14] In the first year after implantation, the risk is between 1% and 3%. After the first year the rate drops to about 0.5% per year. Contamination of the valve may occur at the time of implantation or it may develop later by hematogenous seeding.

Pathophysiology

- Newly replaced valves are not yet endothelialized, which puts them at greater risk for the development of a sterile platelet fibrin thrombus. This thrombus provides a place for bacteria to adhere. This most commonly occurs at the interface with the cuff and the native tissue and frequently perivalvular leaks will be present at diagnosis.
- Biofilm formation plays a large role in the pathogenesis of PVE. Biofilms are polysaccharide-enclosed matrices which protect the infecting organism from host defenses such as phagocytosis. Also, biofilms provide protection from antibiotic exposure. Finally, many organisms in biofilms may lie dormant and many antibiotics require cell division to work effectively.

DIAGNOSIS

- Microbiologic diagnosis of PVE is the same as that for native valve IE. Physicians should have a high index of suspicion for PVE in a patient with fevers and a prosthetic valve. Extension into the myocardium is more common in PVE, and electrocardiography (ECG) abnormalities may be more common.
- Approximately 50% of patients with *Staph. aureus* bacteremia and 40% of patients with coagulase-negative staphylococci bacteremia go on to develop endocarditis.[14]
- **TEE is required in all cases of suspected PVE**.
  - o TTE is inadequate to evaluate PVE due to decreased sensitivity and specificity when prosthetic valve material is present.
  - o The initial TEE may be negative early in PVE or in cases where a small abscess is present.
  - o If initial TEE is negative and suspicion remains high, a repeat TEE should be performed several days later.

TREATMENT

Medications
- The basic principles of medical management of PVE are similar to those of treating native valve IE. Treatment should be with **high-dose, parenteral, bactericidal antibiotic**s.
- Empiric antibiotics should be started after blood cultures if the patient is acutely ill or clinically unstable. If the patient is clinically stable and there is a suspicion for subacute endocarditis, antibiotics need not be given until the culture results are known.
- Empiric antibiotic choice for either early or late PVE should initially include vancomycin 15 mg/kg IV q12h, **PLUS** rifampin 300 mg IV or PO q8h × 6 weeks, **PLUS** gentamicin 1 mg/kg IV q8h.
- Culture-driven antibiotic therapy for PVE is detailed in Table 4-4.[13]
- For non-HACEK group, gram-negative organisms, PVE antipseudomonal penicillin or cephalosporin plus aminoglycoside is recommended. An ID consultation is also recommended.
- Fungal endocarditis should be treated initially with amphotericin B. The mortality of fungal endocarditis is high and early surgical evaluation is suggested.
- Patients with mechanical valves on long-term oral anticoagulation with warfarin should have warfarin held and IV heparin initiated upon the diagnosis of IE, as surgery may be required. Also, all antiplatelet agents should be held. If the patient develops neurologic symptoms, heparin should be stopped until intracranial hemorrhage is ruled out.

Surgical Management
- Patients with PVE are less likely to be cured with antibiotics alone than are patients with native valve IE. A cardiac surgeon should be contacted early in patients with suspected or confirmed PVE.
- Indications for valve surgery in PVE include symptomatic congestive heart failure, instability of the prosthetic valve, persistent bacteremia despite adequate effective antibiotics, vegetation >10 mm, persistent fevers despite antibiotics for ≥10 days, or PVE with fungus, *Pseudomonas*, *Staph. aureus*, or most *Enterococcus* spp.

TABLE 4-4	TREATMENT OF PROSTHETIC VALVE ENDOCARDITIS CAUSED BY SPECIFIC ORGANISMS		
Organism	**Antibiotic regimen**	**Duration**	**Notes**
Viridians Streptococci or Streptococcus bovis			
MIC <0.12 µg/mL	• Penicillin G 12–18 MU IV q24h or ceftriaxone • With or without gentamicin • Vancomycin if PCN allergic	6 wk	Including gentamicin does not improve cure rates and should be used with caution
MIC ≥0.12 µg/mL	• Penicillin G 4MU IV q4h or ceftriaxone **PLUS** gentamicin • Vancomycin if PCN allergic	4 wk	
Enterococcus species (same as native valve endocarditis)			
Penicillin-susceptible	• Ampicillin **PLUS** gentamicin • Vancomycin	4–6 wk	Substitute streptomycin 7 mg/kg q12h for high-level gentamicin resistance
Penicillin-resistant	• β-Lactamase producing: ampicillin–sulbactam **PLUS** gentamicin • Intrinsically resistant: Vancomycin **PLUS** gentamicin	6 wk	
Vancomycin- and ampicillin-resistant	• Linezolid or daptomycin • Quinupristin/ dalfopristin ± doxycycline	≥8 wk	Consult infectious diseases specialist
Staphylococcus species			
Methicillin-sensitive *Staph. aureus* and coagulase-negative staphylococci	Oxacillin/nafcillin **PLUS** rifampin **PLUS** gentamicin	≥8 wk total with 2 wk of gentamicin	
Methicillin-resistant *Staph. aureus* and coagulase-negative staphylococci	Vancomycin **PLUS** rifampin **PLUS** gentamicin		

HACEK organisms and culture-negative IE	Ceftriaxone or ampicillin-sulbactam or ciprofloxacin	4 wk	HACEK = *Haemophilus* spp., *Actinobacillus, Cardiobacterium, Eikenella*, and *Kingella*

IE, infective endocarditis; MIC, minimum inhibitory concentration; PCN, penicillin.

Dosing: Ceftriaxone 2 g IV q24h; gentamicin 2 g qd or 1 mg/kg q8h; vancomycin 1 g IV q24h; ampicillin–sulbactam 3 g IV q6h; ampicillin 2 g IV q4h, oxacillin 2 g IV q4h; rifampin 300 mg PO q8h; cefazolin 2 g IV q8h; daptomycin 6 mg/kg/d; linezolid 600 mg IV q12h; ciprofloxacin 400 mg IV q12h.

Baseline and weekly audiometry recommended for patients receiving aminoglycosides >7 d.

Monitor aminoglycoside and vancomycin levels. Goal vancomycin trough levels are near to 15 μg/mL.

Adapted from Baddour LM, Wilson WR, Bayer AS, et al. Infective endocarditis: diagnosis, antimicrobial therapy, and management of complications: a statement for healthcare professionals from the Committee on Rheumatic Fever, Endocarditis, and Kawasaki Disease, Council on Cardiovascular Disease in the Young, and the Councils on Clinical Cardiology, Stroke, and Cardiovascular Surgery and Anesthesia, American Heart Association: endorsed by the Infectious Diseases Society of America. *Circulation.* 2005;111:e394-e434.

- Intracerebral hemorrhage is a contraindication to cardiac surgery but cerebral embolism without evidence of hemorrhage is not.
- TEE is of the utmost importance to fully evaluate for dysfunction of the prosthetic valve.
- Postoperative antibiotics should be continued for a full course, starting from the time of surgery.

INFECTION OF IMPLANTED CARDIAC DEVICES

GENERAL PRINCIPLES

- The implanted cardiac devices most associated with infection are permanent pacemakers (PPMs), implanted cardioverter–defibrillators (ICD), and left ventricular assist devices (LVADs). Any implanted foreign material, such as cardiac stents, patches, and peripheral vascular grafts, may be infected; however, the rate of infection of these devices is much lower.
- Implanted electrophysiologic cardiac devices (PPM and ICD) are being implanted at an increased rate in the United States. Cardiac device infection is rising at an even greater rate than the rate of implantation.
- LVAD infections can include surgical site infections, sternal infection, deep organ infection, or blood stream infection.

Epidemiology

- The overall rate of device infection is between 0.13% and 19.9%. The higher rate was from the era of intra-abdominal implantation.[15] The current rate is likely closer to 1%.
- Risk factors for the development of cardiac device infections include fever within 24 hours of device implantation, lack of prophylactic antibiotic use, temporary pacing before permanent device placement, presence of a tunneled venous catheter, diabetes mellitus, renal failure, malignancy, operator inexperience, prior device infection, use of more than two leads, and anticoagulation.
- The rate of implantation of electrophysiologic cardiac devices (PPM and ICD) increased by 42% in the United States between 1990 and 1999. The rate of device infections rose by 124% over that same period.[16,17] The reason for this is likely the changing demographics of the patients receiving device implantation. Patients currently receiving devices are older and frequently have more comorbid medical conditions.
- The reported rate of LVAD infection varies from 13% to 80%.[15]

Etiology

- **Staphylococci account for the vast majority of PPM and ICD infections.** Coagulase-negative staphylococci account for 42% of cases and *Staph. aureus* accounts for 29%. The remaining cases are due to gram-negative bacilli (9%), other gram-positive cocci (4%), polymicrobial infection (7%), fungi (2%), and culture negative (7%).[18]
- **Staphylococci account for approximately half of all LVAD infections.**
  - ○ **Other frequently encountered organisms include enterococci, *Enterobacter* spp., and *P. aeruginosa*.**
  - ○ Also of note, infection with *Candida* spp. is not uncommon. The presence of colonization with *Candida* is very common but actual infection is less frequent.
  - ○ Infection due to resistant organisms is common in LVAD infections as the patients who receive LVADs are chronically ill and have frequent hospitalizations, putting them at risk for nosocomial infection.

Pathophysiology

- The pathogenesis of PPM and ICD infections is most commonly **contamination of the device with skin flora at the time of implantation or manipulation** (such as generator change).
- Alternatively implanted cardiac devices may be secondarily infected by **seeding of the device during bacteremia from a distant source of infection** (i.e., vascular catheter infection, skin and soft tissue infections, urinary tract infections, pneumonia, or intra-abdominal infections).
- **Biofilm formation** plays a large role in the pathogenesis of cardiac device infections. Biofilms are polysaccharide-enclosed matrices that protect the infecting organism from host defenses such as phagocytosis. Also biofilms provide protection from antibiotic exposure. Finally, many organisms in biofilms may lie dormant and many antibiotics require cell division to work effectively.
- LVADs are driven by a pump which may be extracorporeal or may be implanted in the abdomen. All LVADs have either a cannula or a driveline that runs transcutaneously. For this reason, **the risk of infection is very high with LVADs.**

Prevention

- The best way to prevent cardiovascular device infection is by practicing **meticulous aseptic technique with device implantation**. Skin preparation should be done with 2% chlorhexidine.
- **Antibiotic prophylaxis** with an appropriate antistaphylococcal agent should be given 30 to 60 minutes before surgery. MRSA coverage should be considered in patients with known MRSA colonization or in areas with high rates of MRSA.
- Antibiotic prophylaxis for patients with implanted cardiac devices prior to dental procedures or other medical procedures is not recommended

DIAGNOSIS

Clinical Presentation

- The presentation can vary depending upon the portion of the device that is infected and the organism causing the infection.
- The most common presentation is local infection at the site of the PPM or ICD implantation. Local infection may manifest itself as cellulitis overlying the pocket, abscess formation, surgical wound dehiscence, sinus tract formation, device migration, or erosion through the skin.
- Patients may also present with occult bacteremia with no evidence of infection at the insertion site.
- The final presentation is with symptoms of endocarditis. The symptoms of device-related endocarditis and other forms of endocarditis are very similar. Systemic septic embolism is rare, but pulmonary embolism is more common due to the right-sided location of implanted cardiac devices.
- Patients with cardiac device infections due to *Staph. aureus* usually present more acutely than those with infection due to coagulase-negative staphylococci.
- If there is obvious inflammation overlying the implanted device, the diagnosis can be readily made.
- A minimum of two blood cultures should be obtained prior to the initiation of antibiotics.
- If there is drainage from the site, it should be swabbed and sent for culture. If a fluid pocket is present over the device, this can be aspirated for culture, although this is not routinely done otherwise.
- Other laboratory findings are nonspecific and may include leukocytosis, anemia, or elevated inflammatory markers.
- **Patients with an ICD or PPM and occult bacteremia should be evaluated for the presence of cardiac device infection, even in the absence of inflammation at the insertion site**.
  - ○ Patients with *Staph. aureus* bacteremia and no evidence of inflammation at the insertion site have been found to have device involvement in up to half of cases.[19]
  - ○ The implantation site can be evaluated for involvement by ultrasound, looking for fluid collection. If fluid is present it can be aspirated for culture, although this carries the risk of introducing infection into a sterile fluid collection. The formation of a sterile fluid collection after 1 month of implantation would be unusual.
  - ○ Indium-labeled leukocyte scan or gallium scanning may help differentiate an inflammatory fluid collection from a noninflammatory one.
- The **Duke criteria** may be used to diagnose implanted cardiac device–related endocarditis (Table 4-2).[9,10] Echocardiography plays a vital role in the diagnosis of device-related

endocarditis. TTE is poorly sensitive for device-related endocarditis and, therefore, TEE should be used. Device-related endocarditis cannot be effectively ruled out with TTE alone.

- Patients with *Staph. aureus* bacteremia, or persistent bacteremia with another organism, and no evidence of infection at the device insertion site (after a thorough evaluation) should be evaluated for evidence of cardiac lead or valve involvement. This should be done with TEE.
- Clinical manifestations of LVAD infection are often different than for other implanted cardiac devices.
  - **Driveline exit site infection is the most common presentation of LVAD infections**.[20, 21] Bacteremia and sepsis may also be apparent at the time of presentation.
  - Less commonly patients may present with dysfunction of the LVAD, manifesting as worsening symptoms of heart failure. This is due to mechanical disruption of the lumen of the device from infection.
  - Diagnosis is made through physical examination of the percutaneous entry site of the driveline or cannula. Blood cultures as well as cultures of any drainage or aspirated fluid collection should be sent for microbiological confirmation.
  - Indium-labeled leukocyte scans have been used to determine the extent of infection.

TREATMENT

- The basic management of implanted electrophysiologic cardiac devices is presented in Figure 4-2.[18]
- **Device removal is required in all cases of suspected or confirmed PPM or ICD infection**.
  - Trials of conservative management with antibiotics alone have had an unacceptably high failure rate.
  - The best strategy is a combination of complete removal of the implanted device AND the cardiac leads combined with parenteral antibiotics.
  - Even if blood cultures are negative, the best strategy is removal of the entire device. In one study of 105 patients with implanted cardiac device infection, 79% had positive cultures of the intravascular portion of the leads, while only 5 patients had bacteremia. Samples of the explanted device and the cardiac leads should be sent for culture and sensitivity testing.
- In some cases, removal of the device and the cardiac leads may either be impossible or it may carry too high a risk of complications. In these cases, as much of the device as possible should be removed. If the device cannot be removed at all, indefinite suppression with oral antibiotics should be considered, after a full treatment course of IV antibiotics.
- Patients with bacteremia with no evidence of pocket inflammation and without evidence of cardiac lead or valve involvement on TEE can usually be managed with antibiotics alone and retention of the implanted device.
- **The antibiotic of choice should be tailored to the results of culture and sensitivity data**. Empiric antibiotics should be directed toward the most likely causative organisms. **Vancomycin is the drug of choice in most cases**.
- Compared with other implanted cardiac devices, **the removal of an LVAD is very complicated, expensive, and frequently unfeasible**.
  - Local debridement of abscesses should be performed when possible.
  - LVAD infections with blood stream involvement should be treated initially with parenteral antibiotics. Successful suppression of symptomatic infection has been

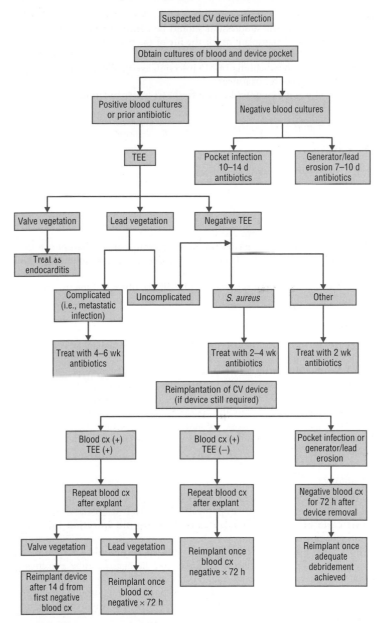

FIGURE 4-2 Management of implanted cardiovascular device infections.

This algorithm applies to patients who have had complete device explantation. Duration of antibiotics should be from the time of device removal.

CV, cardiovascular; cx, culture; TEE, transesophageal echocardiogram.

Adapted from Sohail MR, Uslan DZ, Khan AH, et al. Management and outcome of permanent pacemaker and implantable cardioverter-defibrillator infections. *J Am Coll Cardiol.* 2007;49:1851-1859.

achieved with parenteral antibiotics followed by long-term suppression with oral antibiotics. Antibiotic suppression should be continued until the device is removed at the time of transplant or for the life of the patient when the LVAD is for "destination therapy."
- o Some patients with overwhelming LVAD infection eventually do require removal of the LVAD for successful treatment.
- o LVAD infection is not a contraindication for heart transplantation.

MEDIASTINITIS

GENERAL PRINCIPLES

Definition
- Mediastinitis refers to infection involving the structures of the mediastinum. There are acute and chronic forms.
- Primary infection involving the mediastinum is rare and acute mediastinitis is usually due to the spread of infection from another space, trauma, or following a thoracic surgical procedure.
- Chronic or fibrosing mediastinitis is manifest by diffuse fibrosis of the tissues of the mediastinum.

Epidemiology
- The incidence of mediastinitis after surgery requiring median sternotomy is between 0.5% and 4.4%.[22]
- The incidence is higher in patients who undergo heart transplantation.
- Risk factors for the development of mediastinitis following cardiac surgery are numerous and include obesity, diabetes mellitus, chronic obstructive pulmonary disease, renal failure, cigarette smoking, peripheral vascular disease, use of internal mammary artery for bypass, length of surgery, length of time on cardiopulmonary bypass, need for blood transfusion, length of preoperative hospitalization, and length of ICU stay.

Pathophysiology
- Prior to the advent of cardiothoracic surgery, the most common causes of mediastinitis were esophageal rupture and spread of infection from the oropharynx. Now **most cases of mediastinitis are caused by wound infection following cardiothoracic surgery**.
- Mediastinitis from **esophageal rupture is now most commonly iatrogenic** and may be due to esophageal endoscopic procedure, nasogastric tube placement, esophageal stenting, esophageal dilation, and endotracheal intubation. Other causes of esophageal rupture are spontaneous (also called Boerhaave syndrome), swallowed foreign bodies, penetrating trauma, blunt force trauma, excessive vomiting, and rupture secondary to neoplasm.
- Mediastinitis due to **spread from head and neck infections** occurs by spread along fascial planes into the mediastinum. Head and neck infections that may lead to mediastinitis include Ludwig angina (usually caused by infection of the second or third mandibular molar spreading to the submandibular space and then tracking along the parapharyngeal space or carotid sheath into the mediastinum),

odontogenic infection, tonsillitis, pharyngitis, parotitis, epiglottitis, and Lemierre syndrome (septic thrombophlebitis of the jugular vein and superior vena cava).
- Rarely, mediastinitis may occur following infection of other structures in the chest or abdomen. Mediastinitis has occurred following pneumonia, empyema, infection of the bony structures of the thorax, pancreatitis, and subphrenic abscess.
- Fibrosing mediastinitis may be caused by infection. It is unclear how much of the pathophysiology is due to infection and how much is to an aberrant inflammatory response. It can also be caused by radiation therapy, sarcoidosis, and silicosis.

Etiology

- The bacteriology of mediastinitis depends on if it is postoperative, or secondary to esophageal rupture or spread from head and neck infections.
- Postoperative mediastinitis is most commonly due to contamination of the surgical wound with the patient's endogenous flora. The causative organisms are most commonly gram-positive cocci. ***Staphylococcus epidermidis*, followed by *Staph. aureus*, is the most common causative organism for postoperative mediastinitis**. Gram-negative organisms and fungal organisms are less likely causes.
- Mediastinitis due to esophageal perforation or spread from head and neck infections is frequently polymicrobial and may include anaerobes, gram-negative bacilli, and gram-positive oral flora. Common organisms include Viridans group streptococci, *Peptostreptococcus* spp., *Bacteroides* spp., and *Fusobacterium* spp.
- **The most common underlying infections in chronic or fibrosing mediastinitis are *Histoplasma capsulatum* and tuberculosis**. It has also been described due to *Nocardia asteroides*, *Actinomyces* spp., *Coccidioides immitis*, and *Blastomyces dermatitidis*.

DIAGNOSIS

Clinical Manifestations

- Postoperative patients may complain of out-of-proportion chest pain, which may be pleuritic in nature or may radiate to the neck. This will frequently be accompanied by fevers. Patients may complain of dyspnea, dysphagia, or odynophagia. Instability of the sternotomy fusion is frequently present.
- Mediastinitis stemming from an infection in the head and neck will involve mouth, throat, or neck pain as the earliest manifestation. They may also have facial swelling or neck swelling.
- Physical examination may reveal fever, tachycardia, crepitus, edema or erythema of the chest, and instability of the sternal fusion. Hamman sign is a crunching sound which is synchronous to the heart rhythm due to air in the mediastinum.
- **Lemierre syndrome** usually occurs following bacterial pharyngitis, although it has been described following otitis, mastoiditis, sinusitis, and dental infections.
  - The bacteria migrate along tissue planes to the carotid sheath.
  - The syndrome is characterized by antecedent infection followed by persistent fevers and septic pulmonary embolism.
  - This may be accompanied by neck swelling and induration. Fevers and bacteremia may persist despite adequate antibiotic therapy.
  - The diagnosis can be confirmed by CT scan of the neck or ultrasound demonstrating thrombosis of the jugular vein.
- Patients may also present with signs and symptoms of sepsis.
- Chest radiography may reveal widening of the mediastinum or air in the superior mediastinum. It is important to check a lateral film as some signs may not be

apparent on frontal or posterior views. Chest radiography is less useful in poststernotomy mediastinitis as mediastinal air may be a normal postoperative finding.

- CT scan may be useful to determine the extent of infection or in cases where diagnosis is uncertain. CT scan is essential for the diagnosis of odontogenic or pharyngeal infections. Findings are usually fluid collections, with or without gas present, which track along soft tissue planes. The diagnosis of Lemierre syndrome can be confirmed by CT scan of the neck or ultrasound demonstrating thrombosis of the jugular vein.
- Esophageal rupture may be diagnosed with esophagography using water-soluble contrast material.
- Bacteremia is common in mediastinitis due to *Staph. aureus* or gram-negative bacilli. Blood cultures should be obtained in all cases of suspected mediastinitis, preferably before antibiotics are administered.
- Symptoms of **chronic mediastinitis** can range from chronic cough, dyspnea, wheezing, and hemoptysis to pulmonary hypertension and cor pulmonale.
  - Many patients are asymptomatic.
  - Chronic mediastinitis is the most common, nonmalignant cause of **superior vena cava syndrome**.
  - The diagnosis of chronic mediastinitis is made by pathologic examination from tissue biopsy.

TREATMENT

Acute Mediastinitis

- **Combined medical and surgical treatment is essential in most cases of mediastinitis**. One exception is esophageal microperforation. If microperforation is diagnosed early, it can sometimes be managed by careful monitoring, nasopharyngeal suction, parenteral nutrition, and broad-spectrum antibiotics.
- Postoperative mediastinitis usually requires aggressive surgical debridement and drainage. Initial antibiotics should be broad spectrum and have activity against streptococci as well as gram-negative organisms. Final antibiotic choice should be tailored to the organisms identified in cultures. Duration depends on the extent of infection. **Sternal osteomyelitis is common and, therefore, a prolonged treatment course is usually warranted**.
- Mediastinitis due to spread from head and neck infections should be treated with surgical debridement and drainage along with antibiotics. Frequently surgery is a combined effort with head and neck surgeons and cardiothoracic surgeons. The antibiotics chosen should have activity against oral anaerobes and gram-negative organisms. Traditionally, penicillin G was the drug of choice but with emerging resistance of some mouth anaerobes, combination therapy with β-lactam, β-lactamase inhibitors, carbapenems, or metronidazole or clindamycin combined with gram-negative coverage is usually chosen. Anaerobic coverage should be continued for the duration of therapy, even if no anaerobes are identified in culture, as they are frequently difficult to grow in culture.

Lemierre Syndrome

- Lemierre syndrome is septic thrombophlebitis of the internal jugular vein and or the superior vena cava. Most commonly it occurs in young patients in the second or third decade of life. The most common causative organism is *Fusobacterium necrophorum*, although cases due to *Bacteroides* spp., *Peptostreptococcus* spp., *Staph. aureus*, streptococci, and *Bacteroides fragilis* have been described.

- Empiric therapy should be directed toward oral anaerobes and should include a β-lactam/β-lactamase combination or a carbapenem. Vancomycin should be considered especially if the patient has or has recently had a central venous catheter. Antibiotics should be tailored to the causative organism.
- There remains much controversy regarding the role of anticoagulation. Some authors suggest using anticoagulation only when there is evidence of thrombus extension.[23]
- Surgery may be warranted if an abscess is present, empyema develops, or if the patient fails to improve despite adequate antibiotic therapy.

Chronic Mediastinitis

- There is no definitive or curative treatment for fibrosing mediastinitis.
- Antibiotics and antifungal agents and corticosteroids are usually not indicated, as there is typically no active infection.
- Airway stents can be placed by bronchoscopy and vascular stents percutaneously.
- Sometimes surgery may be required to remove scar tissue in severely symptomatic patients.

ACUTE RHEUMATIC FEVER

GENERAL PRINCIPLES

- Acute rheumatic fever (ARF) is a nonsuppurative sequela of streptococcal pharyngitis. Most cases of ARF are self-limited; however, damage to the cardiac valves may persist and lead to long-term sequela such as progressive cardiac failure, valvular stenosis, and predisposition to endocarditis.
- Patients who recover from ARF are predisposed to future episodes of ARF following subsequent streptococcal infections.

Epidemiology

- The incidence of ARF in the United States and Western Europe has been in steady decline over the past 100 years. This is likely due to the increased antibiotic use for streptococcal pharyngitis and improved general hygiene standards.
- ARF remains a major cause of morbidity and mortality in the developing world. An estimated half-million people worldwide are affected each year. ARF is a disease associated with overcrowding and is more common in lower socioeconomic groups.
- ARF should also be considered in people traveling to endemic regions.
- ARF most commonly affects children between ages 5 and 15 but can occur in adults as well. Recurrent episodes are not uncommon in adults following an acute streptococcal infection.

Etiology

- ARF is a nonsuppurative sequela of Group A streptococcal pharyngitis. It is not known to occur following Group A streptococcal skin infections, implying that the abundant lymphoid tissue in the pharynx may play a role in the pathogenesis.

- The exact mechanism of ARF is not completely understood. It is known that some strains of Group A streptococci are more rheumatogenic than others. There are several theories regarding the pathogenesis of ARF. The first theory is that ARF is caused by the direct toxic effects of a streptococcal toxin. A second theory is that it is caused by a "serum sickness" leading to deposition of antigen–antibody complexes. The third theory, and the theory which garners the most attention, is that ARF occurs as an autoimmune response induced by **molecular mimicry of Group A streptococcal antigens**.

DIAGNOSIS

- Symptoms of ARF usually occur between 1 and 5 weeks following an episode of acute streptococcal pharyngitis.
- **Polyarthritis is the most common symptom** that occurs in about 75% of cases. Clinically evident carditis occurs in 40% to 50% of cases, whereas chorea, subcutaneous nodules, and erythema marginatum are less common, occurring less than 15% of the time.[24]
- Most of the symptoms of ARF are self-limited and resolve without sequela. Carditis is the exception to this.
- Carditis can potentially lead to chronic heart failure and it can rarely be fatal in the acute episode.
- The joint involvement ranges from arthralgias to true arthritis with swelling, erythema, and severe pain. Arthritis is frequently migratory. The most commonly affected joints are the knees, ankles, elbows, and wrists with the joints of the hands being less frequently involved. Typically it resolves within 4 weeks.
- Sydenham chorea is characterized by rapid involuntary movements associated with emotional lability.
- Subcutaneous nodules are firm, painless nodules that tend to occur overlying bony prominences.
- Erythema marginatum is a nonpainful, nonpruritic, erythematous eruption that commonly occurs on the trunk or proximal extremities. The erythema tends to migrate in patterns likened to smoke rings, progressing with the development of central clearing.
- ARF is a clinical diagnosis that is made by using the **Jones criteria**, which are divided into major and minor criteria.
  - The **major criteria** are as follows:
    - Carditis
    - Polyarthritis
    - Sydenham chorea
    - Subcutaneous nodules
    - Erythema marginatum
  - The **minor criteria** are as follows:
    - Arthralgias
    - Fever
    - Elevated acute phase reactants (e.g., ESR and CRP)
    - Heart block (P-R segment prolongation on electrocardiogram)
  - In order to make the diagnosis there must be **evidence of a recent Group A streptococcal infection** (positive throat culture, positive rapid streptococcal antigen test, and elevated antistreptolysin O) in addition to either **two major criteria or one major criterion and two minor criteria**.

TREATMENT

- **Treatment of ARF is essentially supportive.** There are no therapies that prevent the progression to chronic disease. Mild to moderate disease, without carditis, is usually treated with analgesics alone. If carditis is present and there is no evidence of heart failure, **aspirin** is used. If there is evidence of heart failure, **corticosteroids** are used.
- Chorea may be treated with sedative medications or atypical antipsychotics.
- If ARF results in chronic heart failure, it is treated conventionally as heart failure from other causes.
- Recurrent episodes of ARF are common following an acute case. Prophylaxis against subsequent Group A streptococcal infections may be warranted in many situations (Table 4-5).
- The duration of prophylaxis is variable based on the extent of the patient's acute illness and their risk of subsequent Group A streptococcal infections (Table 4-5).

TABLE 4-5 SECONDARY PREVENTION OF RHEUMATIC FEVER

Agents	Dosage	Route
Benzathine penicillin G	600,000 U for children <27 kg, 1.2 million U for children >27 kg every 4 wk	Intramuscular
Penicillin V	250 mg twice daily	Oral
Sulfadiazine	0.5 g daily for children <27 kg, 1 g daily for children >27 kg	Oral
Macrolide or azalide	For individuals with penicillin/ sulfa allergy—dose variable	Oral

Indication	Duration
Rheumatic fever with carditis and residual heart disease (persistent valvular disease)	10 y or until age 40, whichever is longer; sometimes lifetime prophylaxis
Rheumatic fever with carditis but without residual heart disease (no valvular disease)	10 y or until age 21, whichever is longer
Rheumatic fever without carditis —	5 y or until age 21, whichever is longer

Adapted from Gerber MA, Baltimore RS, Eaton CB, et al. Prevention of rheumatic fever and diagnosis and treatment of acute Streptococcal pharyngitis: a scientific statement from the American Heart Association Rheumatic Fever, Endocarditis, and Kawasaki Disease Committee of the Council on Cardiovascular Disease in the Young, the Interdisciplinary Council on Functional Genomics and Translational Biology, and the Interdisciplinary Council on Quality of Care and Outcomes Research: endorsed by the American Academy of Pediatrics. *Circulation.* 2009;119:1541-1551.

MYOCARDITIS

GENERAL PRINCIPLES

- Myocarditis is defined as inflammation of the myocardium. Inflammation may be infectious or noninfectious in etiology. The spectrum of illness ranges from asymptomatic cases to sudden death. In fact, myocarditis is **a major cause of sudden death in patients under age 40**.
- The diagnosis of myocarditis should be considered in anyone presenting with new onset heart failure, or new arrhythmias, especially in the setting of an acute febrile illness or viral upper respiratory syndrome. **Frequently patients may not remember an antecedent infection**, so the absence of prior acute illness does not rule out infectious myocarditis.
- Myocarditis has been identified histologically in 10% to 20% of cases of idiopathic dilated cardiomyopathy.[25]

Etiology

- Numerous viral, bacterial, parasitic, and fungal agents are known to cause myocarditis. Table 4-6 lists potential etiologic agents.
- Although almost any infectious agent can cause myocarditis, viral agents are the most common in the United States and Western Europe. Many cases of idiopathic myocarditis are presumed to be viral in nature.
- **Members of the Enterovirus family, specifically Coxsackie B virus, are the most commonly identified viral pathogens**.
- Bacteria may cause inflammation or infection of the myocardium via toxin production or by direct extension from endocarditis.
  - ○ *Corynebacterium diphtheriae.* Myocardial involvement is the most common cause of death in cases of diphtheria infection. Diphtheritic myocarditis is toxin mediated and not due to direct invasion by the organism.
  - ○ *Rickettsia* spp. Myocarditis is not uncommonly seen with rickettsial infections.
  - ○ *Borrelia burgdorferi.* Up to 10% acute cases of Lyme disease (caused by *B. burgdorferi*) can present with myocardial involvement, usually in the form of conduction abnormalities.[26] Most cases of Lyme myocarditis resolve entirely.
- In South America, the most common infectious agent causing myocarditis is *Trypanosoma cruzi*, the causative agent of **Chagas disease**.
  - ○ Chagas disease is one of the most common causes of dilated cardiomyopathy worldwide. Heart failure is the main feature of chronic Chagas disease.
  - ○ The agents of African trypanosomiasis, *Trypanosoma gambiense* and *Trypanosoma rhodesiense*, may also cause heart failure, although CNS involvement is most common.

DIAGNOSIS

- A high index of suspicion is required to make the diagnosis. Patient history may reveal symptoms of a recent viral infection involving the upper respiratory tract or the gastrointestinal tract. The presenting symptoms are indistinguishable from other more common causes of heart failure and can include dyspnea on exertion, orthopnea, cough, pink frothy sputum production, and peripheral edema.

TABLE 4-6 INFECTIOUS CAUSES OF MYOCARDITIS

Viruses

Coxsackie A and B	Influenza A and B	Lymphocytic choriomeningitis virus
Echoviruses	Respiratory syncytial virus	
Enteroviruses	Rabies virus	Lassa virus
Adenovirus	Dengue virus	Cytomegalovirus
Varicella-Zoster virus	Chikungunya virus	Epstein-Barr virus
Poliovirus	Yellow fever virus	Herpes simplex virus
Mumps virus	Argentine hemorrhagic fever (Junin virus)	Hepatitis B and C
Measles virus		Parvovirus B19
Rubella virus	Bolivian hemorrhagic fever (Machupo virus)	Human immunodeficiency virus
Variola virus		
Vaccinia virus		

Bacteria

Corynebacterium diphtheriae	*Staphylococcus aureus*	*Chlamydophila pneumoniae*
Clostridium perfringens	*Listeria monocytogenes*	*Rickettsia rickettsii*
Neisseria meningitides	*Vibrio cholera*	*Rickettsia prowazekii*
Salmonella spp.	*Mycobacterium tuberculosis*	*Rickettsia tsutsugamushi*
Shigella spp.	*Legionella pneumophila*	*Coxiella burnetii*
Campylobacter jejuni	*Mycoplasma pneumoniae*	*Ehrlichia* spp.
Brucella	*Chlamydia psittaci*	*Borrelia burgdorferi*
Streptococcus pyogenes		*Tropheryma whippelii*

Fungi

Aspergillus spp.	*Blastomyces dermatitidis*	*Cryptococcus neoformans*
Candida spp.	*Coccidioides immitis*	*Histoplasma capsulatum*

Parasites

Trypanosoma cruzi	*Trypanosoma rhodesiense*	*Toxoplasma gondii*
Trypanosoma gambiense	*Trichinella spiralis*	*Toxocara canis*

- Infectious myocarditis should be strongly considered in younger patients and patients without prior history or risk factors for heart disease.
- Physical examination may reveal signs of heart failure. Peripheral edema, jugular venous distension, crackles on auscultation of the lungs, and the presence of the third heart sound may be physical examination clues.
- Electrocardiogram will usually give a clue to myocardial involvement. Abnormalities may include conduction abnormalities, supraventricular tachycardia, ventricular arrhythmias, ectopy, heart block, and ischemic changes.

- Lab abnormalities may also be present including an elevation of cardiac enzymes. These enzymes usually peak early in infection and may return to normal after a few days. Leukocytosis may or may not be present.
- **Identification of the exact viral agent responsible is not routinely done**. Antibody titers to specific infective agents can be followed to document a four-fold rise in the convalescent titer. Serum can be sent for PCR for viral agents, although with the exception of testing for treatable viruses such as influenza or human immunodeficiency virus (HIV). It is not clear that there is a clinical benefit to extensive testing.
- Echocardiography is an important component in the diagnosis of myocarditis. Although echocardiography will not reveal the cause of myocardial dysfunction, it may rule out other causes of heart failure such as hypertrophic cardiomyopathy and valvular disease. In general, the cardiac dysfunction caused by myocarditis is diffuse and involves both ventricles. Serial echocardiography may be important to monitor for either resolution or progression.
- Other imaging modalities have been used, such as cardiac MRI and indium 111–labeled antimyosin antibody scintigraphy, when the diagnosis is not established by echocardiography.
- Endomyocardial biopsy is the "gold standard" for diagnosis but this is not routinely done. There are histopathologic criteria for the diagnosis of myocarditis, the Dallas criteria; however, the sensitivity and specificity of evaluating a single sample of myocardium has been questioned.[27]

TREATMENT

- **Supportive care is mainstay of treatment of myocarditis**.
- If the causative agent of infectious myocarditis is identified and if there is specific treatment available, then this should be initiated as soon as the diagnosis is made. Unfortunately, there are few antiviral agents available for the most common causes of infectious myocarditis.
- Treatment with diuretics, afterload reduction, and possible inotropic agents may be needed short term for heart failure management.
- Treatment with immunosuppression with glucocorticoids or cyclophosphamide has not been supported unless an autoimmune etiology is suspected.
- Nonsteroidal antiinflammatory drugs (NSAIDs) should generally be avoided, as they have been shown to worsen outcomes in animal models.
- Many patients with viral myocarditis recover completely with supportive care alone.
- Vaccination is a useful method for preventing infectious myocarditis caused by agents for which there are vaccines available.

PERICARDITIS

GENERAL PRINCIPLES

- Pericarditis, or inflammation of the pericardium, can be classified into several different types of clinical syndromes: acute, relapsing, tamponade, chronic, or constrictive.

- Most infectious etiologies have an acute presentation.
- Pericarditis, like myocarditis, may be infectious or noninfectious in etiology.
- **There is frequently overlap in the syndromes of pericarditis and myocarditis**, and likewise, there is overlap in many of the agents that can cause infectious pericarditis.

Etiology

- **The etiology of pericarditis is most commonly idiopathic or due to viral infection**. Many idiopathic cases of pericarditis are likely due to viral infection that has gone undiagnosed. **The most common viral causes are enteroviruses**, as in myocarditis.
- There are no clinical distinctions between idiopathic and viral pericarditis.
- Pathogens associated with pericarditis are listed in Table 4-7.
- Bacterial causes of pericarditis, or purulent pericarditis, are usually due to extension from head and neck infections, mediastinitis, or postoperative infections. Anaerobic bacteria may cause pericarditis by direct extension from esophageal rupture or mediastinitis, or they may seed the pericardium via the bloodstream. *Neisseria meningitidis* can cause pericarditis by direct bacterial invasion or through a reactive immune process. Primary pulmonary infection with *Mycobacterium tuberculosis* can progress to constrictive pericarditis in up to 1% of cases.[28]
- Fungal causes of pericarditis are rare and can develop from disseminated histoplasmosis, coccidioidomycosis, or even candidiasis. Pericarditis due to *Aspergillus* spp., *Candida* spp., or *Cryptococcus neoformans* is usually seen only in severely immunocompromised patients. The most common risk factor for fungal pericarditis is prior cardiothoracic surgery.
- Parasitic infection is a very rare cause of pericarditis.

DIAGNOSIS

- A high index of suspicion is required for the diagnosis of pericarditis.
- The presenting symptoms are varied according to the causative agent of pericarditis.
  - Viral pericarditis is most commonly associated with chest pain. Pain is commonly retrosternal and may be aggravated by breathing, swallowing, and lying flat. Pain relief by sitting up and leaning forward is classic for pericarditis. Frequently, symptoms will be accompanied by fevers and upper respiratory symptoms. If a large pericardial effusion is present, patients may also have symptoms of heart failure.
  - Bacterial pericarditis is usually accompanied by severe systemic infection or local infection involving the head, neck, chest, mediastinum, and thorax.
  - Tuberculous pericarditis is frequently insidious in nature. Chest pain may or may not be a predominate feature. Constitutional symptoms are commonly seen, including fevers, cough, night sweats, and weight loss.
  - Pleural effusions are common in HIV-infected patients but these are usually asymptomatic.
- Physical examination may reveal fevers and tachycardia. The classic finding on physical examination is the pericardial friction rub. The rub associated with pericarditis may be evanescent and difficult to perceive. If the pericardial effusion is large enough, there may be signs of cardiac tamponade, including jugular venous distension and pulsus paradoxus of more than 10 mm Hg.

TABLE 4-7	INFECTIOUS CAUSES OF PERICARDITIS

Viruses

Coxsackie A and B	Variola virus	Cytomegalovirus
Echoviruses	Vaccinia virus	Epstein-Barr virus
Adenovirus	Influenza A and B	Herpes simplex virus
Varicella-Zoster virus	Lymphocytic choriomeningitis virus	Hepatitis B
Poliovirus		Human immunodeficiency virus
Mumps virus	Lassa virus	

Bacteria

Streptococcus pneumoniae	Pseudomonas	Nocardia asteroides
Other Streptococcus spp.	Campylobacter spp.	Actinomyces spp.
Staphylococcus aureus	Brucella melitensis	Other anaerobic bacteria
Neisseria meningitidis	Listeria monocytogenes	Legionella pneumophila
Neisseria gonorrhea	Mycobacterium tuberculosis	Mycoplasma pneumoniae
Haemophilus influenzae		Chlamydophila pneumoniae
Salmonella spp.	Nontuberculous mycobacteria	Coxiella burnetii
Yersinia enterocolitica		Borrelia burgdorferi
Francisella tularensis		

Fungi

Aspergillus spp.	Blastomyces dermatitidis	Cryptococcus neoformans,
Candida spp.	Coccidioides immitis	Histoplasma capsulatum

Parasites

Entamoeba histolytica	Toxocara canis	Paragonimus spp.
Toxoplasma gondii	Schistosoma spp.	

- Chest radiography may be normal or if there is presence of an effusion greater than 250 mL, enlargement of the cardiac silhouette may be present.
- ECG is crucial in making the diagnosis of acute pericarditis. The classic ECG finding is diffuse ST-segment elevations.
- Echocardiography is useful to determine the size of the effusion, to evaluate for tamponade, and to evaluate for underlying myocardial dysfunction or myocarditis.
- It is frequently difficult to identify the viral agent responsible for viral pericarditis. Virus can be potentially isolated by testing a specimen from a throat swab or from the stool. Acute and convalescent antibody titers can be evaluated for a fourfold increase.
- If the effusion is large enough to require drainage, the entire volume of fluid should be drained and sent for evaluation. Fluid should be evaluated for cytology and a

spun sediment should be ordered and stained for acid-fast bacilli. Viral isolation from the pericardial fluid is uncommon, even if viral etiology is highly suspected. Viral-specific PCR could potentially increase the proportion of cases of pericarditis where the etiology is elucidated. Pericardiocentesis is rarely indicated in cases of presumed viral or idiopathic pericarditis and it adds little to the diagnostic yield.

- Evaluation of the pericardial fluid by pericardiocentesis or pericardiotomy is not routinely indicated. If tamponade is present or if the pericardial fluid persists for longer than 3 weeks, evaluation of the fluid may be indicated. Pericardiotomy with biopsy is preferable to pericardiocentesis with regard to the potential diagnostic yield but pericardiotomy is not readily available in most situations.
- Cardiac tamponade is more common in noninfectious causes of pericardial effusions. Bacterial, tuberculous, and fungal pericardial effusions are more likely to cause hemodynamic complications and will likely require drainage.

TREATMENT

- Rest and symptomatic treatment with analgesics are the mainstays of treatment for **viral and idiopathic pericarditis**
  - ○ **NSAIDs** are useful for the treatment of the chest pain associated with pericarditis. NSAIDs should be avoided if there is a significant component of myocarditis, as they can worsen outcomes in animal models.
  - ○ Steroids should be avoided as in myocarditis.
  - ○ **Colchicine** 0.6 mg twice daily has shown some benefit in acute pericarditis and may be useful to prevent recurrent episodes; however, prospective double-blind studies are lacking.[29] Colchicine does have, however, multiple contraindications and serious side effect and use should be monitored carefully.
- **Purulent pericarditis** should be diagnosed aggressively, as untreated purulent pericarditis is uniformly fatal.
  - ○ Pericardiocentesis should be performed and empiric **antibiotics** should be given and appropriate antibiotics continued once the causative agent is identified.
  - ○ Cardiothoracic surgery should be notified for emergent drainage, as these effusions usually reaccumulate rapidly and must be surgically drained.
- **Tuberculous pericarditis** should be treated with **standard four-drug antituberculosis treatment**.
  - ○ Effusions should be drained if tamponade develops.
  - ○ Tuberculous pericarditis is an exception to the above recommendation to avoid steroids. **Steroids** have been shown to reduce the risk of death, rapid reaccumulation of the effusion, and the development of constrictive pericarditis. In addition to antituberculosis therapy, patients should be given prednisone 60 mg daily for 4 weeks, 30 mg daily for 4 weeks, 15 mg daily for 2 weeks, and 5 mg daily for 1 week.[30]

REFERENCES

1. Honda H, Krauss MJ, Jones JC, et al. The value of infectious diseases consultation in *Staphylococcus aureus* bacteremia. *Am J Med.* 2010;123:631-637.
2. Mermel LA, Allon M, Bouza E, et al. Clinical practice guidelines for the diagnosis and management of intravascular catheter-related infection: 2009 update by the Infectious Diseases Society of America. *Clin Infect Dis.* 2009;49:1-45.

3. Edgeworth J. Intravascular catheter infections. *J Hosp Infect.* 2009;73:323-330.

4. Goede MR, Coopersmith CM. Catheter-related bloodstream infection. *Surg Clin North Am.* 2009;89:463-474, ix.

5. Grady NP, Alexander M, Burns LA, et al. *Guidelines for the Prevention of Intravascular Catheter-Related Infections, 2011.* Bethesda, MD: Centers for Disease Control and Prevention; 2011.

6. Yahav D, Rozen-Zvi B, Gafter-Gvili A, et al. Antimicrobial lock solutions for the prevention of infections associated with intravascular catheters in patients undergoing hemodialysis: systematic review and meta-analysis of randomized, controlled trials. *Clin Infect Dis.* 2008;47:83-93.

7. Snaterse M, Rüger W, Scholte Op Reimer WJ, Lucas C. Antibiotic-based catheter lock solutions for prevention of catheter-related bloodstream infections: a systematic review of randomized controlled trials. *J Hosp Infect.* 2010;75:1-11.

8. Wilson W, Taubert KA, Gewitz M, et al. Prevention of infective endocarditis: guidelines from the American Heart Association: a guideline from the American Heart Association Rheumatic Fever, Endocarditis, and Kawasaki Disease Committee, Council on Cardiovascular Disease in the Young, and the Council on Clinical Cardiology, Council on Cardiovascular Surgery and Anesthesia, and the Quality of Care and Outcomes Research Interdisciplinary Working Group. *Circulation.* 2007;116:1736-1754.

9. Durack DT, Lukes AS, Bright DK. New criteria for diagnosis of infective endocarditis: utilization of specific echocardiographic findings. Duke Endocarditis Service. *Am J Med.* 1994;96:200-209.

10. Fournier PE, Casalta JP, Habib G, et al. Modification of the diagnostic criteria proposed by the Duke Endocarditis Service to permit improved diagnosis of Q fever endocarditis. *Am J Med.* 1996;100:629-633.

11. Bashore TM, Cabell C, Fowler V Jr. Update on infective endocarditis. *Curr Probl Cardiol.* 2006;31:274-352.

12. McDonald JR. Acute infective endocarditis. *Infect Dis Clin North Am.* 2009;23:643-664.

13. Baddour LM, Wilson WR, Bayer AS, et al. Infective endocarditis: diagnosis, antimicrobial therapy, and management of complications: a statement for healthcare professionals from the Committee on Rheumatic Fever, Endocarditis, and Kawasaki Disease, Council on Cardiovascular Disease in the Young, and the Councils on Clinical Cardiology, Stroke, and Cardiovascular Surgery and Anesthesia, American Heart Association: endorsed by the Infectious Diseases Society of America. *Circulation.* 2005;111:e394-e434.

14. Knoll BM, Baddour LM, Wilson WR. Prosthetic valve endocarditis. In: Mandell GL, Bennett JE, Dolin R, et al., eds. *Mandell, Douglas, and Bennett's Principles and Practice of Infectious Diseases.* 7th ed. Philadelphia, PA: Churchill Livingstone; 2009:1113-1126.

15. Baddour LM, Bettmann MA, Bolger AF, et al. Nonvalvular cardiovascular device-related infections. *Circulation.* 2003;108:2015-2031.

16. Uslan DZ. Infections of electrophysiologic cardiac devices. *Expert Rev Med Devices.* 2008;5:183-195.

17. Uslan DZ, Baddour LM. Cardiac device infections: getting to the heart of the matter. *Curr Opin Infect Dis.* 2006;19:345-348.

18. Sohail MR, Uslan DZ, Khan AH, et al. Management and outcome of permanent pacemaker and implantable cardioverter-defibrillator infections. *J Am Coll Cardiol.* 2007;49:1851-1859.

19. Uslan DZ, Dowsley TF, Sohail MR, et al. Cardiovascular implantable electronic device infection in patients with *Staphylococcus aureus* bacteremia. *Pacing Clin Electrophysiol.* 2010;33:407-413.

20. Zierer A, Melby SJ, Voeller RK, et al. Late-onset driveline infections: the Achilles' heel of prolonged left ventricular assist device support. *Ann Thorac Surg.* 2007;84:515-520.

21. Topkara VK, Kondareddy S, Malik F, et al. Infectious complications in patients with left ventricular assist device: etiology and outcomes in the continuous-flow era. *Ann Thorac Surg.* 2010;90:1270-1277.

22. Van Schooneveld TC, Rupp ME. Mediastinitis. In: Mandell GL, Bennett JE, Dolin R, et al., eds. *Mandell, Douglas, and Bennett's Principles and Practice of Infectious Diseases.* 7th ed. Philadelphia, PA: Churchill Livingstone; 2009:1173-1182.

23. Armstrong AW, Spooner, Sanders JW. Lemierre's syndrome. *Curr Infect Dis Rep.* 2000;2:168-173.

24. Bisno AL. Nonsuppurative poststreptococcal sequelae: rheumatic fever and glomerulonephritis. In: Mandell GL, Bennett JE, Dolin R, et al., eds. *Mandell, Douglas, and Bennett's Principles and Practice of Infectious Diseases.* 7th ed. Philadelphia, PA: Churchill Livingstone; 2009:2611-2622.

25. Knowlton KU, Savoia MC, Oxman MN. Myocarditis and pericarditis. In: Mandell GL, Bennett JE, Dolin R, et al., eds. *Mandell, Douglas, and Bennett's Principles and Practice of Infectious Diseases.* 7th ed. Philadelphia, PA: Churchill Livingstone; 2009:1153-1171.

26. Ciesielski CA, Markowitz LE, Horsley R, et al. Lyme disease surveillance in the United States, 1983–1986. *Rev Infect Dis.* 1989;11(suppl 6):S1435-S1441.

27. Aretz HT, Billingham ME, Edwards WD, et al. Myocarditis. A histopathologic definition and classification. *Am J Cardiovasc Pathol.* 1987;1:3-14.

28. Larrieu AJ, Tylers GF, Williams EH, Derrick JR, Recent experience with tuberculous pericarditis. *Ann Thorac Surg.* 1980;29:464-468.

29. Lotrionte M, Biondi-Zoccai G, Imazio M, et al. International collaborative systematic review of controlled clinical trials on pharmacologic treatments for acute pericarditis and its recurrences. *Am Heart J.* 2010;160:662-670.

30. American Thoracic Society, CDC, Infectious Diseases Society of America. Treatment of tuberculosis. *MMWR Recomm Rep.* 2003;52(RR-11):1-77.

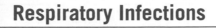

Respiratory Infections

5

Michael J. Durkin, Thomas C. Bailey, and Michael A. Lane

ACUTE PHARYNGITIS

GENERAL PRINCIPLES

- Acute pharyngitis is one of the most common syndromes seen by primary care physicians.
- Pathogenesis may include inflammatory mediators, direct invasion of pharyngeal cells, and lymphoid hyperplasia.

Etiology

- Table 5-1 presents pathogens that can cause pharyngitis in typical patients.
- In patients with HIV, *Candida albicans*, cytomegalovirus (CMV), and sexually transmitted infections such as *Neisseria gonorrhoeae* and herpes simplex virus should be considered.

DIAGNOSIS

Clinical Presentation

- Patients typically have upper respiratory tract infection (URI) symptoms that begin with a prodrome of fever, malaise, and headache.
- Patients may have tonsillar exudates and anterior cervical lymphadenopathy.
- They should not have any signs of a lower respiratory tract infection such as productive cough or abnormal lung sounds.

Diagnostic Criteria

- There are no diagnostic criteria for nonspecific pharyngitis.
- Clinical diagnosis of group A streptococcal (GAS) pharyngitis can be aided by the modified **Centor Diagnostic Criteria** (Table 5-2).[1-3]
- These criteria should be used in conjunction with rapid streptococcal antigen tests to diagnose streptococcal pharyngitis.

Diagnostic Testing

- Throat cultures are the gold standard for GAS pharyngitis; however, it can take days to receive results.
- Rapid streptococcal antigen testing takes minutes and is often done in the office while a patient is waiting. Newer assays have 90% to 99% sensitivity and 90% to 99% specificity.[1] Rapid tests should be performed in patients with 2 to 3 Centor criteria.

TABLE 5-1	ETIOLOGIES OF PHARYNGITIS
Viral	**Bacterial**
Adenovirus	Group A β-hemolytic streptococci
Rhinovirus	*Chlamydia pneumoniae*
Coronavirus	*Mycoplasma pneumoniae*
Influenza	*Haemophilus influenzae*
Parainfluenza	*Corynebacterium diphtheriae*
Respiratory syncytial virus	*Treponema pallidum*
Herpes simplex virus	*Neisseria gonorrhoeae*
Coxsackievirus	*Mycobacterium tuberculosis*
Human immunodeficiency virus	*Arcanobacterium haemolyticum*
Epstein-Barr virus	*Yersinia enterocolitica*
Cytomegalovirus	*Fusobacterium necrophorum*
Measles virus	*Coxiella burnetii*
Rubella virus	**Other**
Echovirus	*Candida albicans*
Human metapneumovirus	Kawasaki disease, Stevens-Johnson syndrome, Behçet's Syndrome

- Serologic tests, such as antistreptolysin O (ASO) and antideoxyribonuclease B, should only be performed in cases of suspected rheumatic fever and not routinely used for possible GAS pharyngitis.
- No further testing needs to be performed for patients with <2 Centor criteria.[1-3]

TABLE 5-2	CENTOR CRITERIA TO DIAGNOSE GROUP A β-HEMOLYTIC STREPTOCOCCAL PHARYNGITIS
Criteria	**Point**
Tonsillar exudates	1
Tender anterior cervical adenopathy	1
History of fever (>38°C [100.4°F])	1
Absence of cough	1
Age 3–14	1
Age 15–44	0
Age ≥45	−1
Score	**Action**
0 criteria	No testing,[a] no antibiotics
1 criterion	May choose to test
2 or 3 criteria	Perform testing, antibiotics if positive
4–5 criteria	Empiric antibiotics

[a]Throat culture or rapid antigen detection testing.

Adapted from McIsaac WJ, White D, Tannenbaum D, Low DE. A clinical score to reduce unnecessary antibiotic use in patients with sore throat. *CMAJ.* 1998;158:75-83.

TABLE 5-3	SUGGESTED ADULT REGIMENS FOR STREPTOCOCCAL PHARYNGITIS

Penicillin V 500 mg PO bid or tid for 10 d

Amoxicillin 875 mg PO bid or 500 mg PO tid for 10 d

Cephalexin 500 mg PO bid for 10 d

Azithromycin 500 mg PO once then 250 mg PO daily for 4 d (some communities have high levels of resistance)

Clindamycin 300 mg PO tid for 10 d

TREATMENT

- Most causes of pharyngitis do not require treatment.
- However, all cases of GAS pharyngitis should be treated (Table 5-3) for the following reasons:
  - ○ Reduce risk of complications including rheumatic fever and peritonsillar abscess
  - ○ Prevent transmission of GAS pharyngitis to other people
  - ○ Reduce duration and severity of symptoms

COMPLICATIONS

- There are few complications for most causes of pharyngitis.
- However, GAS pharyngitis may lead to the following:
  - ○ Acute rheumatic fever (Table 5-4)
  - ○ Peritonsillar abscess and retropharyngeal abscess
- Rheumatic heart disease is common in developing countries but uncommon in the United States. It may manifest years after initial symptoms of rheumatic fever.
- Throat cultures are negative in most patients with rheumatic fever, so ASO and other titers may be beneficial.
- Antibiotic treatment does not affect the risk of developing post-streptococcal glomerulonephritis.

TABLE 5-4	RHEUMATIC FEVER	
Epidemiology	Primarily affects children	
History/exam	**Major criteria:**	**Minor criteria:**
	Migratory arthritis	Fever
	Sydenham chorea	Elevated acute phase reactants
	Erythema marginatum	
	Subcutaneous nodules	Prolonged PR interval
	Carditis	Arthralgias
Diagnosis (Jones criteria)	Serologic evidence of group A streptococcal infection **plus** two major manifestations **or** one major manifestation **plus** two minor manifestations	

ACUTE EPIGLOTTITIS

GENERAL PRINCIPLES

- Acute epiglottitis causes inflammation of the epiglottis and surrounding structures.
- **All cases of epiglottitis should be considered a respiratory emergency** as inflammation of the epiglottis can lead to **airway obstruction**.
- Although historically a disease primarily of children, the *Haemophilus influenzae* type b (Hib) vaccination has reduced childhood risk significantly.
- Pathogens originate from the posterior nasopharynx.
- Bacteria (*Haemophilus influenzae*, *Staphylococcus aureus*, group A β-hemolytic *Streptococcus*, and *Streptococcus pneumoniae*) are the most common causes but viruses and fungi can also cause epiglottitis.
- Epiglottitis results from either transient bacteremia and seeding of the epiglottis or from direct spread from adjacent structures. It is important to consider a possible primary source for infection elsewhere such as pneumonia.

DIAGNOSIS

Clinical Presentation

- Sore throat, odynophagia, and fever are the most common symptoms.
- Drooling, muffled voice, tripod posture, and respiratory distress may be present in patients with epiglottitis.
- Patients may have anterior cervical lymphadenopathy and tenderness to palpation. The oropharyngeal exam may be normal in adults.
- **Inspiratory stridor** is a classic presentation and a sign of impending respiratory failure.
- **Manipulation of a tenuous airway should only be performed by subspecialists as it can precipitate airway compromise**.
- Direct laryngoscopy performed by a subspecialist can assist both in confirming the diagnosis and in assessing the airway.[4]

Differential Diagnosis

- The differential diagnosis includes mononucleosis, *Corynebacterium diphtheriae*, *Bordetella pertussis*, croup, and pharyngeal abscesses such as Ludwig angina.
- Noninfectious causes such as amyloidosis, sarcoidosis, tumors, angioedema, airway irritants, and foreign bodies should also be considered.

Diagnostic Testing

- Blood cultures and throat cultures are often negative but should still be obtained.
- Neck radiographs are often normal and are not necessary to make the diagnosis of epiglottitis. If radiographs are performed, findings may include an enlarged epiglottis or "thumb print sign" and normal subglottic space. Consider lateral view of the neck when you are uncertain about the diagnosis.[4]
- Direct laryngoscopy by subspecialists can assist in the diagnosis and severity of disease.[4]

TREATMENT

- **Airway stabilization** should be considered before all else in patients with epiglottitis (Table 5-5).[5,6] Treatment should be guided by severity of airway compromise.
- After airway management has been established, antibiotics should be initiated.
  - ○ Empiric antibiotic coverage consists of a third-generation cephalosporin, such as ceftriaxone 2 g every 24 hours.
  - ○ Vancomycin or clindamycin may be added if there is concern for methicillin-resistant *S. aureus* (MRSA).
  - ○ Antibiotic treatment duration is often 7 to 10 days but may be extended for patients with bacteremia, meningitis, or immunodeficiency.
  - ○ If possible, antibiotic coverage should be narrowed based on culture results.
- The use of steroids and epinephrine is currently a controversial therapy.
- Rifampin (RIF) postexposure prophylaxis for household contacts is recommended by the American Academy of Pediatrics in cases of known Hib exposure if one of the contacts is an unvaccinated child <4 years old.[7]

TABLE 5-5	FRIEDMAN EPIGLOTTITIS STAGING	
Stage	**Signs and symptoms**	**Airway management**
I	No respiratory distress Respiratory rate <20/min	Close intensive care unit observation
II	Mild respiratory distress Respiratory rate 20–30/min	Intubation by anesthesia or with bronchoscopy (with equipment for emergent tracheostomy at bedside) or formal tracheostomy in operating room
III	Moderate respiratory distress Respiratory rate >30/min Stridor, retractions, perioral cyanosis Pco_2 >45 mm Hg	Immediate intubation or cricothyroidotomy
IV	Severe respiratory distress Severe stridor, retractions Cyanosis, delirium, loss of consciousness, hypoxia Respiratory arrest	Immediate intubation or cricothyroidotomy

Adapted from Ng HL, Sin LM, Li MF, et al. Acute epiglottitis in adults: a retrospective review of 106 patients in Hong Kong. *Emerg Med J*. 2008;25:253-255.

RHINOSINUSITIS

GENERAL PRINCIPLES

- Rhinosinusitis results in inflammation of the mucosa of the nose and paranasal sinuses.
- Sinusitis can be classified by
  - Duration (acute ≤1 month, chronic >12 weeks)
  - Location (maxillary, sphenoid, ethmoid, and frontal)
  - Type of organism—viral, bacterial, fungal, and noninfectious

Pathophysiology

- Paranasal sinuses are outpouchings of the nasal mucosa. They are lined with mucoperiosteum and cilia, which sweep mucus toward the ostia.
- Acute rhinosinusitis (ARS) is a result of impaired mucociliary clearance and obstruction of the ostia.
- This results in stagnant secretions and decreased ventilation, creating an ideal culture medium for bacteria.
- **Viruses** (e.g., rhinoviruses, adenovirus) are the most common cause of acute sinusitis.[8]
- The most common **bacterial** etiologies (often secondary) in acute sinusitis include
  - *S. pneumoniae*
  - *H. influenzae*
  - *Moraxella catarrhalis*
- *S. aureus*, coagulase-negative *Staphylococcus*, and anaerobic bacteria are more common in chronic rhinosinusitis (CRS) but **CRS is more often an inflammatory process.**
- *S. aureus* is increasing in prevalence in sinusitis patients with nasal polyps.
- *Pseudomonas aeruginosa* infection frequently occurs in patients with cystic fibrosis.
- Fungal causes include *Mucor*, *Rhizopus*, and *Aspergillus.*
  - Risk factors for fungal sinusitis include neutropenia, diabetes mellitus, HIV, and other immunocompromised states.
  - In immunocompetent hosts, the presence of fungi is more likely to represent an allergic reaction to environmental fungi rather than a true infection.
- Vasculitis is an uncommon noninfectious cause of rhinosinusitis.

DIAGNOSIS

Clinical Presentation

- The diagnosis of rhinosinusitis is usually entirely clinical and **the differentiation between viral and bacterial infections can be difficult**.
- Multiple studies regarding the utility of symptoms and signs for diagnosing acute sinusitis have sometimes reached differing conclusions. A few have used the true gold standard (i.e., sinus puncture and culture) but more have used a surrogate standard (e.g., sinus plain films and computed tomography [CT]). Radiography cannot differentiate viral from bacterial sinusitis.
- ARS symptoms within the first 7 to 10 days of illness typically indicate a viral rhinosinusitis.

- Acute bacterial sinusitis is unlikely in patients with URI symptoms for <10 days.
- **The prominent symptoms of acute bacterial rhinosinusitis are nasal conges-tion, purulent rhinorrhea, facial–dental pain, postnasal drainage, headache, and cough.**
- Signs of ARS include sinus tenderness, purulent nasal discharge, erythematous mucosa, pharyngeal secretions, and periorbital edema.
- Cough is more prominent in chronic sinusitis.

Diagnostic Testing

- Viral cultures are almost never obtained in routine clinical practice.
- Bacterial cultures of the nasal cavity or of purulent secretions are not helpful.
- Invasive sinus cultures may be performed by an otolaryngologist if there is concern for atypical pathogens or intracranial extension.
- Radiographic imaging is not necessary for the diagnosis in the majority of patients. When performed, **limited sinus CT** has become the most widely used radiographic study for the diagnosis of sinusitis. Findings consistent with sinusitis are
  - Mucosal thickening >4 mm
  - Air-fluid level
  - Complete sinus opacification
  - Absence of all three has a high sensitivity in ruling out disease

TREATMENT

- **Most cases of ARS are caused by viruses and are expected to significantly improve without antibiotic treatment within 10 to 14 days.** Treatment should, therefore, be symptomatic for most patients.
- Trials of the efficacy of antibiotics in ARS have been of variable quality and differing outcome measures. Most of the randomized trials did not definitively enroll only subjects with bacterial infections. Nonetheless, taken together, there may be a **mod-est benefit from antibiotic treatment**.
- Uncomplicated acute bacterial rhinosinusitis may be treated with or without antibiotics.[9-12]
  - **Patients without severe or prolonged symptoms may be managed initially with symptomatic treatment alone** and followed for resolution. Worsening of symptoms during this time should prompt a reconsideration of antibiotic therapy.
  - Individual clinical judgment should be exercised when making the decision to forgo or prescribe antibiotic therapy.
- Appropriate **first-line antibiotics for uncomplicated acute bacterial rhinosinus-itis include amoxicillin, sulfamethoxazole–trimethoprim, and azithromycin** with a duration of 10 to 14 days.[9-14] Significant differences between groups of anti-biotics, including newer more expensive ones, have not been demonstrated.[10,12,14,15]
- The optimal duration of antibiotic therapy is unclear.[13]
- Alternative antibiotic therapy should be considered in patients who worsen or do not improve during the initial 7 days of therapy.[9,10,13,14] Reasonable second-line choices include high-dose amoxicillin–clavulanate, oral fluoroquinolones, and second- or third-generation cephalosporins.
- While evidence is somewhat limited, the addition of **intranasal steroids** may have modest positive benefit in the treatment of ARS.[9,13,16]

- There are no controlled trials of systemic steroids and these are not routinely recommended.
- **Analgesics** should be prescribed to those with significant pain.[10]
- Data to support the use of decongestants, antihistamines, mucolytics/expectorants, and sinus irrigation are lacking but they are at least theoretically beneficial and often recommended.[9,13]

COMPLICATIONS

- Orbital cellulitis, brain abscess, meningitis, cavernous thrombosis, osteomyelitis, and mucocele are all possible but quite uncommon.
- CRS is typically caused by colonizing rather than pathogenic bacteria. Antibiotics are controversial as patients often do not respond clinically to them and biofilms are frequent. Fungal pathogens are often found in cultures of patients with chronic sinusitis but it is unclear if these are pathogenic.

ACUTE BRONCHITIS

GENERAL PRINCIPLES

- Acute bronchitis is inflammation of the large and mid-sized airways characterized by the sudden onset of cough with or without production of phlegm and accompanying upper respiratory and constitutional symptoms.
- A specific etiology is found in the minority of patients. The most common pathogens (usually viruses) are listed in Table 5-6. Less than 10% of cases are due to bacteria.[17]
- The pathophysiology involves direct invasion of epithelial cells of the tracheobronchial tree by pathogens, with resultant release of inflammatory mediators. Patients then develop airway hypersensitivity leading to cough and, occasionally, wheezing.

TABLE 5-6	COMMON PATHOGENS IN ACUTE BRONCHITIS
Viral	**Bacterial**
Parainfluenza	*Bordetella pertussis*
Influenza	*Mycoplasma pneumoniae*
Respiratory syncytial virus	*Chlamydophila pneumoniae*
Rhinovirus	
Coronavirus	
Adenovirus	

DIAGNOSIS

Clinical Presentation

- Cough for at least 5 days is necessary to diagnose acute bronchitis. **Coughing may last up to 3 weeks for an episode of acute bronchitis**. Purulent sputum production is also common (up to half of patients) and does not signify a more serious infection such as pneumonia.
- Normal vital signs are common in bronchitis, whereas abnormal vital signs are more concerning for pneumonia.
- Listen for wheezes, rales, and rhonchi on physical exam.

Differential Diagnosis

The differential diagnosis includes pneumonia, influenza, gastroesophageal reflux, postnasal drip, smoking, toxic inhalations, and angiotensin-converting enzyme inhibitors, asthma, chronic bronchitis, and chronic obstructive pulmonary disease exacerbation.

Diagnostic Testing

- **Routine sputum cultures are not recommended** as bacterial pathogens rarely cause acute bronchitis.
- Patients with severe paroxysmal cough or cough >2 weeks should have nasopharyngeal (NP) swab done for culture or polymerase chain reaction (PCR) testing to evaluate for pertussis.
- Influenza testing should be considered based on seasonal patterns of influenza and patient presentation.
- Chest radiography should not be performed routinely in the absence of abnormal vital signs or concerning physical exam findings.
- The diagnosis of tracheobronchitis in hospitalized patients can be challenging. Patients will often have signs of pneumonia with fever, leukocytosis, and purulent sputum production. However, they will have a clear chest radiograph.
- Quantitative or semiquantitative sputum cultures in symptomatic patients can be obtained to guide therapy.
- To differentiate between tracheobronchitis and pneumonia, see Figure 5-1.

TREATMENT

- **Multiple studies have shown no benefit in antimicrobial therapy for generally healthy patients with acute outpatient non–pertussis-related bronchitis**.[18] Refer to Figure 5-1 for a management algorithm.
- Symptom management is the cornerstone of therapy. This often includes nonsteroidal antiinflammatory drugs, acetaminophen, dextromethorphan, or codeine.
- If clinical suspicion for pertussis is high and patient presents within the first 2 weeks of symptoms, consider azithromycin 500 mg PO once, then 250 mg PO daily for 4 days to reduce the risk of transmission.
- In cases of tracheobronchitis, treatment should be based on sputum culture results.

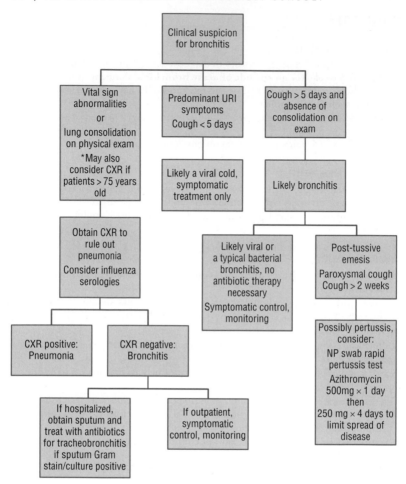

FIGURE 5-1 Differentiating acute bronchitis from pneumonia.

CXR, chest radiograph; NP, nasopharyngeal; URI, upper respiratory tract infection.

COMMUNITY-ACQUIRED PNEUMONIA

GENERAL PRINCIPLES

- Community-acquired pneumonia (CAP) is defined as infection of the pulmonary parenchyma in patients who have not spent any significant amount of time in the hospital, dialysis centers, nursing homes, or clinics recently.
- The rate of CAP is between 5 and 6 per 1,000 persons per year and costs billions of US dollars per year.[19]

TABLE 5-7	PNEUMONIA PATHOGENS
Bacteria	**Viruses**
Streptococcus pneumoniae	Influenza virus A
Haemophilus influenzae	Influenza virus B
Mycoplasma pneumoniae	Parainfluenza virus
Legionella spp.	Respiratory syncytial virus
Chlamydophila pneumoniae	Adenovirus
Staphylococcus aureus	
Enterobacteriaceae	
Association	**Organism**
Aspiration	Gram-negative, oral anaerobes
Lung abscess	Community-acquired methicillin-resistant *S. aureus,* oral anaerobes, fungal, *Mycobacterium tuberculosis,* atypical mycobacteria
Bat/bird droppings	*Histoplasma capsulatum*
Bird fanciers	*Chlamydophila psittaci*
Rabbit exposure	*Francisella tularensis*
Farm animals	*Coxiella burnetii*
HIV	*Pneumocystis jiroveci, Cryptococcus neoformans,* mycobacteria
Cruise ship	*Legionella* spp.
Bioterrorism	*Bacillus anthracis, Yersinia pestis, Francisella tularensis*

- Prior to antibiotics, Sir William Osler called it "the captain of the men of death." Even with antibiotics, pneumonia still can carry a significant risk of death.
- Common pneumonia associations and pathogens are listed in Table 5-7.

Prevention

- All patients should be offered the influenza vaccine prior to discharge from the hospital.
- Patients aged 65 or older, and those with certain medical conditions, should receive the pneumococcal vaccination.

DIAGNOSIS

Clinical Presentation

- CAP is a clinical diagnosis requiring a combination of history, physical exam, and an infiltrate on chest radiograph.
- The presentation of CAP is extremely variable. Frequently, patients will present with productive cough, fever, dyspnea, and pleuritic chest pain. However, delirium,

headache, myalgias, nausea, and vomiting can be seen in elderly individuals or in cases of atypical or "walking" pneumonia.
- Pneumonia can present with abnormalities in any or all of the vital signs. Extremes in vital signs portend a worse prognosis, as shown in the Pneumonia Severity Index (Table 5-8).[20]
- Physical exam findings consistent with pneumonia are the same as lung consolidation such as tactile fremitus, dullness to percussion, decreased breath sounds, rales, and egophony.

Differential Diagnosis

The differential diagnosis for CAP includes heart failure, pneumonitis, pulmonary edema, septic emboli, malignancies, foreign body inhalation, and pulmonary infarction.

Diagnostic Testing

Laboratories
- Sputum for Gram stain and culture should be strongly considered for all patients.[21]
- Blood cultures are usually done on hospitalized patients and should be obtained prior to empiric antibiotics if possible.
- Labs that may be helpful in selected patients include
  - Urine *Legionella* antigen
  - Urine pneumococcal antigen
  - NP swab for viral studies
  - Sputum for acid-fast staining if there is a clinical suspicion for mycobacterial infection

Imaging
- Chest radiography should be performed on all patients suspected of having CAP.
- The location of the infiltrate may help indicate the causative organism.
  - *S. pneumoniae* and *Legionella* pneumonia typically cause lobar infiltrates.
  - "Atypical" and viral pneumonias are typically diffuse or bilateral.
  - Aspiration pneumonia location depends on the position of the patient when they aspirated. It may present as a cavitary lesion if longstanding.
  - *Pneumocystis* pneumonia may have a negative chest radiograph but a CT scan will usually show evidence of disease.

Diagnostic Procedures
Bronchoscopy, CT scan, and thoracentesis are further diagnostic procedures and studies that are typically reserved for severe or nonresponding CAP.

TREATMENT

- The initial step in determining treatment is deciding whether a patient with CAP requires hospitalization or can be safely treated as an outpatient.
- There are two commonly used prediction tools to help assess risk of mortality.
  - The Pneumonia Severity Index, commonly known as the PORT score, was the first indicator used to evaluate for severity of CAP in patients presenting to the emergency department. It has been well validated but requires a lengthy number of laboratory tests (Table 5-8).[20]

| TABLE 5-8 | PNEUMONIA SEVERITY INDEX |

Characteristic	Points
Sex	
Male	0
Female	−10
Demographic factors	
Age	1 per year
Nursing home resident	10
Comorbidities	
Neoplasia	30
Liver disease	20
Heart failure	10
Cerebrovascular disease	10
Renal disease	10
Physical exam	
Altered mental status	20
Respiratory rate ≥30/min	20
Systolic blood pressure <90 mm Hg	20
Temperature <35°C (95°F) or ≥40°C (104°F)	15
Heart rate ≥125/min	10
Labs	
Arterial pH <7.35	30
Blood urea nitrogen ≥30 mg/dL	20
Sodium <130 mmol/L	20
Glucose ≥250 mg/dL	10
Hematocrit <30%	10
Po_2 <60 mm Hg	
Radiographic findings	
Pleural effusion	10

Total points	Class	Mortality (%)	Management
0	I	0.1	Outpatient
≥70	II	0.6	Outpatient
71–90	III	0.9	Brief inpatient
91–130	IV	9.3	Inpatient
>130	V	27.0	Inpatient

—
Adapted from Fine MJ, Auble TE, Yealy DM, et al. A prediction rule to identify low-risk patients with community-acquired pneumonia. *N Engl J Med*. 1997;336:243-250.

TABLE 5-9	CURB-65 SCORE	
Characteristics	**Points**	
Confusion	1	
Urea nitrogen >20 mg/dL	1	
Respiratory rate >30/min	1	
Blood pressure, systolic <90 mm Hg	1	
Age ≥**65**	1	
Total points	**Mortality (%)**	**Management**
0	0.7	Outpatient
1	3.2	Outpatient
2	3	Inpatient
3	17	Consider intensive care unit
4	41.5	Consider intensive care unit
5	57	Consider intensive care unit

Adapted from Lim WS, van der Eerden MM, Laing R, et al. Defining community acquired pneumonia severity on presentation to hospital: international derivation and validation study. *Thorax.* 2003;58:377-382.

○ The CURB-65 or the more simplified CRB-65, which requires no blood tests, is designed to help risk-stratify patients presenting to clinic to either outpatient or inpatient treatment (Table 5-9).[22]
- Other findings consistent with poor prognosis include thrombocytopenia, leukopenia, multilobar infiltrates, septic shock requiring vasopressors, and invasive mechanical ventilation.
- Antibiotics are the mainstay of therapy for CAP since most cases are caused by bacterial pathogens. However, it is important to consider that some cases are caused by viral pathogens and will not respond to antibiotic therapy.

Medications
- Treatment options for CAP are presented in Table 5-10.[21]
- Antibiotic changes should be made according to susceptibilities from your laboratory or culture data as soon as possible to provide the narrowest spectrum antibiotics for a particular pathogen.
- Changing from IV to PO antibiotics should also be constantly reevaluated. Patients can be switched from an IV to a PO regimen and discharged from the hospital when clinically stable or improving.

TABLE 5-10	TREATMENT OF COMMUNITY-ACQUIRED PNEUMONNIA

Category	First line Alternative	Antibiotic selection
Outpatient, no comorbidities	Macrolide (azithromycin) **or** Doxycycline	Azithromycin is the preferred macrolide because of tolerability
Outpatient, with comorbidities	Respiratory FQ (moxifloxacin) **or** PO β-lactam (amoxicillin/ clavulanate or cefpodoxime) **PLUS** macrolide or doxycycline	Use respiratory FQ in areas with higher macrolide resistance
Inpatient, non-ICU	IV β-lactam (ceftriaxone or ertapenem) **PLUS** macrolide or doxycycline **or** Respiratory FQ (moxifloxacin/levofloxacin)	Be aware that there are increasing rates of FQ resistance in certain communities
Inpatient, ICU	IV β-lactam (ceftriaxone, ampicillin–sulbactam) **PLUS** azithromycin **or** respiratory FQ	• For penicillin allergic patients, use a respiratory FQ and aztreonam
	If concern for MRSA, add vancomycin or linezolid If concern for *Pseudomonas,* change β-lactam to cefepime, meropenem, or piperacillin–tazobactam	Daptomycin should not be used for MRSA pneumonia
Aspiration	Clindamycin **or** PO amoxicillin/clavulanate **or** IV ampicillin/sulbactam	Anaerobe coverage is required for community-acquired aspiration pneumonia for oral anaerobes

FQ, fluoroquinolone; ICU, intensive care unit; MRSA, methicillin-resistant *Staphylococcus aureus.*

Adapted from Mandell LA, Wunderink RG, Anzueto A, et al. Infectious Diseases Society of America/ American Thoracic Society consensus guidelines on the management of community-acquired pneumonia in adults. *Clin Infect Dis.* 2007;44(suppl 2):S27-S72.

- Duration of therapy for CAP should be a minimum of 5 days provided that the patient has been afebrile for over 48 hours and has clinically improved and if known that the pathogen was susceptible to the chosen antibiotic.
- **Antibiotics should be administered as soon as CAP is diagnosed as there is evidence that delay in antibiotic therapy leads to higher patient mortality.**

COMPLICATIONS

- **Lack of clinical response** is the most common complication of pneumonia. Causes may include the following:
  - ○ **Wrong antibiotic** (e.g., resistant organism, incorrect choice, and insufficient dose)
  - ○ **Wrong diagnosis** (e.g., drug fever, heart failure, pulmonary embolism, vasculitis, and malignancy)
  - ○ **Complication** (e.g., empyema, acute respiratory distress syndrome [ARDS], secondary infection, superinfection, meningitis, and endocarditis)
- Consider further work-up as follows:
  - ○ Testing for mycobacteria, *Legionella*, varicella-zoster virus, herpes simplex virus, and CMV
  - ○ Bronchoscopy, sometimes with biopsy, for routine, mycobacterial, and fungal staining and culture
  - ○ Thoracentesis
  - ○ CT scan with contrast
- **Parapneumonic effusions are common.** Typically, such effusions are relatively small and resolve with proper antibiotic treatment. Diagnostic thoracentesis is indicated if the effusion is free-flowing and layers >1 cm on a lateral decubitus film.
- The characteristic of pleural fluid are presented in Table 5-11.
  - ○ **Uncomplicated parapneumonic effusions** are exudative and usually sterile.
  - ○ **Complicated parapneumonic effusions** result from persistence of bacterial invasion of the pleural space, though cultures are often negative. Biochemical features include a pH <7.2 and low glucose (<60 mg/dL) and high lactate dehydrogenase levels. Chest tube drainage is generally required.
  - ○ **Empyema** signifies gross purulence in the pleural space but cultures are sometimes still negative. Management of empyema requires chest tube placement and often surgical decortication.

NOSOCOMIAL PNEUMONIAS

GENERAL PRINCIPLES

- Nosocomial pneumonias are more likely to be caused by resistant pathogens and therefore are treated differently than CAP.
- There are three categories of nosocomial pneumonias.[23]
  - ○ **Health care–associated pneumonia** diagnosis requires one of the following:
    - ■ Hospitalization for ≥2 days within the last 90 days
    - ■ Nursing home or long-term care facility resident

TABLE 5-11 **PLEURAL FLUID CHARACTERISTICS**

Characteristic	Transudate	Uncomplicated parapneumonic effusion	Complicated parapneumonic effusion
Appearance	Clear	Variable	Variable[a]
WBC count (cells/mm^3)	<1,000	Variable	Variable
WBC differential	Variable	Predominately neutrophils	Predominately neutrophils
Protein (g/dL)	<3.0	>3.0	>3.0
Glucose (mg/dL)	Same as serum	>60	40–60
pH	Greater than serum	>7.2	7.0–7.2
LDH (units/mL)	<200	<1,000	>1,000
Bacteria	Absent	Absent	Absent[a]

WBC, white blood cell; LDH, lactate dehydrogenase.

[a]Empyema may have bacteria present on Gram stain; the pleural fluid will appear grossly purulent.

■ Received IV therapy, wound care, or chemotherapy within the past 30 days
■ Attendance at a hospital or hemodialysis clinic within the past 30 days
○ **Hospital-acquired pneumonia (HAP)**: develops ≥48 hours after admission to a hospital
○ **Ventilator-associated pneumonia (VAP)**: any pneumonia that develops >48 to 72 hours after intubation.

Epidemiology

• Nosocomial pneumonia is the second most common hospital-acquired infection after urinary tract infections.[23]
• HAP alone increases hospital stay by 7 to 9 days and costs an additional $40,000 per patient.
• 50% of all antibiotics prescribed in the intensive care unit are for HAP.
• Attributable mortality due to HAP is 33% to 50%.
• Patients with late-onset HAP and VAP are more likely to be infected with multi-drug-resistant (MDR) organisms than patients with early-onset disease (within first 4 days of hospitalization).

Etiology

• The organisms are often drug-resistant pathogens including MRSA, *Escherichia coli*, *Klebsiella*, *Serratia*, *Stenotrophomonas*, *Burkholderia*, *Pseudomonas*, and *Acinetobacter*. However, community organisms such as *S. pneumoniae* and *Haemophilus* are not uncommon.

- Viruses, atypical bacteria, and fungal pathogens rarely are a cause of nosocomial pneumonia in immunocompetent patients. However, these pathogens should be kept in the differential diagnosis in immunocompromised hosts, in patients who do not respond to therapy or are very ill, and during influenza season.

Pathophysiology

- In order for these infections to occur, pathogens must invade the lower respiratory tract, usually by aspiration or micro-aspiration.
- The oral flora dramatically changes within a few days of hospitalization to a predominately gram-negative spectrum, often with the drug-resistant pathogens mentioned above.

Risk Factors

- Conditions that increase the risk of aspiration
- Use of proton pump inhibitors or H2 blockers for stress ulcer prophylaxis
- Intubation increases the risk of micro-aspiration despite an inflated endotracheal tube cuff
- Heavily sedated and paralyzed patients have a higher risk of developing pneumonia
- Repeated intubation and extubation increase the risk of infection
- Poorly controlled hyperglycemia

Associated Conditions

- One important associated condition to consider is ARDS.
- ARDS patients should follow a low tidal volume, high positive end-expiratory pressure protocol to minimize additional barotrauma.

DIAGNOSIS

Clinical Presentation

- The diagnosis of nosocomial pneumonia is difficult because the findings are often nonspecific and extremely variable.
- Patients will frequently present with productive cough, fever, dyspnea, and pleuritic chest pain.
  - The diagnosis should also be considered in patients with new or progressive infiltrates on chest radiography, fever or hypothermia, purulent sputum, leukocytosis, change in oxygenation, tachypnea, and hypotension.
- These finding are especially important in patients who may suffer from delirium and dementia or are currently intubated.

Differential Diagnosis

- The differential diagnosis of nosocomial pneumonia includes aspiration pneumonitis, ARDS, septic emboli, heart failure, pulmonary hemorrhage, vasculitis, malignancy, and tracheobronchitis.
- Tracheobronchitis and HAP may have a very similar presentation but a new lung infiltrate is not expected in the former.

Diagnostic Testing

Laboratories

- The goal of diagnostic testing is twofold: (1) isolate the organism to narrow the antibiotic spectrum and (2) confirm pneumonia as the diagnosis.[23]
- Blood cultures, although positive less than 25% of the time, may identify concomitant bacteremia. Tracheal aspirate/sputum (76% sensitivity, 75% specificity) should be considered before bronchoscopy.
- Bronchoscopy (69% sensitivity, 82% specificity) should be considered in patients unable to provide adequate sputum sample and should be strongly considered when diagnosis is in question.
- Other labs to consider include urine pneumococcal antigen, urine *Legionella* antigen (only detects serogroup 1), NP swab for viral pathogens, and urine *Histoplasma* antigen.

Imaging

- Chest radiography is required to differentiate between tracheobronchitis and pneumonia.
- CT scan of the chest should be considered if the diagnosis is in question.

Diagnostic Procedures

Bronchoscopy is the hallmark diagnostic procedure in pneumonia. Bronchoalveolar lavage, bronchial washings, and biopsy may be performed based on the clinical setting. These are often sent for fungal, bacterial, mycobacterial, and viral studies.

TREATMENT

- The treatment of nosocomial pneumonia is present in Table 5-12.[23]
- Treatment duration should be 7 days for most cases.
- *Pseudomonas* infection should be treated for 15 days if isolated or strongly suspected.
- Once patients are started on antibiotics, respiratory cultures should be monitored closely.
  - If negative, consider narrowing spectrum to the antibiotics recommended for those not at risk for MDR organisms (Table 5-12)[23]
  - If positive, narrow antibiotic spectrum after 72 hours based on culture results
- New laboratory tests (e.g., procalcitonin, N-terminal pro–B-type natriuretic peptide, and TREM-1) are under investigation to decrease antibiotic use even further.

LUNG ABSCESS

GENERAL PRINCIPLES

- A lung abscess consists of a collection of necrotic lung tissue contained within a cavity occurring as a result of progressive infection of the lung parenchyma.
- Organisms associated with lung abscesses are listed in Table 5-13.
- Aspiration is a key event in many cases of lung abscess. Predisposing conditions that should be considered include alcohol and sedative use, seizures, strokes, and neuromuscular disease.

| TABLE 5-12 | TREATMENT OF NOSOCOMIAL PNEUMONIA |

Category	Empiric therapy	Additional information
HCAP/HAP/VAP **NOT** at risk for MDR pathogens and hospitalized **<5 d**[a]	Third-generation cephalosporin (ceftriaxone) **or** Ampicillin–sulbactam or piperacillin–tazobactam **or** Respiratory FQ (moxifloxacin/levofloxacin) **or** Non-antipseudomonal carbapenem (ertapenem)	Azithromycin should be considered for atypical organism coverage in very ill patients or those with a high suspicion for atypical organisms or *Legionella* who are not on respiratory FQ
HCAP/HAP/VAP **AT RISK** for MDR pathogens or hospitalized for **≥5 d**	Antipseudomonal cephalosporin (cefepime or ceftazidime) **or** Antipseudomonal carbapenem (imipenem or meropenem) **or** Antipseudomonal penicillin with β-lactamase inhibitor (piperacillin–tazobactam)[b] **PLUS** Antipseudomonal FQ (ciprofloxacin/levofloxacin)[b] **or** Aminoglycoside (gentamicin, tobramycin, amikacin) **PLUS** Anti-MRSA agent (linezolid or vancomycin)	Potential ESBL organisms (e.g., *Escherichia coli, Klebsiella*) should be treated with a carbapenem For patients allergic to penicillin consider FQ and aminoglycoside Aztreonam Meropenem (<1% cross-reactivity) Inhaled antibiotics (e.g., colistin and aminoglycosides) have been used in selected populations and should be used only after consultation with a subspecialist

[a]Choice of agent should be based on pattern of causative organisms and susceptibilities in each health care setting.

[b]Double coverage for *Pseudomonas* or other resistant organisms may be considered in empiric therapy based on local antibiogram and severity of illness.

HCAP, health care–associated pneumonia; HAP, hospital-acquired pneumonia; VAP, ventilator-associated pneumonia; MDR, multidrug resistant; FQ, fluoroquinolone; ESBL, extended spectrum β-lactamase; MRSA, methicillin-resistant *Staphylococcus aureus*.

Adapted from Niederman MS, Craven DE, Bonten MJ, et al. Guidelines for the management of adults with hospital-acquired, ventilator-associated, and healthcare-associated pneumonia. *Am J Respir Crit Care Med*. 2005;171:388-416.

TABLE 5-13	**CAUSES OF LUNG ABSCESS**

Bacterial	**Fungal**
Gram-positive anaerobic cocci from oral mucosa such as *Peptostreptococcus*	*Histoplasma*
	Coccidioides
Pigmented gram-negative bacilli (*Prevotella, Porphyromonas, and Bacteroides*)	*Blastomyces*
	Cryptococcus
Fusobacterium spp. (Lemierre syndrome)	*Aspergillus*
	Rhizopus
Staphylococcus aureus (from both necrotizing pneumonia and hematogenous spread from septic emboli)	**Parasitic**
	Entamoeba
	Echinococcus
Pseudomonas	**Polymicrobial**
Klebsiella	**Noninfectious**
Legionella	Bronchogenic carcinoma
Nocardia	Granulomatosis with polyangiitis (GPA) (formerly known as Wegener's)
Burkholderia	
Streptococcus milleri	Rheumatoid nodules
Mycobacterium	Sarcoidosis
Rhodococcus	Pulmonary infarction
Actinomyces	Congenital pulmonary cysts

DIAGNOSIS

Clinical Presentation

- Patients may present with fever, productive cough, putrid sputum, or chest pain. They may also have weight loss, night sweats, and hemoptysis. These symptoms may also be concerning for malignancy or tuberculosis (TB).
- Decreased breath sounds and hyper-resonance in the area of the cavitation may be appreciated. Poor dentition, malodorous breath, and purulent sputum are classic findings on physical exam but are often not present.

Diagnostic Testing

Laboratories
- Blood cultures are rarely positive in classic aspiration pneumonia, particularly in the case of suspected anaerobic infection.
- Respiratory isolation and sputum testing for TB should be performed in all patients with cavitary lung lesions.
- Sputum cultures should be obtained as they may grow more common aerobic sources of infection. Be aware that oral contamination is common and culture results may be misleading.

Imaging
- Chest radiography is obviously necessary in diagnosis. The lower lobes are usually involved if the aspiration occurred while in an upright position, but can be seen in the upper lobes if supine at the time of aspiration. Cavitation is usually solitary. Multiple cavitary lesions suggest a different process or necrotizing pneumonia rather than lung abscess.
- CT scan is not required for the diagnosis of lung abscess; however, the improved resolution may assist in ruling out malignancies or processes affecting the pulmonary parenchyma. CT scan also will help to diagnose an associated empyema, a common complication of lung abscess.

Diagnostic Procedures
Bronchoscopy is rarely done in classic lung abscess as it is unlikely to yield positive results for anaerobic organisms. It may be helpful if atypical organisms including fungi, parasites, mycobacteria, or malignancy are suspected.

TREATMENT

Medications
- Recommended antibiotic regimens for lung abscess:
  - **Clindamycin** 600 mg IV q8h
  - **Ampicillin–sulbactam** 3 g IV q6h
- Alternative regimens:
  - Ertapenem 1 g IV q24h
  - Moxifloxacin 400 mg IV or PO q24h
- Clindamycin is more efficacious than penicillin (PCN) because of increasing PCN resistance.
- Metronidazole monotherapy is not effective due to the presence of microaerophilic nonculturable organisms.
- For suspected resistant organisms consider using
  - Meropenem or piperacillin–tazobactam for gram-negative coverage
  - Vancomycin or linezolid for MRSA coverage
- Treatment duration is controversial.
  - IV antibiotics can be converted to PO as patients become afebrile and are able to tolerate PO.
  - Imaging may be obtained at regular intervals to monitor for treatment and duration. Some experts recommend continuing antibiotic therapy until the lesion is clear and appears stable.
- Anaerobic coverage should be continued in all cases of lung abscess regardless of culture results.
- Aspiration pneumonia in patients who have been hospitalized more than a few days is much more likely to be due to resistant gram-negative organisms than oral anaerobes because of a change in colonized oral flora. These patients often do not need anaerobic coverage.

Other Nonpharmacologic Therapies
- Drainage is important to resolve lung abscess. Postural drainage and chest physiotherapy are used.

• Barium swallow study should be considered to evaluate for aspiration if no clear cause is identified.

Surgical Management

• Rarely, surgical resection is required to treat lung abscesses that do not resolve despite antibiotic therapy.
• Percutaneous catheter drainage is an alternative to resection and may be used in severe or difficult to treat cases. Bronchopleural fistula and pneumothorax are complications that may occur with a percutaneous approach.

COMPLICATIONS

• Complications include pleural effusion/empyema and hemoptysis.
• Any persistent fluid accumulation with lung abscess or layering >1 cm on decubitus radiograph on the involved side should be aspirated to evaluate for empyema.
  ○ Most patients with complicated pleural effusions should have a chest tube placed.
  ○ All patients with empyema require chest tube drainage and may benefit from other surgical procedures.
  ○ Antibiotic therapy is the same as lung abscess.

INFLUENZA

GENERAL PRINCIPLES

Definition
Influenza is an acute febrile respiratory illness caused by the influenza viruses.

Classification
• Influenza A: severe illness and associated with pandemics
• Influenza B: severe illness in immunocompromised or elderly
• Influenza C: mild illness

Epidemiology
• Influenza causes between 250,000 and 500,000 deaths globally every year.[24]
• Influenza is predominantly seasonal:
  ○ Northern hemisphere: November to April
  ○ Southern hemisphere: May to September
• Antigenic drift:
  ○ Caused by point mutations in hemagglutinin or neuraminidase of circulating strains
  ○ Can lead to epidemics
  ○ Vaccine changed annually to account for antigenic drift
• Antigenic shifts:
  ○ Caused by complete change in hemagglutinin and/or neuraminidase
  ○ Can lead to pandemics
• Spread person to person by contact with respiratory secretions. Infection and replication occur solely in the respiratory tract.

TABLE 5-14	INFLUENZA VACCINE	
Vaccine type	Live attenuated	Inactivated
Administration	Intranasal	Intramuscular
Age	2–49 y	≥6 mo
Contraindications	**Avoid in immunocompromised, chronic cardiovascular and pulmonary disease, diabetes, renal insufficiency, HIV, neurologic dysfunction, and** pregnant women	Acceptable for immunocompromised patients with neurologic dysfunction, pregnancy, or HIV
	Severe allergy to eggs or other vaccine component	Severe allergy to eggs or other vaccine component

Adapted from Fiore AE, Shay DK, Broder K, et al. Prevention and control of seasonal influenza with vaccines: recommendations of the Advisory Committee on Immunization Practices (AICP) 2009. *MMWR Recomm Rep.* 2009;58:1-52.

Prevention

- Vaccination (Table 5-14)[25]:
  - The efficacy of influenza vaccination is 50% to 90% depending on the outbreak and circulating strains.[24]
  - Inactivated vaccine should be administered to all age groups, especially high-risk groups.
  - High-risk patients:
    - Nursing home residents, health care workers, and those >65 years old
    - Those with active pulmonary, cardiovascular, liver, renal, or neurologic disease
    - Immunocompromised individuals: diabetes, malignancy, HIV, transplant, on immunosuppressants, pregnant
  - Contraindications to vaccination[25]:
    - Severe allergy to eggs or vaccine components
    - Patients who developed Guillain-Barré syndrome within 6 weeks of prior influenza immunization
    - Avoid in acute febrile illness until symptoms resolve
- Droplet precautions and routine hand washing for hospitalized patients.
- Chemoprophylaxis after exposure should be administered to the following groups:
  - High-risk individuals within 2 weeks of vaccine administration or unable to receive vaccine
  - Close contact with people at high risk for influenza complications
  - Residents of institutions experiencing influenza outbreaks

DIAGNOSIS

Clinical Presentation

- High-grade fever, cough, coryza, and headache are common presenting symptoms. Systemic symptoms are common in influenza and rare in other upper respiratory tract viral infections. Systemic symptoms may last up to 2 weeks.
- High temperature is suggestive of influenza. Abnormalities such as hypoxia and tachypnea are uncommon and could be signs of another illness or a complication of influenza such as bacterial pneumonia.

Diagnostic Testing

- Viral culture is the gold standard but very slow.
- Rapid testing is readily available and commonly used.
  - Rapid antigen testing (lower sensitivity)
  - Immunofluorescence microscopy (direct or indirect) has variable sensitivity and specificity based on manufacturers
  - PCR

TREATMENT

- Medications for influenza are presented in Table 5-15.
- **Medications are only effective if administered within 24 to 48 hours of onset of symptoms**.
- They may be beneficial in hospitalized patients suffering from complications or a severe case in influenza.
- Resistance evolves rapidly. Updated recommendations can be found annually at the Centers for Disease Control and Prevention influenza web site.

TABLE 5-15	ANTIVIRALS FOR INFLUENZA[a]	
Type	**Drug**	**Additional information**
M2 inhibitors	Amantadine (PO) Rimantadine (PO)	Ineffective for influenza B. High levels of resistance in the United States preclude use for influenza A
Neuraminidase inhibitors	Oseltamivir (PO) Zanamivir (inhaled) Peramivir (IV)[b]	Treat both influenza A and B

[a]Resistance emerges and changes rapidly; always check recent recommendations from the Centers for Disease Control and Prevention (CDC).
[b]Not FDA approved.

TUBERCULOSIS

GENERAL PRINCIPLES

Epidemiology
- TB is one of the most common infectious causes of death worldwide. About one-third of the world's population is infected with latent TB.
- Only a small fraction of immunocompetent patients with latent TB will progress to active TB. The **lifetime** risk of progression is 10%.
- In poorly controlled HIV and other patients with impaired immune systems, the **annual** progression rate from latent to active TB is 10%.

Pathophysiology
- TB is spread by aerosolized droplets from patients with active pulmonary TB.
- The mycobacteria proliferate in alveolar macrophages and are transported to hilar lymph nodes and are subsequently spread to almost any other part of the body, especially the upper lobes of the lung, the pleura, lymph nodes, bones, and genito-urinary and central nervous systems.

Risk Factors and Associated Conditions
- Patients at high risk of TB exposure include immigrants from high-prevalence countries, homeless, IV drug users, migrant farm workers, and prisoners.
- Risk of progression to active TB if infected include HIV/AIDS patients, alcoholics, immunocompromised patients, diabetics, and patients who have received anti-tumor necrosis factor agents.

DIAGNOSIS

Clinical Presentation
- In active pulmonary TB, patients may present with cough (usually nonproductive and 3 weeks or more in duration), fevers, chills, night sweats, and weight loss. Hemoptysis may occur in advanced disease.
- Latent TB patients are asymptomatic.
- Physical exam findings are often nonspecific in TB.

Diagnostic Criteria
- The diagnosis of active pulmonary TB is made with laboratory findings of acid-fast organisms on sputum with a positive nucleic acid amplification test for *Mycobacterium tuberculosis* complex or culture growing *M. tuberculosis.*
- Culture-negative pulmonary TB is diagnosed with active TB symptoms, no alternative diagnosis, and improvement on TB therapy. TB skin testing (PPD) cannot be used to rule out TB in active infection.
- Latent TB is diagnosed with a positive PPD (Table 5-16) or interferon-γ release assay (preferred in patients who have had bacillus Calmette-Guérin vaccine).

Differential Diagnosis
- The differential diagnosis includes non-tuberculous mycobacterial infections, fungal infections, malignancies, lung abscess, septic emboli, and antineutrophil cytoplasmic antibody–associated vasculitis, which can all cause cavitary pulmonary lesions and symptoms suggestive of TB.

TABLE 5-16	TUBERCULIN SKIN TEST INTERPRETATION
Reaction size (mm)	**Risk group**
≥5	HIV, close contact with active TB case, CXR consistent with TB, immunosuppressed, receiving anti-TNF agents
≥10	Dialysis, diabetes, <90% IBW, IVDU, lymphoma, leukemia, head/neck cancer, children ≤4 y old, foreign born from countries of higher incidence, high-risk patients, i.e., health care workers, incarcerated, homeless
≥15	Otherwise healthy persons without risk factors for TB

TB, tuberculosis; CXR, chest radiograph; TNF, tumor necrosis factor; IBW, ideal body weight; IVDU, intravenous drug use.

Diagnostic Testing

Laboratories
- Sputum via natural cough, sputum induction, or bronchoscopy is the gold standard to diagnose TB.[26]
- A nucleic acid amplification test should be performed on all patients who have an acid-fast positive sputum sample.
- For patients with confirmed or suspected TB, the minimum requirements to remove a patient from respiratory isolation are (1) three negative sputum smears for acid-fast bacilli (AFB) obtained on separate days, (2) treatment for TB for at least 2 weeks, **and** (3) symptomatic response to therapy.
- Sputum for AFB smear and culture should be obtained every 2 weeks until a smear-negative specimen is obtained and then daily until three negative specimens are obtained. Thereafter, sputum specimens for AFB smear and culture should be obtained monthly until culture negative.
- All patients with confirmed or suspected TB should have HIV testing.
- Baseline labs for liver transaminases, alkaline phosphatase, creatinine, and platelet count should be obtained. These do not need to be reassessed unless abnormalities are detected or patients are at high risk for subsequent abnormalities.
- Baseline visual acuity and color differentiation should be performed and monitored monthly for all patients treated with ethambutol (EMB).

TREATMENT

- Directly observed therapy is considered the standard of care.[26]
- Culture-positive pulmonary TB treatment regimens are listed in Table 5-17.[26]
- Culture-negative pulmonary TB treatment algorithm is listed in Figure 5-2.
- Radiographic evidence of improvement should be seen on chest radiography by 2 months.

TABLE 5-17 TUBERCULOSIS TREATMENT REGIMEN

8-Wk initial phase			Continuation phase			
Regimen	Drugs	Administration	Regimen	Drugs	Administration (d/wk)	Minimum duration (wk)	Additional notes
1 (HIV and standard)	INH/RIF/PZA/EMB	7 d/wk or 5 d/wk × 8 wk	1a (any CD4)	INH RIF	5–7	18	Preferred for HIV and standard patients
			1b (CD4 > 100)	INH RIF	2	18	
2 (standard regimen)	INH/RIF/PZA/EMB	5–7 d/wk × 2 wk then 2 d/wk × 6 wk	2a	INH RIF	2	18	Avoid use in HIV patients
3 (3 d/wk)	INH/RIF/PZA/EMB	3 d/wk × 8 wk	3a	INH RIF	3	18	Alternative regimen
4 (3-drug)	INH/RIF/EMB	5–7 d/wk × 8 wk	4a	INH RIF	5–7	31	Seek expert advice prior to initiating
			4b	INH RIF	2		

INH, isoniazid; RIF, rifampin; PZA, pyrazinamide; EMB, ethambutol.

Adapted from Centers for Disease Control and Prevention. Treatment of tuberculosis. American Thoracic Society; CDC; Infectious Diseases Society of America. *MMWR Recomm Rep.* 2003;52:1-77.

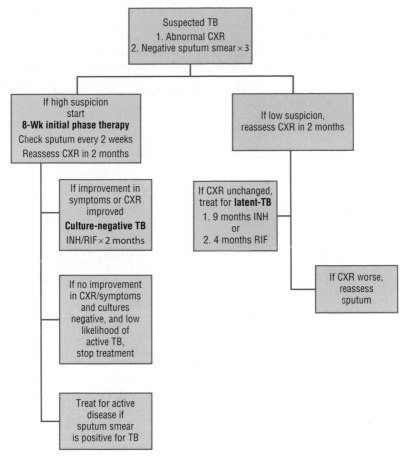

FIGURE 5-2 Management algorithm for suspected culture-negative tuberculosis.

TB, tuberculosis; CXR, chest radiograph; INH, isoniazid; RIF, rifampin.

- Monthly clinical evaluation should be performed to assess adherence and adverse effects including visual disturbances for EMB.
- All patients with HIV on highly active antiretroviral therapy (HAART) and suspected TB should have an experienced HIV clinician assess proper drug therapy, as there are complex drug reactions particularly with RIF and rifapentine.
- Extrapulmonary TB should be treated with 6- to 9-month regimens, which include isoniazid (INH)/RIF, except for meningitis, which requires 9 to 12 months of therapy. Steroids should also be added in patients with tuberculous meningitis or pericarditis.

- Pyrazinamide and EMB dosing regimens must be modified in patients with end-stage renal disease on hemodialysis. TB regimens in patients with hepatic dysfunction should be carefully selected as well. Often patients without significant transaminitis can be on hepatotoxic drugs with close monitoring.
- Pyridoxine supplementation (25 to 50 mg daily) is recommended for patients on INH.
- Side effects from medications are not uncommon. Common side effects are listed in Table 5-18.

TABLE 5-18	MANAGEMENT OF ANTITUBERCULOSIS THERAPY SIDE EFFECTS	
Side effect	**Drug**	**Treatment**
Nausea/GI upset	RIF RPT	Check HFP. Continue meds and administer with food if HFP normal
Drug-induced hepatitis (AST 3× ULN and symptoms or AST 5× ULN without symptoms)	INH RIF **PZA**	Stop INH/RIF/PZA, substitute with second-line medications: EMB, SM, amikacin, kanamycin, capreomycin, FQ
		Consider hepatitis testing
		Obtain hepatotoxin exposure history
		Restart INH, RIF, and PZA in sequential order after transaminases improve
Fever, worsening radiographic findings, or symptoms in an HIV patient	HAART	Rule out secondary process
		Exacerbation likely from immune reconstitution inflammatory syndrome if HAART recently started
		Continue treatment, symptomatic relief
		For severe cases, prednisone has been used

GI, gastrointestinal; RIF, rifampin; RPT, rifapentine; HFP, hepatic function panel; AST, aspartate aminotransferase; ULN, upper limit of normal; INH, isoniazid; PZA, pyrazinamide; EMB, ethambutol; SM, streptomycin; FQ, fluoroquinolone; HAART, high-active antiretroviral therapy.

Adapted from Centers for Disease Control and Prevention. Treatment of tuberculosis. American Thoracic Society; CDC; Infectious Diseases Society of America. *MMWR Recomm Rep.* 2003;52:1-77.

REFERENCES

1. Choby BA. Diagnosis and treatment of streptococcal pharyngitis. *Am Fam Physician.* 2009;79:383-390.
2. Centor RM, Witherspoon JM, Dalton HP, et al. The diagnosis of strep throat in adults in the emergency room. *Med Decis Making.* 1981;1:239-246.
3. McIsaac WJ, White D, Tannenbaum D, Low DE. A clinic score to reduce unnecessary antibiotic use in patient with sore throat. *CMAJ.* 1198;158:75-83.
4. Frantz TD, Rasgon BM, Quesenberry CP. Acute epiglottitis in adults: analysis of 129 cases. *JAMA.* 1994;272:1358-1360.
5. Carey MJ. Epiglottitis in adults. *Am J Emerg Med.* 1996;14:421-424.
6. Ng HL, Sin LM, Li MF, et al. Acute epiglottitis in adults: a retrospective review of 106 patients in Hong Kong. *Emerg Med J.* 2008;25:253-255.
7. *Haemophilus influenzae* infections. In: Pickering LK, Baker CJ, Kimberlin DW, Long SS, eds. *Red Book 2009: Report of the Committee on Infectious Diseases.* 28th ed. Elk Grove Village, IL: American Academy of Pediatrics; 2009:314-321.
8. Fokkens W, Lund V, Mullov J. EP3OS 2007: European position paper on rhinosinusitis and nasal polyps 2007. A summary for otorhinolaryngologists. *Rhinology.* 2007;45:97-101.
9. Dykewicz MS, Hamilos DL. Rhinitis and sinusitis. *J Allergy Clin Immunol.* 2010;125: S103-S115.
10. Rosenfeld RM. Clinical practice guideline on adult sinusitis. *Otolaryngol Head Neck Surg.* 2007;137:365-377.
11. Hickner JM, Bartlett JG, Besser RE, et al. Principles of appropriate antibiotic use for acute rhinosinusitis in adults: background. *Ann Intern Med.* 2001;134:498-505.
12. Ahovuo-Saloranta A, Borisenko OV, Kovanen N, et al. Antibiotics for acute maxillary sinusitis. *Cochrane Database Syst Rev.* April 2008;(2):CD000243.
13. Slavin RG, Spector SL, Bernstein IL, et al. The diagnosis and management of sinusitis: a practice parameter update. *J Allergy Clin Immunol.* 2005;116:S13-S47
14. Piccirillo JF, Acute bacterial sinusitis. *N Engl J Med.* 2004;351:902-910.
15. Piccirillo JF, Mage DE, Frisse ME, et al. Impact of first-line vs second-line antibiotics for the treatment of acute uncomplicated sinusitis. *JAMA.* 2001;286:1849-1856.
16. Zalmanovici A, Yaphe J. Intranasal steroids for acute sinusitis. *Cochrane Database Syst Rev.* October 2009;(4):CD0051.
17. Gonzales R, Sande MA. Uncomplicated acute bronchitis. *Ann Intern Med.* 2000;133:981-991.
18. Smucny J, Fahey T, Becker L, Glazier R. Antibiotics for acute bronchitis. *Cochrane Database Syst Rev.* 2004;(4):CD0000245.
19. Marrie TJ, Huang JQ. Epidemiology of community-acquired pneumonia in Edmonton, Alberta: an emergency department based study. *Can Respir J.* 2005;12:139-142.
20. Fine MJ, Auble TE, Yealy DM, et al. A prediction rule to identify low-risk patients with community-acquired pneumonia. *N Engl J Med.* 1997;336:243-250.
21. Mandell LA, Wunderink RG, Anzueto A, et al. Infectious Diseases Society of America/ American Thoracic Society consensus guidelines on the management of community-acquired pneumonia in adults. *Clin Infect Dis.* 2007;44(suppl 2):S27-S72.
22. Lim WS, van Der Eerden MM, Liang R, et al. Defining community acquired pneumonia severity on presentation to hospital: an international derivation and validation study. *Thorax.* 2003;58:377-382.
23. Niederman MS, Craven DE, Bonten MJ, et al. Guidelines for the management of adults with hospital-acquired, ventilator-associated, and healthcare-associated pneumonia. *Am J Respir Crit Care Med.* 2005;171:388-416.

24. Monto AS, Whitley RJ. Seasonal and pandemic influenza: a 2007 update on challenges and solutions. *Clin Infect Dis.* 2008;46:1024-1031.

25. Fiore AE, Shay DK, Broder K, et al. Prevention and control of seasonal influenza with vaccines: recommendations of the Advisory Committee on Immunization Practices (AICP) 2009. *MMWR Recomm Rep.* 2009;58:1-52.

26. Centers for Disease Control and Prevention. Treatment of tuberculosis. American Thoracic Society; CDC; Infectious Diseases Society of America. *MMWR Recomm Rep.* 2003;52:1-77.

Infections of the Gastrointestinal and Hepatobiliary Tract

6

Zhuolin Han and Erik R. Dubberke

INFECTIONS OF THE ORAL CAVITY

HERPETIC GINGIVOSTOMATITIS

GENERAL PRINCIPLES

- Herpetic gingivostomatitis is caused by herpes simplex virus (HSV)-1 and occasionally by HSV-2.
- It is a disease of children and adults, but can also occur in infants.

DIAGNOSIS

Clinical Presentation

- Herpetic gingivostomatitis ranges from a few painful ulcers without systemic manifestations to fever, sore throat, malaise, and regional lymphadenopathy.
- Primary infection is more severe than recurrent disease.
- Pain occurs 1 to 2 days before the onset of oral lesions, which are 2- to 4-mm small ulcers with an erythematous base. Symptoms persist for 2 to 3 days, although the vesicles may take 1 to 2 weeks to resolve.

Differential Diagnosis

The differential diagnosis includes herpangina, varicella, herpes zoster, hand-foot-and-mouth disease, aphthous ulcers, Behçet syndrome, cyclical neutropenia, and erythema multiforme.

Diagnostic Testing

Direct immunofluorescence, polymerase chain reaction (PCR), or viral culture may be done on samples from the ulcers.

TREATMENT

Treatment is effective if started early. Acyclovir 400 mg PO q8h for 7 to 10 days is used.

HERPANGINA

GENERAL PRINCIPLES

- Herpangina is caused by coxsackieviruses and echovirus, which produce characteristic oropharyngeal vesicles at the junction of the hard and soft palate.
- The disease primarily affects children and teenagers and occurs in epidemics during summer.

DIAGNOSIS

Clinical Presentation
- The disease is usually mild, but fever, neck pain, sore throat, and headache can occur.
- Lesions consist of multiple small white papules on an erythematous base, which spontaneously rupture in 2 to 3 days and seldom persist for >1 week. These lesions are more vesicular and less inflamed than in herpetic gingivostomatitis.
- Cervical lymphadenopathy is unusual.

Differential Diagnosis
The differential diagnosis includes HSV, hand-foot-and-mouth disease, and infectious mononucleosis.

Diagnostic Testing
- The diagnosis is made by culture of a sterile swab of the vesicles.
- PCR is more sensitive than culture and is used widely.

TREATMENT

Therapy consists of topical analgesia only.

ORAL CANDIDIASIS
See Chapter 13.

SALIVARY GLAND INFECTIONS

GENERAL PRINCIPLES

- Salivary gland infections are usually viral in origin, including mumps virus, parainfluenza, coxsackievirus, echovirus, Epstein-Barr virus (EBV), and HIV, although bacterial infections also occur.
- Risk factors for bacterial parotitis include advanced age, diabetes, dehydration, anticholinergic medication or diuretic use, and poor oral hygiene.
- *Staphylococcus aureus*, *Streptococcus pyogenes*, *Streptococcus viridans*, *Haemophilus influenzae*, and, rarely, mycobacteria are involved.

DIAGNOSIS

Clinical Manifestations
- Viral parotitis is associated with gradual onset of painful swelling of the parotid glands, either unilateral or bilateral.
- Mumps is sometimes associated with orchitis and/or meningoencephalitis.
- Bacterial parotitis usually begins with the rapid onset of pain, swelling, and induration.
- Manual palpation of the gland is painful and can result in discharge of pus from the duct.

Diagnostic Testing
- Culture of secretions for viral and bacterial pathogens should be sent.
- A rise in convalescent antibody titers for mumps virus is diagnostic.
- Nontuberculous mycobacterial infection of the parotid gland presents with unilateral painless indurated swelling. It can be differentiated from malignancy by fine needle aspiration with cytology and culture.

TREATMENT

- Viral parotitis is managed symptomatically.
- Bacterial infections need treatment with antibiotics such as oxacillin 2 g IV q4h for methicillin-sensitive *S. aureus* or vancomycin for methicillin-resistant *S. aureus* (MRSA).
- Drainage of the duct should be assisted by manual massage. Surgical drainage is rarely necessary.
- Management includes resection for nontuberculous mycobacterial infection and standard antituberculosis therapy for infection caused by *Mycobacterium tuberculosis*.

ESOPHAGEAL INFECTIONS

CANDIDAL ESOPHAGITIS
See Chapter 13.

VIRAL ESOPHAGITIS

GENERAL PRINCIPLES

- HSV-1, cytomegalovirus (CMV), and varicella zoster virus (VZV) are common viral causes.
- Viral esophagitis usually occurs in immunocompromised patients, but HSV-1 can sometimes occur in immunocompetent hosts.
- HSV infects the squamous epithelium of the esophagus, inducing the characteristic painful herpetic vesicles with an erythematous base.
- CMV infects subepithelial fibroblasts and endothelial cells.

DIAGNOSIS

Clinical Presentation

- Abrupt onset of severe odynophagia is a common presenting symptom of HSV esophagitis. Patients may also present with nausea, vomiting, and persistent retrosternal pain. Herpes labialis or skin involvement may precede or occur concurrently with esophageal infection.
- Symptoms are more gradual in CMV esophagitis. Nausea, vomiting, fever, epigastric pain, diarrhea, and weight loss may be present, whereas dysphagia and odynophagia are less common.
- VZV esophagitis is extremely rare. Concurrent shingles is helpful in diagnosing VZV esophagitis.

Differential Diagnosis

- Less common infections include cryptococcosis, histoplasmosis, tuberculosis, and cryptosporidiosis.
- Noninfectious causes include lymphoma, Kaposi sarcoma, squamous cell carcinoma, peptic esophagitis, aphthous ulcers, tablet mucositis, corrosive ingestion, mucositis from chemotherapy, and idiopathic ulcerative esophagitis in AIDS.

Diagnostic Testing

- Diagnosis is made by endoscopy with viral culture or PCR and cytologic or histologic exams of brushings and biopsy from ulcer edge (HSV) and ulcer base (CMV).
- Vesicular herpetic lesions in the mid- to distal esophagus are seen early, which slough off and leave discrete, circumscribed ulcers with raised edges.
- CMV is associated with extensive, large, shallow ulcers in the distal esophagus.

TREATMENT

- HSV is treated with acyclovir 400 mg PO five times a day, famciclovir 250 mg PO tid, or valacyclovir 500 mg PO tid for 14 to 21 days. For those who cannot swallow, IV acyclovir 5 mg/kg q8h should be used. In immunocompetent patients, spontaneous resolution can occur after 1 to 2 weeks.
- CMV is treated with ganciclovir at an induction dose of 5 mg/kg IV q12h for 21 to 28 days or until signs and symptoms have resolved. Oral valganciclovir 900 mg bid can be used if oral intake is possible. Foscarnet is an alternative for ganciclovir-resistant CMV esophagitis.
- VZV esophagitis can be treated with acyclovir or famciclovir.

INFECTIONS OF THE STOMACH

HELICOBACTER PYLORI GASTRITIS

GENERAL PRINCIPLES

- *Helicobacter pylori* infection causes chronic active gastritis, is the main cause of duodenal and gastric ulcers, and is a risk factor for gastric adenocarcinoma and lymphoma.

- Other infectious causes of gastritis are rare and occur in immunocompromised patients.
- *H. pylori* is a spiral, gram-negative, urease-producing bacillus.
- *H. pylori* infection has been associated with >90% of duodenal ulcers and 80% of gastric ulcers. Chronic infection is associated with a two- to sixfold increase in gastric cancer and MALT (mucosa-associated lymphoid tissue) lymphoma.

DIAGNOSIS

Clinical Presentation

- Patients may have chronic active gastritis, chronic persistent gastritis, or atrophic gastritis.
- The majority of patients are asymptomatic.
- Symptoms may include epigastric discomfort with a burning sensation. Less commonly, nausea, vomiting, and anorexia occur. Bleeding may occur, leading to signs and symptoms of anemia.

Diagnostic Testing

- Testing for *H. pylori* should be performed only if treatment is planned.
- Proton pump inhibitors (PPIs) should be stopped for at least 2 weeks and antibiotics for at least 4 weeks before all tests except serology.
- Noninvasive tests include antibody tests, the urea breath test, and the stool antigen test; the latter two are also useful in assessing the success of treatment.
  - IgG antibody to *H. pylori* has a sensitivity and specificity of 85% and 79%, respectively.[1]
  - However, positive serology detects *H. pylori* exposure, not necessarily active infection.
- Endoscopy is performed to obtain mucosal biopsy specimens, to perform rapid urease testing, and for histology and culture.
  - Endoscopy is also used to document healing of gastric ulcers and to rule out malignancy.
  - Endoscopy is mandatory if age >55, anemic, and has weight loss, gastrointestinal (GI) bleeding, or palpable mass.

TREATMENT

- The recommended primary therapies include the following[1]:
  - Clarithromycin-based triple therapy: a PPI, clarithromycin 500 mg bid, and amoxicillin 1 g bid or metronidazole 500 mg bid.
  - Bismuth quadruple therapy: a PPI or H2 blocker (ranitidine 150 mg PO bid), bismuth 525 mg PO qid, metronidazole 250 mg PO qid, and tetracycline 500 mg PO qid.
- Treatment duration is 10 to 14 days.
- Eradication rates are 70% to 85% in clarithromycin-based triple therapy and 75% to 90% in bismuth quadruple therapy. If treatment is a failure, retreat with a different regimen.[1]
- Treatment failures are associated with poor patient compliance and antibiotic resistance, especially with previous antibiotic exposure.
- Side effects and the importance of compliance should be discussed.

INTESTINAL INFECTIONS

ACUTE INFECTIOUS DIARRHEA

GENERAL PRINCIPLES

- Diarrhea is defined as three or more loose or watery stools per day or a definite decrease in consistency and increase in frequency based upon an individual baseline.
- Infectious diarrhea can be caused by viruses, bacteria, and less commonly protozoa.
- Acute diarrhea is an episode of diarrhea of ≤14 days in duration and is usually of an infectious etiology.
- Viral infections are the most common cause.
- If diarrhea lasts >3 days, bacteria are the likely etiology.

DIAGNOSIS

Clinical Manifestations

- A careful history and physical exam is important. History of antibiotic use, recent or remote travel, duration of diarrhea, amount of weight loss, water supply, hobbies or occupation, pets, drugs, family exposure, and diet should be elicited.
- Infectious diarrhea can be noninflammatory or inflammatory.
- The majority of the cases are **noninflammatory**, with no blood or fecal leukocytes, suggesting an enterotoxic bacterial, viral, or noninvasive parasitic process. Pathogens include enterotoxigenic *Escherichia coli*, enteroaggregative *E. coli*, enteroinvasive *E. coli*, *Vibrio cholerae*, and viruses.
- **Inflammatory** diarrhea involves the colon and occasionally the distal small intestine.
  ○ Symptoms include fever, low-volume stools with blood and mucus, chills, abdominal cramping, and tenesmus. Fever, tenesmus, and bloody diarrhea are characteristic of dysentery.
  ○ The most common bacterial pathogens for dysenteric syndrome are *Campylobacter*, nontyphoid *Salmonella*, *Shigella*, and Shiga toxin–producing *E. coli*, such as O157:H7.
  ○ *Aeromonas* spp., noncholera *Vibrio*, and *Yersinia enterocolitica* are less common.
- Risk factors for death in diarrheal disease include malnutrition, immunosuppression, extremes of age, and complications such as dehydration, pneumonia, sepsis, and development of hemolytic uremic syndrome (HUS).

Differential Diagnosis

Noninfectious causes of diarrhea include drugs, food allergies, primary GI diseases such as inflammatory bowel disease, thyrotoxicosis, and the carcinoid syndrome.

Diagnostic Testing

- In nonhospitalized patients with mild-to-moderate symptoms (<5 stools/d) and no fever, nausea, vomiting, or cramps, supportive therapy is indicated. Stool culture is unlikely to be clinically helpful, but may help to identify outbreaks.

- All other patients must undergo testing, including exams for fecal leukocytes, stool culture, parasite exam, stool antigen testing, or stool toxin testing.
- Stool exams for **fecal leukocyte and occult blood** are indicated in any patient with fever and moderate-to-severe diarrhea.
  - Numerous leukocytes indicate an invasive enteric pathogen, such as *Shigella*, *Salmonella*, *Campylobacter*, *Y. enterocolitica*, *Aeromonas hydrophila*, *Vibrio parahaemolyticus*, enteroinvasive *E. coli*, or enterohemorrhagic *E. coli*.
  - Mononuclear cells suggest typhoid fever or amebic dysentery.
  - If the exam for fecal leukocytes is positive, stool must be cultured.
- Stool exams for **ova and parasites** are indicated in all patients who have had diarrhea for >2 weeks, have traveled to developing countries, drink well water, have sex with men, or are HIV positive.
  - *Cryptosporidium* outbreaks have been associated with contaminated municipal water supplies and community swimming pools.
  - Special stains are needed for amebic trophozoites, *Cryptosporidium*, *Isospora*, and *Microsporidia*, so specify the organisms of interest.
- **Stool antigen assays** can detect *Isospora*, *Giardia*, *Cryptosporidium*, and *Entamoeba histolytica*.
- **Stool toxin assays** detect *Clostridium difficile* toxin and Shiga-like toxin.
- **Stool cultures** identify common bacterial pathogens such as *Campylobacter* spp., *Salmonella* spp., and *Shigella* spp.
  - The "3-day rule" is applied by most microbiology labs. Patients who develop diarrhea after 3 days of hospitalization are unlikely to have a non–*C. difficile* bacterial or parasitic cause of diarrhea, and stool for cultures and/or ova and parasites is not recommended.
  - The exceptions are patients aged ≥65, comorbid diseases, neutropenia, and HIV infection, who may warrant cultures despite diarrhea onset ≥3 days after hospitalization.
- **Blood cultures** should be obtained in severely ill patients when salmonellosis is suspected or in any immunocompromised patient.
- **Endoscopy** is useful in identifying amebiasis, in ruling out inflammatory bowel disease, and when no pathogen can be identified by other means.

TREATMENT

- Fluid and electrolyte replacement is the mainstay of therapy.
- Dietary alteration is helpful and includes a lactose-free diet, starches and cereals, crackers, and soup.
- Symptomatic therapy with antimotility agents, such as loperamide and bismuth sulfate, may reduce the number of stools. **Antimotility agents should be avoided if dysentery symptoms present**, as they may worsen disease.
- Antimicrobial therapy is appropriate in patients with febrile dysentery.
  - Ciprofloxacin 500 mg PO bid for 3 days is used in adults.
  - A single dose of azithromycin 1 g PO is recommended for quinolone-resistant *Campylobacter* infections.
  - **Antibiotics are contraindicated in diarrhea caused by enterohemorrhagic *E. coli***, such as *E. coli* O157:H7, as they may increase the risk of HUS but do not reduce the duration of diarrhea.[2,3]

CHRONIC INFECTIOUS DIARRHEA

GENERAL PRINCIPLES

- Chronic diarrhea refers to diarrheal symptoms lasting ≥30 days. Most chronic diarrheas are noninfectious. Infectious etiologies are discussed here.
- Small intestinal bacterial overgrowth (SIBO) is caused by an increased number of bacteria in the small intestine due to intestinal stasis.
- Predisposing factors to SIBO include short bowel syndrome, chronic pancreatitis, intestinal fistula, achlorhydria, blind loop syndrome, liver disease, and immunodeficiency.

DIAGNOSIS

- SIBO manifests as watery diarrhea in a small bowel pattern, with large-volume, infrequent stools, bloating, gas, malabsorption, and periumbilical pain.
- Fever and systemic symptoms are not usually present.
- History, radiographic findings, and quantitative aerobic and anaerobic cultures of the upper small bowel contents by upper endoscopy are useful.
- Serum cobalamin is often decreased, while serum folate is elevated.

TREATMENT

- In the case of intestinal stasis, medications enhancing motility can be used.
- Antimicrobial therapy needs to cover aerobes and anaerobes, such as **amoxicillin–clavulanate** 500 mg PO tid or 875 mg bid for 2 weeks. Recurrence is common.
- Surgery and vitamin supplementation may be necessary.

GIARDIASIS

See Chapter 17.

CRYPTOSPORIDIOSIS, MICROSPORIDIOSIS, CYCLOSPORIASIS

See Chapter 13.

FOOD-BORNE ILLNESSES

GENERAL PRINCIPLES

- Food-borne illnesses result from the ingestion of foods contaminated with pathogenic organisms, toxins, or chemicals (Table 6-1).
- Most food-borne illness results in vomiting and/or diarrhea and is commonly called food poisoning.

TABLE 6-1 COMMON ORGANISMS CAUSING FOOD-BORNE ILLNESS

Staphylococcus aureus	Ham, poultry, egg salad, pastries
Bacillus cereus	Fried rice, meats, vegetables
Clostridium perfringens	Beef, poultry, gravy, Mexican food
Escherichia coli O157:H7	Undercooked beef, raw milk
Salmonella	Poultry, beef, egg, dairy products
Shigella	Egg salads, potato salads, lettuce
Campylobacter jejuni	Raw milk, poultry (spring, summer)
Vibrio cholerae	Shellfish
Yersinia enterocolitica	Milk, tofu, pork
Enteroinvasive *E. coli*	Cheese
Enterotoxigenic *E. coli*	Salad, cheese, sausage, seafood, cheese, hamburger
Clostridium botulinum	Vegetables, fruits (especially home-canned), fish

DIAGNOSIS

Clinical Manifestations

- Timing of symptoms and food exposure is important.
  - Nausea, vomiting, and diarrhea within 1 hour of ingestion of seafood suggest seafood neurotoxin disease, Scombroid poisoning, or ciguatoxin poisoning.
    - Scombroid poisoning presents as histamine reactions with flushing, headache, dizziness, urticaria along with GI symptoms and resolves within 12 hours.
    - Ciguatoxin poisoning presents as abdominal cramps and diarrhea with circumoral paresthesia.
  - Nausea and vomiting within 1 to 6 hours of ingestion suggest preformed toxin (*S. aureus* and *Bacillus cereus*). Abdominal cramps and diarrhea without vomiting within 8 to 16 hours of ingestion are usually caused by toxins produced in vivo (*B. cereus* and *Clostridium perfringens*).
  - Abdominal cramps and watery diarrhea within 1 to 3 days suggest enterotoxigenic *E. coli*, *V. parahaemolyticus*, *V. cholerae*, *Campylobacter jejuni*, *Salmonella* spp., and *Shigella* spp. Disease is enterotoxin or cytotoxin mediated. Symptoms usually resolve in 76 to 92 hours but may last >1 week.
  - Bloody diarrhea without fever 3 to 5 days after eating suggests noninvasive enterohemorrhagic *E. coli*, such as *E. coli* O157:H7. Infection is characterized by severe abdominal cramping and diarrhea, which is initially watery but subsequently grossly bloody. There is risk for the development of HUS.
- Associated symptoms
  - Diarrhea followed by fever and systemic complaints such as headache, muscle aches, and stiff neck may suggest infection with *Listeria monocytogenes*.

   ○ *Yersinia* spp. cause watery diarrhea in children aged 1 to 5, but may mimic appendicitis in older children and adolescents.

   ○ Nausea, vomiting, diarrhea, and descending paralysis (beginning with cranial nerve weakness manifested as dysphonia, dysphagia, diplopia, and blurred vision, followed by muscle weakness and respiratory insufficiency) suggest *Clostridium botulinum* toxin ingestion. The sensory system is intact.

     ■ The differential includes Guillain-Barré syndrome, which can develop 1 to 3 weeks after *Campylobacter* spp. infection.

     ■ Guillain-Barré syndrome is usually an ascending weakness/paralysis with sensory findings and abnormal nerve conduction studies.

Diagnostic Testing

- Obtain appropriate specimens from patients (see the section "Acute Infectious Diarrhea: Diagnosis").
- Also, any leftover food should be cultured, as well as the food preparation environment and food handlers, where applicable.
- Botulism is diagnosed by the detection of toxin in food, serum, or stool of patients or *C. botulinum* spores in the stool by culture.

TREATMENT

- Supportive therapy is indicated.
- Treatment is instituted where appropriate (see the section "Acute Infectious Diarrhea: Treatment").
- State health departments should be notified.
- Antitoxin for botulism should be obtained.

TRAVELER'S DIARRHEA

GENERAL PRINCIPLES

- Traveler's diarrhea is defined as three or more unformed stools per day in a person traveling to a developing nation.
- Infection is acquired through ingestion of fecally contaminated food or water.
- **Enterotoxigenic *E. coli* is the most common pathogen**, accounting for up to one-third of cases.
- Other common pathogens include *Salmonella* spp., *Shigella* spp., *Campylobacter* spp., and enteroaggregative *E. coli*.
- Viral causes include noroviruses and rotavirus.
- Parasites are less common and are usually seen in long-term travelers.
- Prevention includes avoiding raw fruits, vegetables, water, and ice cubes. All water should be boiled or bottled. More information can be found at http://www.cdc.gov/travel/ or call 1-877-FYI-TRIP (1-877-394-8747). **Antibiotic prophylaxis breeds resistance** and is recommended only for patients at high risk for morbidity and mortality from diarrhea.

DIAGNOSIS

- Diarrhea, anorexia, nausea, vomiting, and cramping abdominal pain can occur.
- Patients may have low-grade fever.
- The illness is self-limited, usually lasting 3 to 5 days.
- Postdiarrhea irritable bowel syndrome may develop in some patients.

TREATMENT

- Fluid replacement is important.
- Symptomatic treatment with bismuth subsalicylate or loperamide is effective when there is no bloody stool or temperature >38.5°C (101.3°F).
- Antibiotics are usually not required, but are indicated when the symptoms are severe (>4 stools in 24 hours), associated with fever, blood, mucus, or pus in the stool.
- **Ciprofloxacin** 500 mg PO bid for 3 days is the usual treatment. However, fluoroquinolone-resistant *Campylobacter* species are emerging, especially in Southeast Asia and the Indian subcontinent. Azithromycin 1 g PO × 1 dose should be used in these regions.

ENTERIC FEVER (TYPHOID FEVER)

GENERAL PRINCIPLES

- Several enteric infections characterized by abdominal pain and fever are distinct from acute infectious diarrhea. These include enteric fever, mesenteric adenitis (which can mimic appendicitis), and eosinophilia with abdominal cramps/diarrhea.
- Enteric fever, also known as typhoid fever, is an acute systemic illness with fever, headache, and abdominal discomfort caused by *Salmonella typhi* and *Salmonella paratyphi*.
- Typhoid fever is prevalent in Asia, Africa, and Latin America.
- Multidrug-resistant (MDR) strains of *S. typhi* are increasingly prevalent globally.
- Risk factors for typhoid fever include gastrectomy, hypochlorhydria, altered intestinal motility, prior antibiotic therapy, sickle cell anemia, chronic liver disease, and CD4 T-cell deficiency.
- Organisms are ingested, multiply in intestinal lymphoid tissue, and disseminate systemically via lymphatic or hematogenous routes. Incubation period is 5 to 21 days.
- Infection may be food- or waterborne.

Prevention

- A live oral *S. typhi* strain TY21a and a parenteral Vi polysaccharide vaccine are available. Unfortunately, they are not completely effective and do not protect recipients from *S. paratyphi* infection.
- Travelers should be advised about precautions regarding the foods and water they consume, even after they received the vaccine.

- Vivotif Berna is an oral vaccine taken every other day for 4 days at least 2 weeks before departure. It should not be given to pregnant women or patients with immunodeficiency. Oral typhoid vaccine has an efficacy of about 50% to 80%.[4-6]
- Typhim Vi is administered as a single dose intramuscularly. The vaccine is safe for immunocompromised individuals, including HIV-infected patients. Efficacy is similar to oral vaccine.[5,6] Booster doses are given every 2 to 3 years.

DIAGNOSIS

Clinical Manifestations

- Symptoms include insidious onset of fever, headache, and abdominal pain with cough, conjunctivitis, and constipation or diarrhea.
- Diarrhea is rare after the first few days.
- Physical exam may reveal abdominal tenderness, hepatosplenomegaly, rose spots (faint, maculopapular, salmon-colored blanching lesions predominately on the trunk), relative bradycardia, and mental status changes. Rales may be present.
- Complications include pneumonia, endocarditis, osteomyelitis, arthritis, and meningitis.

Differential Diagnosis

- A variety of infections and noninfectious etiologies can present with similar symptoms and the differential diagnosis can be extensive.
- The differential includes infections with *Y. enterocolitica*, *Yersinia pseudotuberculosis*, and *Campylobacter fetus*, as well as typhoidal tularemia.

Diagnostic Testing

- Obtain multiple blood, stool, and urine cultures. Urine and stool cultures are positive in <50% of patients. If cultures are negative, bone marrow can be cultured, as it may be positive even after antibiotics have been started.
- Serology is helpful but a positive test could represent previous infection.
- Chest radiography may occasionally reveal an infiltrate.
- Liver tests are often elevated, with alkaline phosphatase and transaminase levels relatively higher than bilirubin levels.
- Pyuria and proteinuria due to complement-mediated glomerulonephritis can occur.

TREATMENT

- Resistance to antibiotics is increasing. MDR *S. typhi* and *S. paratyphi* are defined as strains resistant to ampicillin, chloramphenicol, and trimethoprim–sulfamethoxazole.
- A fluoroquinolone (e.g., **ciprofloxacin**, 500 mg PO bid for 10 days) or a third-generation cephalosporin can be used (**ceftriaxone**, 2 g IV daily for 1 to 2 weeks).[7,8]
- Increasing fluoroquinolone resistance has been observed in India.
- **Azithromycin** 1 g daily for 5 days is an alternative regimen.[7,8]

ABDOMINAL PAIN OR DIARRHEA WITH EOSINOPHILIA

GENERAL PRINCIPLES

Eosinophilic gastroenteritis may be due to a variety of infectious causes including bacterial overgrowth, Whipple disease, and parasitic infection caused by *Strongyloides stercoralis*, *Ascaris lumbricoides*, *Toxocara* spp. (visceral larva migrans), *Trichinella spiralis*, various nematodes, and *Cystoisospora* (*Isospora*) *belli*.

DIAGNOSIS

Clinical Presentation
- Diarrhea along with abdominal pain, nausea, vomiting, and weight loss can occur.
- Steatorrhea and protein-losing enteropathy may occur, with edema or anasarca.
- GI bleeding, malabsorption, and gastric outlet obstruction may develop.
- Peripheral eosinophilia is present in up to 75% of patients.

Differential Diagnosis
Noninfectious causes include vasculitis, regional enteritis, ulcerative colitis, food allergy, systemic lupus erythematosus, solid tumors, and lymphomas.

Diagnostic Testing
- Stool culture and exam for leukocytes, parasites, and Charcot-Leyden crystals.
- Definitive diagnosis is made by endoscopy with multiple biopsies, as involvement is patchy.

TREATMENT

- Treatment of the underlying infection is usually curative, but corticosteroids may be helpful.
- Strongyloidiasis is treated with ivermectin or albendazole.
- A single dose of albendazole is effective for ascariasis in almost all patients.
- For patients with mild visceral larval migrans, antibiotic treatment is not necessary. For those with moderate-to-severe symptoms, treatment with albendazole may be considered.
- Albendazole may also be used for treatment of trichinellosis with systemic symptoms.
- First-line therapy for *Cystoisospora* infection is trimethoprim–sulfamethoxazole.

ANTIBIOTIC-ASSOCIATED DIARRHEA/COLITIS

GENERAL PRINCIPLES

- *C. difficile* is a spore-forming, gram-positive obligate anaerobe that is present in 3% of healthy adults. However, colonization rates are 10% to 30% of hospitalized patients.

- *C. difficile* infection (CDI) should be suspected in any patient who has diarrhea in association with antibiotic exposure.
- Risk factors for CDI include advanced age, hospitalization, cancer chemotherapy, GI surgery, manipulation of the GI tract such as tube feeding, and acid-suppressing medications. The most important modifiable risk factor is exposure to antimicrobial agents.
- CDI results in acute inflammation of the colonic mucosa. Disease results from spore germination, colonization, overgrowth, and toxin production. Pathogenic strains produce toxin A and B or B alone. About 10% of *C. difficile* strains produce no toxin and are not pathogenic.
- During infection, only the epithelium and the superficial lamina propria are affected, although in more severe cases, deeper tissues are involved. Pseudomembranes may be found throughout the colon but are worst in the rectosigmoid region. The ileum is rarely involved unless there is a previous colostomy/ileostomy.

DIAGNOSIS

Clinical Manifestations

- Infection results in profuse watery or green mucoid, foul-smelling diarrhea with cramping abdominal pain usually beginning 4 to 10 days after starting antibiotic therapy (range 24 hours to 8 weeks).
- The stool may be positive for occult blood.
- Patients may develop toxic megacolon, perforation, and peritonitis.

Differential Diagnosis

- Osmotic diarrhea from antibiotic use is more common than CDI, but not associated with fever or leukocytosis.
- Other differential diagnoses include Crohn disease, ulcerative colitis, ischemic colitis, or infection with other intestinal pathogens, such as *E. coli*, *Salmonella* spp., *Campylobacter* spp., *Yersinia* spp., *E. histolytica*, or *Strongyloides*.

Diagnostic Testing

- Diagnosis is based on detection of *C. difficile* toxin.
- Cytotoxicity cell assays detecting toxin B, enzyme immunoassay detecting toxin A and B or toxin A, and PCR detecting toxin A or B have variable sensitivity and specificity.
- Because of the minimal increase in yield and false-positive results, repeat testing of multiple stools is not recommended.
- *C. difficile* common antigen glutamate dehydrogenase (GDH) is present in all *C. difficile* strains but testing for it must be followed by toxin assay. Nontoxigenic strains do not cause CDI and other bacteria also produce GDH.
- Culture followed by detection of toxigenic isolate is the gold standard but takes up to 4 days.
- Endoscopy may be useful, but pseudomembranous colitis is seen in only about half of patients with CDI.

TREATMENT

- Offending antibiotics should be stopped when possible.
- Antibiotic treatment of CDI is presented in Table 6-2.

TABLE 6-2	*CLOSTRIDIUM DIFFICILE* INFECTION MANAGEMENT	
Type of CDI	**Criteria**	**Treatment**
Mild-to-moderate and first or second episode		Metronidazole 500 mg PO q8h for 10–14 d
≥Third episode		Vancomycin 125 mg PO q6h for 10–14 d, considering tapering or pulsed regimen
Severe	Leukocytosis with >15,000 cells/μL or Creatinine ≥1.5 times the premorbid level	Vancomycin 125 mg PO q6h for 10–14 d
Severe, complicated	Ileus, megacolon, pending perforation, hypotension, or shock	Vancomycin 125–500 mg PO q6h or vancomycin enema + metronidazole 500 mg IV q8h. Request surgical consult

CDI, *Clostridium difficile* infection.

[a]An example of tapering vancomycin regimen: 125 mg PO tid for 1 wk, 125 mg PO bid for 1 wk, 125 mg PO daily for 1 wk, then 125 mg PO three times a week for 2–8 wk.

DIVERTICULITIS

GENERAL PRINCIPLES

- Infection of the diverticula, including extension into adjacent tissues, can result from obstruction from a fecalith.
- Inflammation or micropuncture of diverticula can lead to perforation with pericolic abscess formation, fistula formation, or, less commonly, peritonitis.
- Organisms usually include anaerobes and facultative gram-negative bacilli.

DIAGNOSIS

- Left lower quadrant pain and a change in bowel habits is the typical presentation.[3]
- Fever, chills, nausea, and vomiting can occur.
- Microscopic rectal bleeding occurs in up to 25% of cases.
- Occasionally, shock and peritonitis can develop.
- Computed tomography (CT) scanning is helpful to evaluate for abscess formation.

TREATMENT

- Initial, uncomplicated diverticulitis is primarily a medical disease. NPO, IV fluids, and IV antimicrobial therapy are the mainstay of treatment.

- IV antibiotic regimens are as follows:
  - β-lactam/β-lactamase inhibitor such as ampicillin–sulbactam (3 g q6h) or piperacillin/tazobactam (3.375 g IV q6h)
  - A third-generation cephalosporin such as ceftriaxone (1 g IV q24h) **and** metronidazole (500 mg IV q8-12h)
  - A fluoroquinolone (e.g., ciprofloxacin 400 mg IV q12h **or** levofloxacin 500 mg or 750 mg IV daily) **and** metronidazole (500 mg IV q8h)
  - A carbapenem, such as imipenem (500 mg q6h) or meropenem (1 g q8h) or ertapenem (1 g daily)
- Regardless of the initial empiric regimen, the therapeutic regimen should be revisited once culture results are available.
- Patients who are less ill can be treated with ciprofloxacin 500 mg PO bid **and** metronidazole 500 mg PO tid for 10 days.
- The patient may need percutaneous drainage of an abscess.
- Surgical intervention is indicated if the patient does not respond in 48 to 72 hours and has recurrent attacks at the same location, for complications such as fistula formation, obstruction, or perforation, or if carcinoma is suspected.

PERITONEAL INFECTIONS

PRIMARY PERITONITIS

GENERAL PRINCIPLES

- Primary peritonitis (or spontaneous bacterial peritonitis [SBP]) occurs mostly in patients with liver disease and ascites, although it can occur in patients with other causes of ascites (e.g., heart failure, nephrotic syndrome).
- SBP is almost always monobacterial.
- **The most common organisms are *E. coli* and *Streptococcus pneumoniae*.**
- Prophylactic antibiotic therapy has led to increased infection with viridians *Streptococci*, MRSA, and extended-spectrum β-lactamase-producing gram-negative bacilli.
- Rare etiologies are HSV, histoplasmosis, and coccidioidomycosis.
- An episode of SBP and a low ascetic fluid protein value of <1.5 g/dL are indications for prophylaxis.[9-11]
  - Norfloxacin 400 mg PO daily, ciprofloxacin 750 mg PO weekly, or trimethoprim–sulfamethoxazole DS 1 tab PO daily are used.
  - Short-course prophylaxis with a quinolone or a third-generation cephalosporin (ceftriaxone 1 g IV daily for 7 days) improves survival in patients with variceal hemorrhage, regardless of the presence of ascites.[12]

DIAGNOSIS

Clinical Manifestations
- New onset of abdominal pain with evidence of systemic sepsis in a patient with chronic ascites suggests SBP.

- Presentation can be subtle, with acute deterioration of renal function, unexplained encephalopathy, and borderline fever.
- **A low threshold for paracentesis is appropriate in patients with chronic ascites.**

Diagnostic Testing

- Diagnosis is made by paracentesis, with fluid sent for culture (in blood culture bottles to increase yield), cell count, and differential.
- Blood cultures should be obtained, as bacteremia can be present in up to 75% of patients.
- Definitive diagnosis is made by a positive culture combined with a neutrophil count in the peritoneal fluid >250 cells/mm^3.
- **Since cultures are not always positive, patients with chronic ascites with neutrophil count >250 cells/mm^3 should be treated with antibiotics.**
- A polymicrobial infection plus ascitic fluid protein >1 g/dL, glucose <50 mg/dL, or lactate dehydrogenase (LDH) >serum level suggests secondary peritonitis and the need for emergent imaging to detect GI perforation.

TREATMENT

- Initial therapy usually consists of a third-generation cephalosporin, such as ceftriaxone, 2 g IV daily, or levofloxacin, or a β-lactam/β-lactamase inhibitor. Therapy can be tailored to the results of cultures.
- Treatment should continue for 7 days if blood cultures are negative or 2 weeks if blood cultures are positive.
- Albumin infusions (1.5 g/kg on day 1 and 1 g/kg on day 3) reduce acute renal failure.[13]
- Treatment is successful in most cirrhotic patients, especially if instituted early and gram-positive organisms are found.
- Poor prognosis is associated with renal failure, hyperbilirubinemia, hypoalbuminemia, and encephalopathy.

SECONDARY PERITONITIS

GENERAL PRINCIPLES

- Infection results from perforation of the GI tract with spillage of intestinal contents into the peritoneum or from contiguous spread from a visceral infection or abscess.
- **Secondary peritonitis is typically a polymicrobial infection with intestinal organisms.**

DIAGNOSIS

Clinical Manifestations

- Manifestations include severe abdominal pain, nausea, vomiting, anorexia, fever, chills, and abdominal distension.
- Patients may have abdominal tenderness, hypoactive or absent bowel sounds, rebound, guarding, and abdominal rigidity.

Diagnostic Testing

- Bacteremia is present in 20% to 30% of cases.
- An abdominal series helps rule out free air and obstruction.
- An abdominal CT or ultrasound to evaluate for the source of the infection may be helpful.

TREATMENT

- Broad-spectrum antibiotics that cover both gram-negative aerobic and anaerobic organisms should be started, and treatment should continue for ≥5 to 7 days.
- Ampicillin–sulbactam, 3 g IV q6h, or a third-generation cephalosporin with metronidazole works well (e.g., ceftriaxone 1 to 2 g IV daily and metronidazole 500 mg IV q8h).
- Surgical management of the source, such as repair of perforations and removal of necrotic or infected material, is essential.
- Prognosis depends on the patient's age, duration of peritoneal contamination, presence of foreign material (e.g., bile or pancreatic secretions), the primary intraabdominal process, and the microorganisms involved in infection.

PERITONITIS ASSOCIATED WITH CHRONIC AMBULATORY PERITONEAL DIALYSIS

GENERAL PRINCIPLES

- Peritonitis associated with chronic ambulatory peritoneal dialysis occurs at an average rate of one infection per person undergoing peritoneal dialysis per year.
- Recurrent infection may result in sclerosing peritonitis, which can lead to discontinuation of ambulatory peritoneal dialysis.
- Infections usually originate from contamination of the catheter by skin organisms, usually due to exit site infections or subcutaneous tunnel catheter infections.
- Transient bacteremia or contamination of the dialysate delivery system during bag exchanges can also occur.
- **Common causative organisms are *S. aureus*, *Staphylococcus epidermidis*, *Streptococcus species*, gram-negative bacilli, anaerobes**, and, less commonly, *M. tuberculosis*, *Aspergillus*, *Nocardia*, and *Candida* spp.

DIAGNOSIS

- Patients describe abdominal pain, tenderness, nausea, vomiting, fever, and diarrhea.
- The diagnosis is made by analysis and culture of the dialysate.
- The dialysate is almost always cloudy, with a leukocyte count >100 cells/mm^3 with >50% neutrophils.
- Ascites cultures reveal the organisms >50% of the time.
- Blood cultures are rarely positive.

TREATMENT

- Intraperitoneal antibiotics that cover both gram-positives and gram-negatives should be used.
- First-generation cephalosporin such as cefazolin (vancomycin if there are high rates of MRSA) and an aminoglycoside or a third-generation cephalosporin should be used empirically.
- Antibiotic therapy should be adjusted based on culture results.
- Intraperitoneal antibiotics can be given continuously or intermittently with once-daily exchange. Examples of continuous intraperitoneal antibiotic dosing are as follows:
  - Vancomycin 1.0 g/L dialysate loading dose, then 25 mg/L dialysate maintenance dose
  - Gentamicin 8 mg/L loading, then 4 mg/L maintenance
  - Cefazolin 500 mg/L loading, then 125 mg/L maintenance
  - Cefepime 500 mg/L loading, then 125 mg/L maintenance
- Most patients improve in 2 to 4 days. If symptoms persist >96 hours, reevaluate to rule out a GI source.
- If patients are severely ill or blood cultures are positive, antibiotics can be given parenterally.
- Depending on the organism and the severity of the illness, patients may need their catheters removed. This is especially true in the case of relapsing or refractory peritonitis, fungal peritonitis, and refractory catheter infections.

BILIARY INFECTIONS

CHOLECYSTITIS

GENERAL PRINCIPLES

- In >90% of cases, cholecystitis is caused by impaired biliary drainage due to the impaction of gallstones in the cystic duct.
- Acalculous cholecystitis can occur in acutely ill patients following major surgery or burns.
- **Causative organisms usually consist of normal intestinal flora such as *E. coli*, *Klebsiella*, *Enterobacter*, *Proteus* spp., *Enterococcus* spp., and anaerobes.**

DIAGNOSIS

Clinical Manifestations
- Patients usually describe right upper quadrant abdominal pain that radiates to the right shoulder and scapula. Fever may occur.
- Repeated chills and fever, jaundice, and hypotension suggest cholangitis. Some patients can present with sepsis or altered mental status (especially the elderly).
- Complications of cholecystitis may include empyema, gangrene of the gallbladder, emphysematous cholecystitis, pericholecystic abscess, intraperitoneal abscess, cholangitis, peritonitis, liver abscess, and bacteremia.

Differential Diagnosis

The differential diagnosis includes myocardial infarction, pancreatitis, perforated ulcer, right lower lobe pneumonia, intestinal obstruction, cholangitis, hepatitis, and right kidney disease.

Diagnostic Testing

- Patients may have hyperbilirubinemia and alkaline phosphatase elevation with a mild increase in transaminases.
- Imaging with ultrasound, CT, or technetium hepatoiminodiacetic acid (HIDA) scan is diagnostic.
- Ultrasound and CT may reveal stones, a thickened gallbladder wall, a dilated lumen, or pericholecystic fluid.
- HIDA scan may reveal an occluded cystic duct and the gallbladder may not be visualized.

TREATMENT

- Treatment consists of IV fluid resuscitation and **broad-spectrum antibiotic therapy covering gram-negative bacilli and anaerobes**.
- Monotherapies include ampicillin/sulbactam 3 g IV q6h, piperacillin/tazobactam 3.375 g IV q6h or ertapenem 1 g IV q24h.
- Combination therapies include metronidazole 500 mg IV q8h **plus** a third-generation cephalosporin, such as ceftriaxone 1 g IV q24h, **or** ciprofloxacin 400 mg IV bid.
- Immediate surgery is indicated for emphysematous cholecystitis, perforation, and suspected pericholecystic abscess.
- The timing of surgery in uncomplicated cholecystitis is varied; surgery is usually performed within 6 days of onset of symptoms, but can be delayed for 6 weeks if the patient is responding to medical management. Earlier surgery is associated with fewer complications and hospitalizations.

CHOLANGITIS

GENERAL PRINCIPLES

- Cholangitis is characterized by inflammation or infection involving the hepatic and common bile ducts.
- Infection can be acute, recurrent, idiopathic, or secondary to pancreatitis or cholecystitis.
- Obstruction of the common bile duct results in congestion and necrosis of the walls of the biliary tree followed by proliferation of bacteria.
- Obstruction is often due to gallstones, but can be due to tumor, chronic pancreatitis, parasitic infection, or a complication of endoscopic retrograde cholangiopancreatography (ERCP).
- Organisms are similar to those associated with cholecystitis.

DIAGNOSIS

Clinical Manifestations
- Patients frequently have a history of gallbladder disease.
- The onset is usually acute.
- The classic presentation of Charcot triad is present in about 50% of patients and consists of fever, right upper quadrant pain, and jaundice.
- If confusion and hypotension (Reynold pentad) are also present, there is significant morbidity and mortality.
- Complications of cholangitis include bacteremia, shock, gallbladder perforation, hepatic abscess, and pancreatitis.

Differential Diagnosis
The differential includes cholecystitis, hepatic abscess, perforating ulcer, pancreatitis, intestinal obstruction, right lower lobe pneumonia, and myocardial infarction.

Diagnostic Testing
- Marked leukocytosis, hyperbilirubinemia, and elevated alkaline phosphatase and transaminases are seen and evidence of disseminated intravascular coagulation (DIC) may be present.
- Blood cultures are positive in >50% of patients.
- Ultrasound can be used to evaluate gallbladder size, the presence of stones, and the degree of bile duct dilatation.
- ERCP can confirm the diagnosis and facilitate therapeutic sphincterotomy, stone extraction, and/or stent insertion.

TREATMENT

- Treatment consists of IV fluid resuscitation and broad-spectrum antibiotics.
- Antibiotic regimens are similar to cholecystitis.
- Prompt decompression of the common bile duct is mandatory.

VIRAL HEPATITIS

ACUTE VIRAL HEPATITIS

GENERAL PRINCIPLES

- Acute viral hepatitis is a systemic infection that affects the liver predominantly. There are five major hepatotropic viruses (A, B, C, D, and E) that cause acute hepatitis.
- Hepatitis B, C, and D can also progress to chronic infection, leading to chronic liver disease, cirrhosis, and hepatocellular carcinoma (Table 6-3).

TABLE 6-3	VIRAL HEPATITIS				
	Incubation average (range)	Main route of transmission	Chronic phase	Diagnostic tests	Vaccine
Hepatitis A	4 wk (2–8 wk)	Fecal–oral	No	Anti-HAV IgM: acute infection Anti-HAV IgG: resolved infection, immunity	Havrix 0 and 6–12 mo Vaqta 0 and 6–18 mo
Hepatitis B	2–3 mo (1–6 mo)	Vertical, sexual, blood-borne such as intravenous drug use	Yes	See Table 6-4	0, 1–2, and 4–6 mo
Hepatitis C	6–8 wk (2–26 wk)	Blood-borne	Yes	Anti-HCV; HCV RNA: infection	Not available
Hepatitis D	2–8 wk	Blood-borne	Yes	Anti-HDV with anti-HBc IgM: coinfection with HBV; Anti-HDV with anti-HBc IgG: superinfection with HBV	Vaccine for hepatitis B
Hepatitis E	6 wk (2–8 wk)	Fecal–oral	No	Anti-HEV IgM: acute infection Anti-HEV IgG: resolved infection	Not commercially available

Prevention

- There is no immunization for HCV, HDV, or HEV.
- An HAV vaccine is available and is 85% to 100% effective in preventing disease. Vaccination doses should be given at 0 and 6 to 12 months (Havrix) or 0 and 6 to 18 months (Vaqta). Immunization against HAV should be given to
  - Men who have sex with men
  - People traveling to high-risk areas
  - Patients with chronic liver disease
  - Military personnel
  - IV drug users
- Hepatitis B vaccine is given at 0, 1 to 2, and 4 to 6 months. Immunization is recommended for
  - Sexual partners and household contacts of a person who is hepatitis B surface antigen (HBsAg) positive
  - Persons who are not in a long-term monogamous relationship
  - Persons seeking diagnosis or treatment for a sexually transmitted infection
  - Current or recent IV drug users
  - Staff and residents of care facilities for the developmentally disabled
  - Public safety and health care workers potentially exposed to blood or blood-contaminated body fluids
  - End-stage renal disease patients
  - Chronic liver disease patients
  - HIV-infected patients
  - International travelers to endemic regions (>2%)
- If combined hepatitis A and B vaccine (Twinrix) is used, the doses are given at 0, 1, and 6 months.

DIAGNOSIS

Clinical Manifestations

- Symptoms range from asymptomatic illness to fulminant hepatic failure.
- A large proportion of infections with any of the hepatitis viruses are asymptomatic or anicteric.
  - Hepatitis A causes minor disease in childhood, with >80% of infections being asymptomatic. In adults, infection is more often symptomatic.
  - Infections with HBV, HCV, and HDV can also be asymptomatic.
- Clinically apparent acute hepatitis presents with jaundice or elevated liver enzymes.
- Common symptoms in the preicteric phase include fever, myalgia, nausea, vomiting, diarrhea, fatigue, malaise, and dull right upper quadrant pain.
- About 10% of patients with acute HBV infection and 5% to 10% patients with acute HCV infection present with a serum sickness–like illness, with fever, urticarial or maculopapular rash, and migratory arthritis. This diminishes rapidly after the onset of jaundice.
- Coryza, photophobia, headache, and cough can occur in hepatitis A.
- Fulminant hepatic failure typically presents with hepatic encephalopathy within 8 weeks of symptoms or within 2 weeks of onset of jaundice.
  - Fulminant hepatitis carries a high mortality.
  - Pregnant women with acute HEV infection have a 15% risk of fulminant liver failure and a mortality rate of 10% to 40%.
  - The risk of liver failure in HAV infection increases with age and with preexisting liver disease.

- There are very few specific physical findings in the preicteric phase.
  - Urticaria may be present if a serum sickness–like syndrome develops.
  - In the icteric phase, jaundice and a slightly enlarged and tender liver may be present.
  - A minority of patients may have a palpable spleen tip.
  - Signs of hepatic encephalopathy and asterixis may be present if fulminant hepatic failure develops.

Differential Diagnosis

- EBV, CMV, rubella, measles, mumps, and coxsackie B can cause mild liver enzyme abnormalities but rarely jaundice.
- Disseminated herpes virus infection with hepatic involvement can occur in immunocompromised hosts.
- Yellow fever is a cause of acute hepatitis in Central and South America.
- Elevated transaminases can be seen in rickettsial infection, bacterial sepsis, *Legionella* infection, syphilis, and disseminated mycobacterial and fungal infections.
- Q fever (*Coxiella burnetii*) is associated with jaundice in 5% of patients.
- Noninfectious causes may include many drugs that can cause hepatitis, including acetaminophen, isoniazid, and alcohol.
- Usually, the aspartate transaminase (AST) is elevated out of proportion to the alanine transaminase (ALT) in acute alcohol-related hepatitis.
- Anoxic liver injury can occur from hypotension, heart failure, or cardiopulmonary arrest.
- Cholestatic liver disease and other diseases (e.g., Wilson disease, sickle cell disease, acute Budd-Chiari syndrome, tumor infiltration of the liver, and Gilbert and Dubin-Johnson syndromes) can lead to acute hepatitis.

Diagnostic Testing

- Large elevations of AST and ALT (>eightfold normal) may occur.
- The degree of rise in transaminases does not correlate with the risk of developing hepatic failure.
- Bilirubin, alkaline phosphatase, and LDH may be one to three times normal.
- Findings of DIC can develop with fulminant hepatic failure, along with prothrombin time (PT) elevation and hypoglycemia.

TREATMENT

- Treatment for acute hepatitis is supportive and includes bed rest, a high-calorie diet, avoidance of hepatotoxic medications, and abstinence from alcohol.
- Most patients do not require hospitalization and can be managed at home.
- Patients should be hospitalized for severe dehydration or hepatic failure if the bilirubin level is >15 to 20 mg/dL or if PT is prolonged.
- Transaminases, alkaline phosphatase, bilirubin, and PT should be monitored one to two times per week for 2 weeks and then every other week until normalized.
- Corticosteroids have not been shown to shorten disease course or lessen symptoms; in fact, they may predispose to longer illness and more relapses.
- Patients with fulminant hepatic failure should be considered for liver transplantation.

ACUTE HEPATITIS A

- HAV is an acute, self-limited disease, but can cause fulminant hepatitis in adults. The incubation period ranges from 15 to 50 days (mean 30 days).
- Outbreaks of HAV occur worldwide.
- Infection at a younger age is less severe and leads to immunity.
- **Detection of anti-HAV IgM antibodies together with a typical clinical presentation is diagnostic** of acute hepatitis A infection. IgM is detectable up to 6 months after exposure, and IgG confers lifelong protective immunity.

ACUTE HEPATITIS B

- HBV is the most common cause of chronic viral hepatitis worldwide and is also a major cause of acute viral hepatitis.
- HBV infection is rare in developed countries, occurring in 2% of the population.
  - The incidence is 20% in high-risk areas such as Southeast Asia and sub-Saharan Africa.
  - Vertical transmission is common in high-risk areas.
  - In low-risk countries, sexual or blood-borne transmission through IV drug use is the main mode of transmission.
- The incubation period is usually 28 to 160 days, averaging 2 to 3 months.
- HBV has a more insidious onset and a more prolonged course than HAV. The occurrence of the serum sickness–like syndrome favors the diagnosis of HBV infection.
- The diagnosis rests on serologic testing (Table 6-4).
  - HBsAg: HBsAg appears in serum 1 to 10 weeks after an acute exposure to HBV, prior to the onset of symptoms or elevation of serum ALT. In patients who subsequently recover, HBsAg becomes undetectable after 4 to 6 months. **Persistence of HBsAg for more than 6 months implies chronic infection**.
  - HBsAb (hepatitis B surface antibody): HBsAb appears when HBsAg declines in patients who mount a protective immune response. **It confers immunity in patients with recovered hepatitis B or with previous vaccination**.

TABLE 6-4	SEROLOGICAL MARKERS FOR HEPATITIS B INFECTION					
HBsAg	HBsAb	IgM HBcAb	IgG HBcAb	HBeAg	HBeAb	Interpretation
+	–	+	–	–	–	Acute infection
–	–	+	–	–	–	Window period
–	+	–	–	–	–	Postvaccination: immune
–	+	–	+	–	+	Recovery: immune
+	–	–	+	+	–	High replicative phase
+	–	–	+	–	+	Low, nonreplicative phase

○ HBcAb (hepatitis B core antibody): HBcAb suggests hepatitis B infection. IgM HBcAb could be the only positive antibody in the "window period" (the period of acute hepatitis B infection when both HBsAb and HBsAg may be negative).

○ HBeAg (hepatitis B e antigen): HBeAg serves as a marker for hepatitis B replication and infectivity. **The presence of HBeAg indicates high HBV DNA and high rates of transmission**.

○ HBeAb (hepatitis B e antibody): HBeAb development is a marker for **low HBV DNA and lower rates of transmission in patients without protective immunity**.

ACUTE HEPATITIS C

- HCV infection usually presents as a chronic hepatitis.
- The primary route of transmission is blood exposure, such as transfusion or IV drug use, but up to 20% of patients have no identifiable exposure. Sexual and vertical transmission are rare.
- The incubation period is 2 to 26 weeks, with an average of 6 to 8 weeks.
- The diagnostic screening test is HCV antibody. **The presence of HCV antibody suggests prior exposure to HCV but does not convey immunity**. Seroconversion may not occur early in illness; only 40% of patients with acute HCV infection have HCV antibody compared with >95% of patients with chronic infection.

ACUTE HEPATITIS D

- HDV, also known as delta agent, is an incomplete RNA virus and requires HBsAg to enable replication and infection; therefore, **HDV always occurs in association with hepatitis B infection**.
- The primary route of transmission is parental, either via transfusion or IV drug use. The incubation period is variable.
- HDV is endemic to the Mediterranean basin, the Middle East, and portions of South America.
- The two most common forms of infections are acute HBV and HDV coinfection and acute HDV infection superimposed on chronic HBV infection (superinfection).
- Clinically, HDV tends to be a severe illness with a **high mortality** (2% to 20%). HDV often has a protracted course and frequently leads to cirrhosis.
- Anti-HDV antibody testing should be done only when evidence of HBV infection is found. Antibody is negative in the acute phase, but rises in the convalescent stage.
- Most patients with acute coinfection clear both infections.
- **Superinfection results in chronic HDV infection along with chronic HBV infection**. High titers of HDV antibody indicate ongoing infection.

ACUTE HEPATITIS E

- Epidemiologically, HEV resembles HAV, with fecal–oral transmission and both epidemic and sporadic cases.
- Most cases occur in developing countries, including India, Southeast Asia, Africa, and Mexico, in association with contaminated drinking water.

- Young adults are affected, with high mortality rates in pregnant women. US cases usually have a history of travel to endemic areas. HEV has an incubation period of 2 to 8 weeks, averaging approximately 6 weeks.
- Anti-HEV antibodies may be detected, but in the United States, serologic testing and PCR are available only through the Centers for Disease Control and Prevention. IgM is usually detectable by the onset of symptoms.

CHRONIC HEPATITIS

- Chronic viral hepatitis is defined as **the presence of liver inflammation persisting for ≥6 months and associated with HBV, HCV, or HDV infection**.
- Early referral to a hepatologist for evaluation is recommended.
- **The majority of patients with chronic viral hepatitis are asymptomatic**.
- Patients may complain of lethargy and right upper abdominal pain.
- Extrahepatic manifestations include polyarteritis nodosa (HBV), glomerulonephritis (HBV, HCV), mixed cryoglobulinemia (HCV), or porphyria cutanea tarda (HCV).
- Physical findings occur late in the course of viral infection and indicate the presence of cirrhosis. These include spider angiomata, hepatomegaly, splenomegaly, ascites, jaundice, gynecomastia, testicular atrophy, asterixis, and loss of body hair.
- Testing for HBsAg, anti-HBsAb, anti-HBcAb, HBeAg, anti-HBeAb, and anti-HCVAb should be done.
- Transaminases, bilirubin, alkaline phosphatase, PT, and albumin levels should be measured.
- Histologic confirmation is needed to document the presence and severity of disease and treatment decisions. Histologic severity of disease is an important prognostic indicator for survival.

CHRONIC HEPATITIS B

- The risk of developing chronic HBV infection varies with age and is higher in children <5 years old than in immunocompetent adults.
- Risk factors for progression to cirrhosis include older age, HBV genotype C, high levels of HBV DNA, alcohol consumption, and concurrent infection with HCV, HDV, or HIV.
- Treatment of chronic HBV infection includes interferon (IFN)-α and a nucleoside/nucleotide, both aimed at inhibiting HBV replication; however, the choice of a specific regimen is complex.[14-16] Response is measured by loss of HBeAg, development of HBeAb and cessation of viral replication in HBeAg-positive patients, and viral suppression in HBeAg-negative patients.
- In HBeAg-positive patients, IFN-α works better in those with high pretreatment ALT level, high histologic activity index, low HBV DNA level, and genotype A and B.
- There is no consistent predictor of sustained response among HBeAg-negative patients. Use of IFN-α is restricted to patients with normal synthetic function and elevated transaminases without evidence of decompensated liver disease.
- Several nucleoside/nucleotide agents are available for HBV infection, including lamivudine, adefovir, entecavir, telbivudine, emtricitabine, and tenofovir.
- Patients with coinfection with HIV should be treated with tenofovir plus lamivudine or emtricitabine.

CHRONIC HEPATITIS C

- Patients are frequently asymptomatic and are identified at the time of blood donation or surgery.
- The current treatment for hepatitis C is combination of IFN-α and ribavirin. For those with genotype 1, the addition of a protease inhibitor (telaprevir or boceprevir) improves virologic response.[17,18]
- Predictors of poor response include cirrhosis, male gender, advanced age, HIV, and the presence of HCV genotype 1 or 4.

CHRONIC HEPATITIS D

- Chronic HDV occurs only in the presence of chronic HBV.
- Diagnosis is made by persistence of HDV antigen in the liver or anti-HDV titers.
- The incidence of chronicity is <5% in coinfection but >50% in superinfection.
- IFN-α has limited efficacy and the oral agents used for HBV are not effective for hepatitis D.

OTHER HEPATIC INFECTIONS

PYOGENIC LIVER ABSCESS

GENERAL PRINCIPLES

- Pyogenic liver abscesses are the most common type of visceral abscess. The right lobe is most commonly involved.
- Liver abscesses result from the following:
  - Direct spread from biliary infection. Underlying biliary tract disease such as gallstones or malignant obstruction is present in about 40% to 60% of cases. Enteric gram-negative bacilli and *Enterococci* are predominant, and anaerobes are not generally involved.
  - The portal circulation, usually related to bowel leakage and peritonitis. Mixed flora with aerobic and anaerobic species are often isolated.
  - Hematogenous seeding, cultures usually yield single organisms like *S. aureus* or *Streptococcus* species.

DIAGNOSIS

Clinical Manifestations

- Fevers and chills along with right upper quadrant pain and possibly pleuritic symptoms (depending on the location of abscess) are usual presentations. Fatigue, malaise, and weight loss are common.
- Onset can be insidious; liver abscess was a common cause of fever of unknown origin prior to CT scanning.
- Over half of the patients have tender hepatomegaly.
- Jaundice is not present unless there is ascending cholangitis or extensive involvement with multiple hepatic abscesses.

Diagnostic Testing
- Elevated alkaline phosphatase, mild elevations in the transaminase levels, and leukocytosis are seen.
- Blood cultures are positive in about half of the patients.
- Cultures from liver abscesses are diagnostic.
- Ultrasound and CT are the imaging methods of choice. Gallium scans show increased uptake.

TREATMENT

- Drainage of the abscess is important and may need to be repeated several times, particularly if there are multiple lesions.
  - Drainage can usually be done percutaneously.
  - Surgical drainage is needed for loculated abscesses, underlying disease requiring primary surgical management, and inadequate response to percutaneous drainage after 7 days of treatment.
- Patients should receive broad-spectrum antibiotics.
  - β-lactam/β-lactamase inhibitor **or** third-generation cephalosporin **and** metronidazole are recommended.
  - Fluoroquinolone **and** metronidazole **or** a carbapenem can also be used.
  - Duration of treatment is 4 to 6 weeks. Intravenous antibiotics can be switched to oral therapy (amoxicillin–clavulanate **or** fluoroquinolone **and** metronidazole) after 2 to 4 weeks if the patient has a good response to drainage.
- Follow-up imaging is necessary only with prolonged clinical symptoms or when drainage is not making good progress. Radiological abnormalities resolve much more slowly than clinical and biochemical markers—around 16 weeks for abscesses <10 cm, 22 weeks for abscesses >10 cm.[19]

AMEBIC LIVER ABSCESS

GENERAL PRINCIPLES

- Amebic liver abscesses are the most common extraintestinal manifestation of *E. histolytica*.[20]
- Organisms ascend the portal venous system and establish infection.
- Amebic liver abscess occurs mainly in the developing world. Most cases in the United States are among travelers.
- Amebic liver abscesses typically occur within weeks after returning from an endemic area but can also occur years later.

DIAGNOSIS

Clinical Manifestations
- Clinical differentiation between amebic and pyogenic liver abscess is difficult.
- Patients with amebic abscess may have a history of diarrhea and may lack spiking fevers.
- Frequently, amebic abscesses are solitary and occur in the right lobe of the liver.

Diagnostic Testing

- The workup is the same as with pyogenic abscess; gallium scans do not show increased uptake.
- A definitive diagnosis is made by finding invasive trophozoites on microscopic exam from tissue or pus obtained from the abscess or culture, but the yield is low (about 20% to 30%).
- Serologic testing for antibodies to *E. histolytica* is sensitive. A negative test rules out the diagnosis except in early infection (<1 week).
- Percutaneous aspiration is not recommended except in cases where immediate exclusion of a pyogenic abscess is warranted. Typical amebic pus is described as anchovy paste and is thick, acellular, proteinaceous debris consisting of necrotic hepatocytes and a few leukocytes.

TREATMENT

- Treatment consists of metronidazole 500 to 750 mg PO q8h 7 to 10 days followed by the luminal agents paromomycin 10 mg/kg PO q8h for 10 days or diiodohy-droxyquin (iodoquinol) 650 mg PO q8h for 20 days.
- In contrast to pyogenic liver abscesses, drainage of amebic liver abscesses is not usually necessary. Aspiration is usually reserved for patients with extremely large abscesses to decrease the risk of rupture or no response to antibiotics after 3 to 5 days.
- Complete radiological resolution may take up to 2 years and repeated imaging is not helpful.

REFERENCES

1. Chey WD, Wong BC, Practice Parameters Committee of the American College of Gastroenterology. American College of Gastroenterology guideline on the management of *Helicobacter pylori* infection. *Am J Gastroenterol.* 2007;102:1808-1825.
2. Wong CS, Jelacic S, Habeeb RL, et al. The risk of the hemolytic-uremic syndrome after antibiotic treatment of *Escherichia coli* O157:H7 infections. *N Engl J Med.* 2000;342:1930-1936.
3. Wong CS, Mooney JC, Brandt JR, et al. Risk factors for the hemolytic uremic syndrome in children infected with *Escherichia coli* O157:H7: a multivariable analysis. *Clin Infect Dis.* 2012;Mar 19. [Epub ahead of print]
4. Levine MM, Ferreccio C, Abrego P, et al. Duration of efficacy of Ty21a, attenuated *Salmonella typhi* live oral vaccine. *Vaccine.* 1999;17:S22-S27.
5. Fraser A, Paul M, Goldberg E, et al. Typhoid fever vaccines: systematic review and meta-analysis of randomised controlled trials. *Vaccine.* 2007;25:7848-7857.
6. Fraser A, Goldberg E, Acosta CJ, et al. Vaccines for preventing typhoid fever. *Cochrane Database Syst Rev.* 2007;(3):CD001261.
7. Effa EE, Lassi ZS, Critchley JA, et al. Fluoroquinolones for treating typhoid and paraty-phoid fever (enteric fever). *Cochrane Database Syst Rev.* 2011;(10):CD004530.
8. Thaver D, Zaidi AK, Crichley J, et al. A comparison of fluoroquinolones versus other antibiotics for treating enteric fever: meta-analysis. *BMJ.* 2009;338:b1865.
9. Cohen MJ, Sahar T, Benenson S, et al. Antibiotic prophylaxis for spontaneous bacterial peritonitis in cirrhotic patients with ascites, without gastro-intestinal bleeding. *Cochrane Database Syst Rev.* 2009;(2):CD004791.

10. Saab S, Hernandez JC, Chi AC, Tong MJ. Oral antibiotic prophylaxis reduces spontaneous bacterial peritonitis occurrence and improves short-term survival in cirrhosis: a meta-analysis. *Am J Gastroenterol.* 2009;104:993-1001.

11. Loomba R, Wesley R, Bain A, et al. Role of fluoroquinolones in the primary prophylaxis of spontaneous bacterial peritonitis: meta-analysis. *Clin Gastroenterol Hepatol.* 2009;7:487-493.

12. Chavez-Tapia NC, Barrientos-Gutierre T, Tellez-Avila FI, et al. Antibiotic prophylaxis for cirrhotic patients with upper gastrointestinal bleeding. *Cochrane Database Syst Rev.* 2010;(9):CD002907.

13. Sort P, Navasa M, Arroya V, et al. Effect of intravenous albumin on renal impairment and mortality in patients with cirrhosis and spontaneous bacterial peritonitis. *N Engl J Med.* 1999;341:403-409.

14. Wong DK, Cheung AM, O'Rourke K, et al. Effect of alpha-interferon treatment in patients with hepatitis B e antigen-positive chronic hepatitis B. A meta-analysis. *Ann Intern Med.* 1993;119:312-323.

15. Perrillo R. Benefits and risks of interferon therapy for hepatitis B. *Hepatology.* 2009;49:S103-S111.

16. Woo G, Tomlinson G, Nishikawa Y, et al. Tenofovir and entecavir are the most effective antiviral agents for chronic hepatitis B: a systematic review and Bayesian meta-analyses. *Gastroenterology.* 2010;139:1218-1229.

17. Ghany MG, Strader DB, Thomas DL, et al. Diagnosis, management, and treatment of hepatitis C: an update. *Hepatology.* 2009;49:1335-1374.

18. Butt AA, Kanwal F. Boceprevir and telaprevir in the management of hepatitis C virus-infected patients. *Clin Infect Dis.* 2012;54:96-104.

19. K C S, Sharma D. Long-term follow-up of pyogenic liver abscess by ultrasound. *Eur J Radiol.* 2010;74:195-198.

20. Stanley SL Jr. Amoebiasis. *Lancet.* 2003;361:1025-1034.

Urinary Tract Infections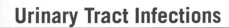

Amelia M. Kasper and Jeffrey P. Henderson

UNCOMPLICATED CYSTITIS IN WOMEN

GENERAL PRINCIPLES

- Uncomplicated bacterial cystitis is one of the most common causes of physician office visits and antibiotic use in women.
- Hallmark symptoms of acute bacterial cystitis are dysuria, frequency, and/or urgency in the setting of bacteriuria, without upper urinary tract symptoms or fever.
- Most episodes of cystitis are self-limited to the lower urinary tract but may progress to pyelonephritis and bacteremia.

Epidemiology

- The high incidence of urinary tract infections (UTIs) results in significant morbidity over the population and a heavy burden on the health care system.
- Approximately 40% to 50% of women in the United States will be diagnosed with UTIs during their lifetimes, with an annual self-reported incidence of about 12% in females and 3% in males.[1-4]
- The estimated incidence of uncomplicated UTI in the United States depends greatly on the population studied. For college-age women, it is estimated to be 0.7 episodes per person-year[4]; 25% to 50% of women have recurrent infection within 1 year of the initial infection.[2]

Etiology

- Most uncomplicated UTIs are believed to originate with urethral ascension of vaginal and bowel flora, although they may be able to persist within bladder tissue.
- 75% to 95% of cases of uncomplicated cystitis are caused by *Escherichia coli.*[3,4] Less commonly, cystitis is associated with *Staphylococcus saprophyticus, Enterococcus, Klebsiella pneumoniae, Proteus mirabilis,* or *Pseudomonas.* Cases due to MRSA are rare.
- Uropathogenic *E. coli* strains have acquired virulence factors, enabling them to adhere to host tissue, acquire host nutrients, and evade host defenses.
- UTIs originating from hematogenous or lymphatic spread of infection are less frequent. Tuberculosis and staphylococcal infections can spread to the urinary tract through hematogenous spread.

Risk Factors

- History of UTIs
- Recent or frequent vaginal intercourse
- Spermicide use, especially when used with a diaphragm
- A childhood or maternal UTI history is associated with recurrent UTI

Prevention

- Since diaphragm use and spermicide use are strongly associated with UTIs, patients with recurrent UTIs may benefit from alternative forms of contraception.
- Cranberry juice and capsules have been shown in small studies to prevent UTIs, possibly by interfering with bacterial adhesion to uroepithelial cells. At present, there is no consensus on an optimal form or dose of cranberry for UTI prevention.[2,4] Notably, cranberry extract may interact with other medications, including warfarin.
- Antibiotic prophylaxis may be considered in women with three or more UTIs per year. Daily low-dose trimethoprim–sulfamethoxazole (TMP-SMX), nitrofurantoin, or ciprofloxacin has been shown to effectively prevent UTIs in patients with recurrent cystitis. Postcoital antibiotics are another option for patients with recurrent UTIs related to sexual activity.[4] Refer to Table 7-1 for more detail.

Pre- or postcoital micturition, front-to-back wiping patterns, and the avoidance of douching have not been proven to prevent UTIs, but are commonly recommended to patients to prevent recurrent UTIs.

TABLE 7-1	EMPIRIC THERAPY FOR URINARY TRACT INFECTIONS	
Disease	**Empiric therapy**	**Notes**
Simple cystitis[5]	*First line:* TMP-SMX DS mg PO bid × 3 d *OR* TMP (if sulfa allergic) 100 mg PO bid × 3 d *OR* nitrofurantoin sustained release 100 mg PO bid × 5 d (avoid if early pyelonephritis suspected). *Alternate:* Fosfomycin 3 g PO × 1 d *OR* pivmecillinam 400 mg PO bid × 5 d (neither recommended for early pyelonephritis). *Second line:* Ciprofloxacin 250 mg PO bid × 3 d *OR* levofloxacin 250 mg PO bid × 3 d	Choose an alternative to TMP-SMX if local resistance is >20% or if used within the prior 3 mo. Consider alternatives to TMP/SMX in older women. Avoid FQs if local resistance is >10%
Cystitis in men[6]	Initial episode can be treated empirically with TMP-SMX for at least 7 d; use ciprofloxacin 500 mg PO q12h *OR* levofloxacin 500 mg PO qd for recurrent episodes, treat 10–21 d.	Consider urologic evaluation for recurrent disease or pyelonephritis
Recurrent cystitis in women[4]	*Postcoital prophylaxis:* TMP-SMX SS × 1 d *OR* nitrofurantoin 100 mg × 1 d *OR* cephalexin 250 mg × 1 d. *Continuous prophylaxis:* TMP-SMX SS qd *OR* qod *OR* nitrofurantoin 50 mg qd *OR* cephalexin 125 mg qd *OR* fosfomycin 3 g every 10 d	Cranberry juice and topical vaginal estrogen in postmenopausal women *may* have a role in preventing recurrent UTI.

		Most non-*Escherichia coli,* non-*Citrobacter* gram negatives such as *Klebsiella, Proteus,* and *Pseudomonas* are nitrofurantoin resistant
Pregnancy (*N Engl J Med.* 2003;349: 259-266)	Nitrofurantoin 100 mg PO qid × 7 d *OR* cephalexin 200–500 mg PO qid ×7 d *OR* cefuroxime axetil 250 mg PO qid ×7 d	Treat all asymptomatic bacteriuria in pregnancy. Screen pregnant women near end of first trimester with urine culture (*Clin Infect Dis.* 2005; 40:643-654)
Complicated UTI[6]	*Mild–moderate illness:* second-generation FQ.[a] *Severe illness, recent FQ, or institutionalized:* cefepime 2 g IV q12h *OR* third-generation cephalosporin[b] OR carbapenem[c] OR piperacillin–tazobactam 3.375–4.5 g IV q6h. Consider adding vancomycin empirically for gram-positive cocci on urine gram stain	Base empiric coverage on local sensitivity patterns and narrow therapy when organism identified. Continue therapy for 10–14 d but can consider shortening if complicating factor is resolved (i.e., removal of indwelling device or stone)
Candiduria[12]	Candida albicans: Fluconazole 100–200 mg PO qd × 5 d. *Critically ill or non-albicans species:* amphotericin B.	Remove catheter if present. Indications to treat: symptoms with pyuria, hardware, pregnancy, prior to GU surgery, or risk of dissemination
Pyelonephritis[5]	*Outpatient:* Ciprofloxacin 500 mg PO BID × 7 d *OR* ciprofloxacin ER 1,000 mg PO qd × 7 d *OR* levofloxacin 750 mg PO × 5 d *OR* TMP-SMX DS PO BID × 14 d (if known to be susceptible). *Inpatient:* second-generation IV FQ[a] OR aminoglycoside[d] OR ampicillin–sulbactam 1–2 g IV q6h *OR* third-generation cephalosporin.[b]	Treat IV until afebrile × 48 h then change to PO to complete 14 d. Consider single-dose IV (1 g ceftriaxone or a 24-h dose of an aminoglycoside) followed by outpatient oral therapy in stable patients, especially

(continued)

TABLE 7-1	(CONTINUED)
Pregnancy: Cefazolin 1 g IV q8h *OR* ceftriaxone 1 g IV *OR* IM q24h *OR* piperacillin 4 g IV q8h	in areas where FQ resistance is >10% or if TMP-SMX is used when susceptibility is unknown. Do not use FQs during pregnancy. Do not use nitrofurantoin

TMP-SMX, trimethoprim–sulfamethoxazole; FQ, fluoroquinolone; GU, genitourinary.

[a]Oral: ciprofloxacin 500 mg PO bid; ofloxacin 200 mg PO bid; levofloxacin 500 mg PO qd; norfloxacin 400 mg PO bid. Parenteral: levofloxacin 500 mg IV qd; ciprofloxacin 400 mg IV q12h.

[b]Cefotaxime 1 or 2 g IV q8h; ceftriaxone 1 g IV qd; ceftazidime 1–2 g IV q8-12h.

[c]Imipenem 500 mg IV q6h; meropenem 1 g IV q8h.

[d]Gentamicin or tobramycin 2 mg/kg loading dose IV, then 1.5–3.0 mg/kg/d or divided dose.

DIAGNOSIS

- Uncomplicated UTI is often clinically diagnosed, based on the classic symptoms of dysuria, increased urinary frequency, urinary urgency, malodorous urine, suprapubic pain, and occasionally hematuria.
  - Women with concurrent vaginal discharge or irritation should be evaluated for causes of vaginitis and cervicitis.
  - For low-risk women with recurrent UTIs and the cluster of classic symptoms, an office visit is not necessary for the diagnosis and treatment of uncomplicated cystitis.
  - Other cases warrant an examination and further testing with possible referral for cystoscopy or urodynamic tests.
- A midstream, clean-catch urine sample should be collected for diagnostic evaluation and plated within 2 hours of collection or refrigerated.
  - Urine dipstick testing for nitrites or leukocyte esterase is a readily available and an inexpensive method to screen for UTIs. The sensitivity of a positive nitrite or leukocyte esterase on urine dipstick is 75%; therefore, negative results should not preclude treatment in a patient who is symptomatic.[2]
  - A patient with positive dipstick in the setting of the recent onset of typical symptoms does not need a urine culture and may be treated empirically.
- Urine culture is warranted in women who have had symptoms for >7 days, persistent symptoms in spite of empiric antibiotics, or recurrent symptoms within a month of treatment. Using a threshold of >10^2 bacteria/mL of urine increases the sensitivity of testing in symptomatic patients, with little effect on specificity.
- A diagnosis can also be made by microscopic examination; this method is less sensitive, but more specific than dipstick testing. Either pyuria (>8 leukocytes/high-power field [HPF]) or bacteriuria (>1 organism per oil-immersion field) is suggestive of UTI.
- Sexually active women with dysuria without pyuria should be evaluated for sexually transmitted infections (see Chapter 11).
- Symptoms that are not responsive to typical short-course antibiotic therapy and not associated with bacteriuria might be categorized instead under the interstitial cystitis or painful bladder syndrome spectrum of disease.

TREATMENT

- Current guidelines recommend a **3-day course of TMP-SMX** (if ≤20% of the local uncomplicated cystitis pathogens are susceptible), trimethoprim alone, a 5-day course of nitrofurantoin, or a single dose of fosfomycin as empiric treatments for uncomplicated cystitis.[5] Longer courses of antibiotics have not been shown to increase bacterial clearance, though recurrence rates may be lower.
  - ○ **Fluoroquinolones should not be used as first-line treatment for uncomplicated UTIs** because of emerging resistance to these important broad-spectrum agents. They should only be used if first-line medications are unavailable or if there is a patient history of drug intolerance.
  - ○ β-lactams (other than pivmecillinam, not available in the United States) should also be considered second-line agents.
  - ○ Empiric coverage for MRSA is not recommended.
  - ○ Even in the setting of high prevalence of TMP-SMX resistance, cure rates using trimethoprim exceed 85%.[4]
- If symptoms do not improve within 48 hours of initiating antibiotics, clinical evaluation and urine culture should be performed. Posttreatment urine cultures are otherwise not necessary.
- Phenazopyridine, a urinary analgesic, may be used for 1 to 2 days to relieve dysuria. Providers should be aware of the relative and absolute contraindications of this medication (renal insufficiency, liver disease, glucose-6-phosphate dehydrogenase deficiency).
- Refer Table 7-1 for further details.

PYELONEPHRITIS

GENERAL PRINCIPLES

Pyelonephritis is typified by flank pain and fever, often in the presence of urinary symptoms and bacteriuria.

DIAGNOSIS

- All patients with symptoms suggestive of pyelonephritis should have urine collected for culture, preferably prior to starting antibiotics.
- Urine testing usually reveals significant pyuria, hematuria, and bacteriuria. Observation of leukocyte casts is of questionable utility in discriminating pyelonephritis from cystitis.
- Hospitalized patients should also have blood cultures drawn; bacteremia is detected in 15% to 20% of hospitalized patients with pyelonephritis.

TREATMENT

- Urine cultures should be sent before initiating treatment.
- Outpatient treatment of uncomplicated acute pyelonephritis can usually be achieved with a 7-day course of oral ciprofloxacin (500 mg bid, or 100 mg extended release

daily) or a 5-day course of levofloxacin (750 mg daily). If the causative organism is susceptible, 14 days of TMP-SMX can be used.[5]

- An initial one-time IV dose of 1 g ceftriaxone or a 24-hour consolidated dose of an aminoglycoside is recommended when fluoroquinolones are used where prevalence of resistance is >10% or if TMP-SMX is used with no culture data.

- If a patient is hospitalized or unable to tolerate oral medications, treat with an intravenous fluoroquinolone, a third- or fourth-generation cephalosporin (and/or an aminoglycoside), an aminoglycoside (and/or ampicillin), an extended-spectrum penicillin (and/or an aminoglycoside), or a carbapenem. These patients should be transitioned to an oral regimen once stable. Adjust antibiotics per culture results.

- Patients who do not respond to treatment within 48 hours should be evaluated for obstruction, intrarenal or perinephric abscesses, and renal calculi by ultrasonography or CT scan.

ASYMPTOMATIC BACTERIURIA

GENERAL PRINCIPLES

Definition

Asymptomatic bacteriuria is defined as the presence of a uropathogen on urine culture without symptoms of UTI or pyuria detected on urinalysis.

Etiology

- In women, *E. coli* is the most common cause of bacteriuria.
- Men have a lower incidence of asymptomatic bacteriuria but often harbor other gram negatives, enterococci, and coagulase-negative staphylococci.
- Stents and other indwelling devices can be colonized by multiple organisms, including urease-producing organisms and *Pseudomonas.*

Risk Factors

- The prevalence of asymptomatic bacteriuria increases with age and is associated with sexual activity.
- Prevalence is 6% among sexually active nonpregnant young women.[2]
- It is uncommon in young men but frequency increases with age and the onset of prostatic hypertrophy.
- A history of neurologic injury with resulting voiding dysfunction, diabetes, hemodialysis, immunosuppression, and the presence of an indwelling urinary catheter are independent risk factors for developing bacteriuria.

DIAGNOSIS

- **Screening is only indicated for select populations** and should not be performed in the absence of symptoms in nonpregnant women, diabetic women, elderly patients, patients with a history of spinal cord injury, or patients with chronic indwelling urinary catheters.
  - ○ **Pregnant women** should be screened between 12 and 16 weeks gestation for bacteriuria because of an increased risk of pyelonephritis, premature labor, and

an association with lower infant birth weights. **Screening for pyuria is not sufficient, and a urine culture is always indicated**. Rescreening later in pregnancy should be considered for individual cases, such as women with urinary tract anomalies, sickle cell syndromes, or a history of preterm labor. Women treated for bacteriuria should be retested periodically throughout pregnancy.

  ○ **Patients undergoing any urologic procedures that are expected to cause mucosal bleeding, including transurethral resection of the prostate, should be screened for bacteriuria**. If present, treatment should be started shortly prior to the procedure. Antibiotics do not need to be continued afterward unless an indwelling catheter is continued postoperatively.

- Asymptomatic bacteriuria in women is defined as isolation of $\geq 10^5$ colony forming units (cfu)/mL of the same bacterial strain in two consecutive clean-voided urine samples. In men, a single clean-catch specimen with $\geq 10^5$ cfu/mL of a single bacterial species is sufficient for diagnosis. If straight catheterization is used to obtain a specimen, bacteriuria can be diagnosed if $\geq 10^2$ cfu/mL of a single bacterial species is isolated.[7]

TREATMENT

- For premenopausal, nonpregnant women, asymptomatic bacteriuria is not associated with long-term adverse outcomes; however, it is associated with an increased risk of symptomatic UTI. Though antibiotics have been shown to lead to bacterial clearance, treatment does not decrease the frequency of symptomatic UTI; therefore, **treatment in this group is not recommended**.
- There is no proven benefit of treating asymptomatic bacteriuria in elderly patients in nursing homes or in the community.
- Patients with diabetes are screened routinely for proteinuria, and asymptomatic bacteriuria is often an incidental finding. Diabetic patients are at a higher risk of acute cystitis and complications from UTIs; however, treatment does not change the frequency of these events and does not improve or preserve renal function. Recolonization is common after therapy is stopped.
- Similarly, there is little evidence for treating asymptomatic bacteriuria in patients with spinal cord injury or chronic indwelling catheters. There is a high rate of bacterial colonization in these populations and a high risk of developing resistant organisms with repeated courses of unnecessary antibiotics.
- **Women who are pregnant with a positive screen for bacteriuria should be treated**, but the optimum length of treatment has not been established. A 5- to 7-day course of nitrofurantoin is considered first-line therapy (see Table 7-1). Trimethoprim, a folic acid antagonist, should be avoided, especially early in pregnancy. Fluoroquinolones should also be avoided.

URINARY TRACT INFECTION IN MEN

GENERAL PRINCIPLES

- UTI and asymptomatic bacteriuria are less common in men.
- Simple cystitis does occur in men, but **recurrent infection should prompt evaluation for anatomic abnormalities**.
- >50% of recurrent UTIs in men are caused by **prostatitis**.

Etiology

- More than 50% of UTIs in men are caused by *E. coli.*
- Other pathogens include *Klebsiella, Proteus, Providencia, Pseudomonas,* enterococci, and other gram-negative enterics.
- Most UTIs in men are thought to originate with urethral ascension of bowel flora. Normal prostatic fluid contains antimicrobial factors that may be protective against UTI in men.

Risk Factors

- Sexual intercourse with a partner colonized with uropathogens[8]
- Insertive anal sex without using a condom
- Lack of circumcision
- Prostatic hypertrophy contributes to a higher incidence of UTI in older men

DIAGNOSIS

- Men with UTI also present with dysuria, increased urinary frequency, urgency, and suprapubic pain. Symptoms are often subtle in elderly men.
- **All men presenting with urinary symptoms should be evaluated with a pretreatment urinalysis and midstream urine culture**.
- Sexually active men should also be evaluated for sexually transmitted infections.
- Other causes of dysuria in men include urethritis, prostatitis, and epididymitis.

TREATMENT

- Young, otherwise healthy men with an initial UTI may be started on empiric treatment with TMP-SMX until culture data are available.
- Men with recurrent UTIs or anatomic abnormalities should be treated empirically with a urinary fluoroquinolone. Continue treatment with a quinolone or TMP-SMX for 10 to 21 days based on susceptibility testing.
- Prophylactic antibiotic use has not been well-studied in men.
- If a patient has upper urinary tract symptoms (e.g., fever, flank pain) and recurrent UTI or his symptoms do not respond within 48 hours of starting antibiotics, urologic referral is warranted.
- See Table 7-1 for details.

ACUTE BACTERIAL PROSTATITIS

GENERAL PRINCIPLES

- Acute bacterial prostatitis (ABP) usually presents with urinary symptoms; fever; chills; pelvic, perineal, or rectal pain; and obstructive symptoms (dribbling, hesitancy). Patients may also have fever or present with septic shock with no localizing urinary symptoms.
- ABP is most often caused by *E. coli* or other gram-negative enterics.[9]
- Complications include urinary retention and prostatic abscess.

Epidemiology

- ABP accounts for 5% of prostatitis cases.
- Most patients are <65 years old or have a history of recent urinary tract manipulation.

Pathophysiology

- Bacteria ascend through the urethra and enter the prostate by urinary reflux through the prostatic ducts.
- Other routes for infection are direct invasion or lymphatic spread of bacteria from the rectum to the prostate.

Risk Factors

- Indwelling catheters, urinary instrumentation, and receptive anal intercourse increase the risk of developing acute prostatitis.
- Patients with HIV or diabetes are at a higher risk of developing prostatic abscesses.

DIAGNOSIS

- Diagnosing ABP can be challenging, and all male patients with UTIs potentially have prostatic involvement.
- The diagnosis is usually based on the presence of systemic symptoms (fever, chills), bacteriuria and pyuria on urine dipstick, and prostate tenderness on rectal examination. Warmth and swelling may also be noted.
- Prostatic massage is contraindicated, since it may lead to translocation of bacteria into the bloodstream.
- Urinalysis of midstream urine will reveal pyuria and bacteriuria. **Consider alternative diagnoses if urinalysis is negative**.
- Peripheral leukocytosis is also common.
- Pretreatment urine and blood cultures should also be drawn whenever possible.
- Prostate-specific antigen levels are often markedly elevated for up to a month following an episode of ABP.
- Ultrasound or pelvic CT should be obtained if prostatic abscess is suspected.

TREATMENT

- Refer Table 7-2 for recommended antibiotic regimens.
- In ABP, intense inflammation facilitates tissue penetration by antibiotics.
- If bladder outlet obstruction develops, patients may require catheterization.
- Pain control, hydration, and a bowel regimen are recommended adjunctive therapies.
- Prostatic abscesses should be evaluated by a surgeon for drainage.

CHRONIC BACTERIAL PROSTATITIS

GENERAL PRINCIPLES

- Chronic prostatitis is a common problem, affecting approximately 8% of men.[10]
- Chronic bacterial prostatitis (CBP) may result from acute prostatitis, but it commonly occurs in men with no prior history of prostatitis. It has a variable clinical course and is often difficult to cure.

TABLE 7-2	DIAGNOSIS AND TREATMENT OF PROSTATITIS BY NATIONAL INSTITUTES OF HEALTH CLASSIFICATION		
Disease	Diagnosis	Treatment	Alternative treatments
ABP[6]	(1) Presence of fever, chills, urinary symptoms (2) UA/UCx with bacteriuria, pyuria (3) Tender prostate on examination (4) Pelvic CT or u/s if no improvement on abx to evaluate for abscess	Outpatient: TMP-SMX 1 tab PO BID × 6 wk *OR* ciprofloxacin 500 mg PO q12h × 6 wk Inpatient: Ampicillin 2 g IV q6h *PLUS* gentamicin 5 mg/kg q8h until afebrile, then switch to PO therapy	
CBP[10]	(1) Treat UTI first, if present (2) 2-glass test (urine, prostatic fluid cultures) (3) If prostate fluid culture (+), then CBP, otherwise, CPPS	**Wait for culture results before starting therapy.** Ciprofloxacin 500 mg PO bid × 4 wk *OR* levofloxacin 500 mg PO qd × 4 wk *OR* norfloxacin 400 mg PO BID × 4 wk *OR* TMP-SMX 1 tab PO bid × 4 wk	Doxycycline 100 mg PO bid × 28 d
CPPS[6]		(1) α-blockers (alfuzosin, terazosin) (2) 4-wk trial of an FQ may be considered (3) 5α-reductase inhibitors (finasteride)	Reassurance, stress management, analgesics. Urology referral is often necessary
Asymptomatic prostatitis	Incidentally discovered inflammation on prostate biopsy or semen analysis	Refer for urologic evaluation	

ABP, acute bacterial prostatitis; TMP-SMX, trimethoprim–sulfamethoxazole; CBP, chronic bacterial prostatitis; UTI, urinary tract infection; CPPS, chronic pelvic pain syndrome; FQ, fluoroquinolone UA, urinalysis; UCx, urine culture; abx, antibiotics.

- Chronic prostatitis accounts for approximately 2 million outpatient visits annually in the United States.[10]
- **Prostatic pain commonly occurs without evidence of bacterial infection, known as chronic pelvic pain syndrome** (CPPS). The etiology of CPPS is unclear; it is likely multifactorial, with a hypothesized infectious component.

Etiology

- *E. coli* is the most common etiologic agent in CBP. Other associated organisms include enterococci, *Ureaplasma*, fungi, and tuberculosis.
- Patients with HIV are at risk of chronic prostatitis from atypical organisms.

Risk Factors

- Men middle-aged or older are at higher risk of developing chronic prostatitis as a complication of prostatic hypertrophy and associated urinary stasis.
- Prostatic calculi may harbor microcolonies of bacteria that lead to chronic infection.

DIAGNOSIS

- Urinalysis and urine cultures should be obtained while the patient is symptomatic.
- The prostate should be evaluated for symmetry and consistency. Irregularities should be further investigated for possible malignancy.
- If the patient has confirmed recurrent UTIs with no anatomic abnormalities or long-term urinary catheterization, CBP is the most likely underlying cause.
- Before further diagnostic evaluation, coexisting UTIs should be treated with nitrofurantoin or a β-lactam antibiotic, which do not penetrate prostate tissue.
- The Meares-Stamey test is the preferred method of diagnosing CBP.
  - Ideally, testing should be postponed until a month after all antibiotic use.
  - Ejaculation should be avoided within 2 days of the test.
  - For the 4-glass Meares-Stamey test, first-void urine, midstream urine, elicited prostatic fluid, and postmassage urine samples are collected and cultured.
  - A 2-glass method culturing midstream urine before massage and elicited prostatic fluid has been shown to correlate with the 4-glass method and is easier to perform.
  - If cultures are positive only in prostatic fluid, or if bacteria counts are more than 10 times higher in prostatic fluid compared with premassage urine, then CBP can be definitively diagnosed.
- Postvoid residual urine should be measured if obstruction is suspected.

TREATMENT

- Treatment of CBP is challenging because of poor penetration of antibiotics into the prostate gland. CBP requires at least 4 weeks of treatment.[10]
- Patients should be reevaluated after treatment. If symptoms are still present or recur, then a further 3 months of therapy is warranted.
- Repeat urine and prostatic fluid cultures should be collected at 6 months.
- Refer to Table 7-2 for details.

EPIDIDYMITIS AND ORCHITIS

GENERAL PRINCIPLES

- Epididymitis results when infection in the urethra spreads retrograde to the epididymis. Orchitis is almost always an extension of epididymitis.
- Epididymitis and orchitis are most common in young, sexually active men but can also be seen in older men with a recent history of urinary tract manipulation.
- Mumps virus infection is a rare cause of orchitis.
- Potential complications include abscess formation, testicular infarction, testicular atrophy, and infertility.
- **The most common causative pathogens in sexually active men are *Neisseria gonorrhoeae* and *Chlamydia trachomatis*. *E. coli* and other gram-negative enterics are the most common pathogens in men >35 years old and those with a history of urinary tract instrumentation.**

DIAGNOSIS

- The most common presenting symptom is a dull unilateral ache in the affected scrotum, which may radiate to the flank. If there is a concomitant urethritis, urinary symptoms or urethral discharge may be present.
- On examination, the epididymis is swollen and very tender. Lifting the ipsilateral testicle may be extremely painful.
- Urinalysis and urine culture should be obtained.
- If there is any suspicion of testicular torsion, a testicular ultrasound should be obtained emergently. Testicular neoplasm is usually not painful, but should also be considered in the differential.

TREATMENT

- Sexually active men should be treated empirically for chlamydia and gonorrhea (see Chapter 11 and Table 7-2).
- If an enteric organism is the likely etiology, treat with levofloxacin 500 mg PO daily or ofloxacin (not available in United States) 300 mg PO bid for 10 days.
- Bed rest, scrotal support, and analgesics may offer symptomatic relief.

CATHETER-ASSOCIATED URINARY TRACT INFECTIONS

GENERAL PRINCIPLES

- **Catheter-associated (CA) UTIs are very common and often completely preventable.**
- Health care providers should be judicious about the use of indwelling urinary catheters and **avoid them whenever possible**.
- The indication for an existing indwelling catheter should be frequently reviewed and the catheter should be removed as soon as it is no longer needed.
- Urinary stents have many of the same risks as urinary catheters. Similarly, they should be removed when no longer needed.

Definition

- A patient is considered to have a CA-UTI when the following conditions are met[11]:
  - ○ The signs or symptoms of UTI are present.
  - ○ Urine collected from a suprapubic or urethral catheter (or from a midstream collection if a catheter had been removed within the past 48 hours) shows bacterial counts of $\geq 10^3$ cfu/mL or ≥ 1 species of bacteria.
- A patient is considered to have CA-asymptomatic bacteriuria when the following conditions are met[11]:
  - ○ Urine collected from a suprapubic or urethral catheter shows bacterial counts of $\geq 10^3$ cfu/mL or ≥ 1 species of bacteria.
  - ○ Urinary symptoms are not present.

Epidemiology

- Up to 25% of inpatients have urethral catheters inserted during their hospital stay.
- CA-bacteriuria is the most common health care–associated infection, affecting 900,000 inpatients in the United States annually.
- An estimated 20% to 30% of patients with CA-bacteriuria eventually develop CA-UTI.
- In hospitalized patients, the urinary tract is the most common source of gram-negative bacteremia; however, bacteremia only develops in 1% to 4% of patients with bacteriuria.

Etiology

- **Besides *E. coli,* other gram-negative enterics, *Pseudomonas aeruginosa*, gram-positives (staphylococci, enterococci), and yeast are common uropathogens in this population**. Multidrug-resistant organisms are of particular concern.
- Bacteria are introduced into the urethra from nonsterile catheter insertion or from translocation through breaks in the closed catheter system, migrating upward intra- or extraluminally.
- Intra- and extraluminal biofilm formation promotes polymicrobial infection and facilitates antibiotic resistance.

Pathophysiology

- Catheterization introduces bacteria into the sterile urinary tract and disrupts the uroepithelium, facilitating bacterial adhesion. The collection system can also be an entry point, through contamination by health care workers' hands or breaches in the closed system.
- The attached uropathogens produce polysaccharides, trapping other bacteria, Tamm-Horsfall proteins, urinary salts, and other nutrients, which eventually mature to form a biofilm. Within the biofilm, bacteria can exchange genes promoting antibiotic resistance.
- Urease-producing organisms (e.g., *Proteus* and some *Pseudomonas*, *Klebsiella*, and *Providencia*) promote the development of catheter encrustations that can eventually obstruct the catheter.

Risk Factors

- **Essentially all patients with an indwelling catheter will develop bacteriuria within 30 days of catheter insertion**.
- Other risk factors for developing bacteriuria include diabetes, advanced age, female sex, elevated serum creatinine at the time of insertion, and catheter insertion outside of the operating room.[11]

Prevention

- Reconsider the need for a urinary catheter daily while a patient is in the hospital.
- Alternatives to urinary catheterization should be considered, especially for women, elderly, and immunocompromised patients.[11,12]
  - A condom catheter is often a reasonable alternative for men, especially for short-term catheterization, but does not eliminate the risk of CA-UTI.
  - Intermittent straight catheterization is a good alternative for both short- and long-term catheterization.
  - There is no consensus on the risk of long-term suprapubic catheters versus long-term urethral catheterization.
  - Consider noninvasive methods (e.g., portable bladder ultrasound) to evaluate residual urine volume rather than repeated catheterization.
- **Indwelling catheters should not be used to manage incontinence, except to promote healing of open decubitus or perineal ulcers**.
- Indwelling catheters should be inserted using sterile technique and frequently monitored to ensure that the catheter remains patent. In the nonacute care setting, clean conditions are sufficient for intermittent catheterization.
- Other strategies to prevent or delay infection include the use of antimicrobial-coated catheters and closed catheter drainage systems.
- Cranberry extract, daily urethral meatal disinfection, catheter irrigation, and routine catheter exchanges have not shown to effectively prevent CA-UTI.
- There is no role for antibiotic prophylaxis for CA-UTI prevention.
- Screening and treating asymptomatic bacteriuria is not recommended for patients with indwelling catheters or who intermittently straight-catheterize.

DIAGNOSIS

- The diagnosis of CA-UTI is based on the following:
  - A positive urinalysis, as above.
  - The signs and symptoms of CA-UTI are often nonspecific and may include fever, rigors, flank pain, and altered mental status. Patients with spinal cord injury may have a sense of foreboding, increased spasticity, and autonomic dysfunction. During the 48 hours after catheter removal, CA-UTI may present as dysuria, urgency, increased urinary frequency, or suprapubic pain.
- In patients with condom catheters, contamination of specimens with skin flora is common, and significant bacteriuria is defined as $\geq 10^5$ cfu/mL. Contamination can be minimized by collecting a midstream sample or a sample from a new catheter after cleaning the glans.
- Before starting antibiotics, a urine culture should be collected from a fresh catheter if possible. If the catheter is no longer present, a midstream sample should be sent prior to treatment.
- The presence or absence of pyuria should not be used to diagnose or rule out CA-bacteriuria or distinguish it from CA-UTI; however, in symptomatic patients without pyuria, diagnoses other than UTI should be considered.
- Patients with urinary catheters should not be screened for asymptomatic bacteriuria.

TREATMENT

- **Removal of the infected catheter is the cornerstone of CA-UTI treatment**. If medically necessary, a new catheter should be placed at the beginning of treatment.

- For CA-bacteriuria, treatment is only indicated for women who are pregnant, patients who are immunocompromised, and patients who will be undergoing urologic procedures.
- For patients who are mildly ill with CA-UTI, treat with levofloxacin 500 mg PO daily for 5 days or ciprofloxacin 500 mg PO q12h for 10 days. A 3-day regimen may be considered for women ≤65 years old if the catheter has been removed and no upper tract symptoms are present.
- Patients who are ill should be treated for at least 7 days. Because CA-UTI is often associated with drug-resistant organisms, empiric therapy with an intravenous antipseudomonal cephalosporin, carbapenem, or penicillin is appropriate until culture and sensitivities are available. If there is delayed response to antibiotic treatment, continue treatment for 10 to 14 days.
- Candiduria should only be treated if there are symptoms with pyuria with no bacterial source **and** the patient is immunocompromised or has a high risk for candidemia. Removal of the catheter is otherwise sufficient treatment for candiduria.

COMPLICATED URINARY TRACT INFECTION

GENERAL PRINCIPLES

UTIs in patients who have urinary tract abnormalities (i.e., anatomical, functional, foreign bodies) or are immunocompromised are considered complicated UTIs.

FUNGURIA

- Funguria is most commonly caused by *Candida albicans*, but is also caused by non *albicans* species and other fungi.
- Treatment for funguria should take into account the risk of invasive fungemia.
- Patients who are otherwise healthy do not require treatment. Urinary catheters should be removed, if present.
- Treat patients who are neutropenic, have a history of a renal transplant, or are scheduled to have a urologic procedure.
- Treat azole-sensitive *Candida* with fluconazole 200 mg daily for 7 to 14 days. If resistant, treat with amphotericin B or flucytosine.[13]
- Providers should have a low threshold for imaging the kidney and urinary tract for abnormalities (e.g., fungus balls, abscess) in patients with funguria.

DIABETES

- Asymptomatic bacteriuria, symptomatic UTIs, and complications from UTIs occur more frequently in patients with diabetes.
- Impaired host immunity and autonomic neuropathy may be contributing factors.
- Proteinuria, advanced age, and history of recurrent UTIs are risk factors for UTIs in diabetic patients.
- **Treatment of asymptomatic bacteriuria does not improve clinical outcomes. Patients with diabetes should not be screened for bacteriuria**.
- Treat funguria regardless of the presence or absence of symptoms in diabetic patients.

- Pyelonephritis and other severe complications, such as perinephric abscess, renal papillary necrosis, renal cortical abscess, and emphysematous pyelonephritis, often present insidiously in diabetic patients. Emphysematous pyelonephritis is a surgical emergency, while emphysematous cystitis can be treated with antibiotics.

ANATOMIC ABNORMALITIES

- Patients with adult polycystic kidney disease (APKD), vesicoureteric reflux, or obstructive uropathy may be at higher risk of developing upper tract disease and subsequent renal failure.
- Antibiotic prophylaxis or treatment of asymptomatic bacteriuria has not been shown to delay renal impairment.
- Infected cysts or pyelonephritis in the setting of APKD requires a long course of an IV fluoroquinolone followed by prophylaxis.
- Urinary tract stones should be removed whenever possible to minimize the need for antibiotics.

RENAL TRANSPLANT

- UTIs are a common infection in patients receiving renal transplants and are associated with graft dysfunction and rejection.
- The recipient should be treated prior to transplant if an infection is present. All patients should receive perioperative antibiotic prophylaxis.
- A course of at least 6 months of low-dose TMP-SMX has been shown to reduce UTIs after renal transplantation.[14] Ciprofloxacin and norfloxacin are alternatives. Prophylaxis may need to be extended indefinitely for patients with anatomical or functional urinary tract abnormalities or those who have recurrent UTIs.
- If the recipient develops urinary symptoms, treat empirically with a fluoroquinolone or TMP-SMX for 10 to 14 days.

REFERENCES

1. Foxman B. Epidemiology of urinary tract infections: incidence, morbidity, and economic costs. *Am J Med.* 2002;113(suppl 1A):5S-13S.
2. American College of Obstetricians and Gynecologists. ACOG Practice Bulletin No. 91: treatment of urinary tract infections in nonpregnant women. *Obstet Gynecol.* 2008; 111:785-794.
3. Foxman B. The epidemiology of urinary tract infection. *Nat Rev Urol.* 2010;7:653-660.
4. Hooton TM. Uncomplicated urinary tract infection. *N Engl J Med.* 2012;366:1028-1037.
5. Gupta K, Hooton TM, Naber KG, et al. International clinical practice guidelines for the treatment of acute uncomplicated cystitis and pyelonephritis in women: a 2010 update by the Infectious Diseases Society of America and the European Society for Microbiology and Infectious Diseases. *Clin Infect Dis.* 2011;52:e103-e120.
6. European Association of Urology. 2008. http://www.uroweb.org/gls/pdf/Urological%20 Infections%202010.pdf.
7. Nicolle LE, Bradley S, Colgan R, et al. Infectious Diseases Society of America guidelines for the diagnosis and treatment of asymptomatic bacteriuria in adults. *Clin Infect Dis.* 2005;40:643-654.

8. Grabe M, Bishop MC, Bjerklund-Johansen TE, et al. *Guidelines on the Management of Urinary and Male Genital Tract Infections*. Arnhem, The Netherlands: European Association of Urology (EAU); 2008:79-88.

9. Etienne M, Chavanet P, Sibert L, et al. Acute bacterial prostatitis: heterogeneity in diagnostic criteria and management. Retrospective multicentric analysis of 371 patients diagnosed with acute prostatitis. *BMC Infect Dis.* 2008;8:12.

10. Schaeffer AJ. Chronic prostatitis and the chronic pain syndrome. *N Engl J Med.* 2006;355:1690-1698.

11. Hooton TM, Bradley SF, Cardenas DD, et al. Diagnosis, prevention and treatment of catheter associated urinary tract infection in adults: 2009 International Clinical Practice Guidelines from the Infectious Diseases Society of America. *Clin Infect Dis.* 2010;50:625-663.

12. Gould CV, Umscheid CA, Agarwal RK, et al. Guideline for prevention of catheter-associated urinary tract infections 2009. *Infect Control Hosp Epidemiol.* 2010;31:319-326.

13. Pappas PG, Kauffman CA, Andes D, et al. Clinical practice guidelines for the management of candidiasis: 2009 update by the Infectious Diseases Society of America. *Clin Infect Dis.* 2009;48:503-535.

14. Fox BC, Sollinger HW, Belzer FO, et al. A prospective, randomized, double-blind study of trimethoprim-sulfamethoxazole for prophylaxis of infection in renal transplantation: clinical efficacy, absorption of trimethoprim-sulfamethoxazole, effects on the microflora, and the cost-benefit of prophylaxis. *Am J Med.* 1990;89:255-274.

Infections of the Bone and Joint

8

Molly F. Sarikonda and Jonas Marschall

ACUTE AND CHRONIC OSTEOMYELITIS

- Osteomyelitis refers to an inflammatory process in bone due to infecting microorganism(s).
- Osteomyelitis can be classified by duration (acute vs. chronic), location (type of bone involved), and origin (hematogenous vs. contiguous).
  - Infection develops over days to weeks (acute osteomyelitis) or months to years (chronic osteomyelitis).
  - Osteomyelitis is described in many different locations, but certain bones are more commonly involved (vertebral bodies and extremities with vascular compromise).
  - The origin of infection can be bacteremia leading to hematogenous seeding or from direct spread from a contiguous focus of infection.
  - See Table 8-1 for specific clinical scenarios associated with less common pathogens.
- Three categories of osteomyelitis will be discussed in detail: (1) hematogenous osteomyelitis; (2) diabetes- and peripheral vascular disease–associated osteomyelitis; and (3) other types of contiguous osteomyelitis
- Osteomyelitis results from a microbial inoculum through the bloodstream or trauma or associated with an implanted foreign body.
- Various bacterial virulence factors facilitate bone infection (e.g., increased bony adherence in *Staphylococcus aureus*).[1]
- Local inflammation, with the release of cytokines, toxic oxygen radicals, and proteolytic enzymes, damages bone and tissue and leads to abscess formation.
- In chronic osteomyelitis, invasion of vascular channels by pus eventually leads to ischemic necrosis and devascularized bony fragments ("sequestra").

HEMATOGENOUS OSTEOMYELITIS

GENERAL PRINCIPLES

Epidemiology

- Hematogenous osteomyelitis commonly affects the vertebral bodies and disk spaces (lumbar>thoracic>cervical) in older adults.[2]
- Other joints (sacroiliac and sternoclavicular) are more common with intravenous drug abuse (IVDA).
- Often both bones and joints are affected.

Etiology

- Bone infection arises from bacteremia (sometimes transient and unapparent).
- Infection is commonly monomicrobial.
  - *S. aureus* and gram-negative rods (including *Pseudomonas*) are most common.[2]

TABLE 8-1	UNUSUAL ORGANISMS ASSOCIATED WITH BONE AND JOINT INFECTIONS	
Organism	**Clinical scenario**	**Special considerations**
Mycobacterium tuberculosis	Exposure to an endemic area or known tuberculosis contact	Most common site of bone involvement is spine. Check for HIV infection
Brucella spp.	Exposure to an endemic area; may have history of ingestion of unpasteurized dairy products or animal exposure	Sacro-ileitis and vertebral osteomyelitis are common sites of focal infection
Salmonella	Sickle cell disease	Infection usually occurs in the long bones
Candida spp.	Intravenous drug use	
Human oral flora (*Eikenella corrodens*, *Peptostreptococcus*, *Fusobacterium*)	Bone inoculation by human mouth (e.g., hand injury while punching person's face), licking intravenous needle prior to IV drug use	Human bites carry a high rate of infection and often require surgical debridement
Group B streptococci	Diabetes, underlying malignancy	
Animal oral flora (*Pasteurella multocida*, *Capnocytophaga* spp., anaerobes)	Cat or dog bite	In setting of deep tissue injury, start empiric antibiotics. Rabies prophylaxis should be considered
Mycoplasma hominis	Septic arthritis in postpartum period or immunocompromised patient	May have history of urinary tract manipulation
Aeromonas spp.	Water contaminating open fracture or wound	*Pseudomonas* is also a common pathogen seen with water contamination

- ○ Methicillin-resistant *S. aureus* (MRSA) is an important emerging pathogen.[3]
- ○ Other organisms include *Streptococcus* spp., coagulase-negative staphylococci or enterococcus.

Risk Factors
- Older age and male sex[4]
- Conditions leading to bacteremia including IVDA, urinary tract infections, and vascular access such as central venous or dialysis catheters
- Preexisting degenerative joint disease

DIAGNOSIS

Clinical Presentation

History
- History should include risk factors for bacteremia (e.g., IVDA and urinary symptoms) and establish presence of local symptoms such as pain, swelling, and drainage.
- Query prior antibiotic use as this may affect organism recovery during culture.
- Systemic symptoms, such as fever, may be present or absent.

Physical Examination
- Examination should include inspection for erythema, tenderness, or fluctuance.
- The presence of a draining sinus tract is indicative of chronic osteomyelitis.
- Determine the presence of neurological complications in vertebral osteomyelitis (present in up to one-third of patients).[5]

Differential Diagnosis

Erosive osteochondrosis, malignancy, gout, soft tissue infection, bursitis, or fracture can all mimic osteomyelitis.

Diagnostic Testing

Laboratories
- Baseline testing, including a complete blood count and renal function and liver function tests, should be performed.
- WBC count may be normal or elevated.
- Elevated inflammatory markers such as erythrocyte sedimentation rate (ESR) and C-reactive protein (CRP) correlate with degree of bone involvement, but are nonspecific.
- **Blood cultures should be obtained and are positive in 58% (range 30% to 78%) of the patients.[2]**
- More invasive procedures may be forgone if an organism is recovered from blood cultures.

Imaging
- MRI is more sensitive and specific (96% and 93%, respectively) than CT scans, radionuclide studies, or plain films.[6]
- Plain films may demonstrate soft tissue swelling, narrowing or widening of joint space, periosteal reaction, and bone destruction.
- MRI or CT scan can detect complications like paraspinal abscess formation.
- MRI is the test of choice for vertebral osteomyelitis in the presence of neurological symptoms. Involvement of the disk space and two adjacent vertebra is a clue to the diagnosis.

Diagnostic Procedures
- Tissue sampling is necessary in most cases of hematogenous osteomyelitis with negative blood cultures.
- If patient is clinically stable, efforts to obtain a microbiological diagnosis prior to antibiotic administration should be undertaken.
- Bone sampling through CT-guided needle or open biopsy should be sent for aerobic and anaerobic bacteria, fungi, and mycobacteria and for histological examination.
- Yield for causative organism is 77% (reported range 44% to 100%) with CT-guided needle or open biopsy and may vary depending on the method of sampling.[2]

TREATMENT

Medications

- **Whenever possible, antibiotic administration should be delayed in the stable patient until tissue diagnosis can be performed**.
- Antibiotics should be directed at the causative organism and generally are administered parentally (Table 8-2).
- Length of treatment should be 6 to 8 weeks from last surgical debridement or last positive blood cultures.

Other Nonpharmacologic Therapies

- Fitted back brace may be needed when vertebral destruction is extensive.
- Physical therapy in vertebral osteomyelitis is useful for improving functionality once neurological stability is ensured.

TABLE 8-2	ORGANISM-DIRECTED THERAPY IN BONE AND JOINT INFECTIONS		
Microorganism	**General considerations**	**First choice**	**Alternative choice**
Methicillin-sensitive *Staphylococcus aureus*	At time of discharge, preference is generally given to antibiotics administered once daily or via continuous infusion due to ease of home infusion	β-Lactam (oxacillin 2 g intravenously every 6 h or 12 g over 24 h via continuous infusion; cefazolin 2 g intravenously every 8 h)	Ceftriaxone 2 g intravenously every 24 h (may be preferred over cefazolin for outpatient administration)
Methicillin-resistant *S. aureus* or coagulase-negative staphylococci	Goal vancomycin troughs are 15–20 µg/mL and twice-daily administration is preferred to once daily	Vancomycin 15–20 mg/kg intravenously every 12 h	Daptomycin 6 g/kg intravenously every 24 h
Vancomycin-intermediate *S. aureus* (VISA)	Data for VISA treatment in bone and joint infections are limited.	Daptomycin 6 g/kg intravenously every 24 h	Linezolid 600 mg orally every 12 h
Streptococcal species	At time of discharge, preference is generally given to antibiotics administered once daily or via continuous infusion due to ease of home infusion	Penicillin G 3–4 million units intravenously every 4 h or 12–18 million units over 24 h via continuous infusion pump	Ceftriaxone 2 g intravenously every 24 h

Enteric gram-negative bacilli (i.e., *Escherichia coli*, *Klebsiella*, and *Proteus* spp.)	Treatment must be based on antibiotic susceptibility testing. Until susceptibility results are available, therapy should be guided by the individual hospital's antibiogram	Fluoroquinolone (ciprofloxacin 750 mg orally every 12 h), third-generation cephalosporin (ceftriaxone 2 g intravenously every 24 h), carbapenem (ertapenem 1 g intravenously every 24 h)	Cefepime 2 g every 12 h
Pseudomonas aeruginosa	Higher or more frequent doses of antibiotic therapy are needed for pseudomonal coverage	Fluoroquinolone (ciprofloxacin 750 mg orally every 12 h); cefepime or ceftazidime intravenously 2 g every 8 h	Piperacillin–tazobactam 4.5 g intravenously every 6 h
Anaerobes	Anaerobic coverage is adequate when carbapenems or piperacillin–tazobactam are included in the regimen and additional added coverage is not necessary	Metronidazole 500 mg by mouth every 8 h	Clindamycin 300–600 mg by mouth every 6–8 h is preferred in cases where oral flora is suspected

Surgical Management

- Surgery is often not necessary in cases of acute, uncomplicated hematogenous osteomyelitis.
- Surgical intervention is required for drainage of a large abscess, spinal stabilization, or relief of spinal compression and intraoperative cultures and pathology can aid with diagnosis.

SPECIAL CONSIDERATIONS

Culture-Negative Osteomyelitis

- Culture-negative hematogenous vertebral osteomyelitis occasionally occurs despite adequate biopsy attempts and is mostly due to previous antibiotic exposure and/or sampling errors.
- If the initial culture is negative, repeat biopsy, proceeding to open biopsy, allowing an antibiotic-free period, and molecular methods should all be considered.
- If culture results are not obtained, coverage for the most likely causative organisms should be attempted.

TABLE 8-3	ANTIBIOTIC DOSING IN HEMODIALYSIS PATIENTS FOR BONE AND JOINT INFECTIONS
Antibiotic	**Dosing**
Vancomycin	20 mg/kg loading dose during the last hour of the dialysis session, then 500 mg during the last 30 min of each subsequent dialysis session
Ceftazidime	1 g after each dialysis session
Cefazolin	20 mg/kg after each dialysis session
Daptomycin	6 mg/kg after each dialysis session

- For empiric treatment and in cases of culture-negative hematogenous osteomyelitis, a combination of vancomycin and a third- or fourth-generation cephalosporin is reasonable.

Dialysis Patients

Care should be taken to choose an antibiotic regimen that can be easily administered during dialysis (Table 8-3).

COMPLICATIONS

- Spinal instability and neurological compromise can occur in vertebral osteomyelitis.
- Associated abscess (psoas and epidural or paraspinal abscess in vertebral osteomyelitis) can necessitate drain placement or open surgical drainage.
- 12% of cases of lumbar vertebral osteomyelitis are complicated by an epidural abscess, with higher rates in thoracic and cervical osteomyelitis.[7]
- Long-term antibiotic therapy can be complicated by line-related infections; *C. difficile*; hematological, renal, or liver toxicity; and other antibiotic-specific adverse events.

MONITORING/FOLLOW-UP

- Clinical reassessment is indicated after 3 to 6 weeks of treatment.
- Concern for treatment failure is warranted if symptoms fail to improve and inflammatory markers (CRP and ESR) are persistently elevated.
- Reimaging is not routinely indicated as it does not correlate well with clinical healing, but can be used for cases that worsen or fail to improve or to ensure resolution of a large abscess.[8]

OUTCOME/PROGNOSIS

- Acute osteomyelitis is generally easier to cure than chronic bone infection.
- Cure rates for vertebral osteomyelitis approach 90%, with mortality <5%.[2]
- Back pain and neurological symptoms persist in a minority of patients with vertebral osteomyelitis, and functional limitations may persist in up to one-third of survivors.[7]

OSTEOMYELITIS ASSOCIATED WITH DIABETES AND PERIPHERAL VASCULAR DISEASE

GENERAL PRINCIPLES

- This type of osteomyelitis develops almost exclusively in the feet of patients at risk, often following a pressure ulcer.
- Polymicrobial with common organisms including *S. aureus*, other gram-positive cocci such as streptococci, and various gram-negative organisms and anaerobic organisms.[9]
- Risk factors for foot infections in the setting of diabetes and/or peripheral arterial disease include vascular compromise, poor glucose control or evidence of diabetic end-organ damage, poorly fitted footwear, and trauma.
- Preventive strategies include the following:
  - Optimize glucose control in diabetics
  - Smoking cessation should be encouraged
  - Ensure appropriate footwear and minimize foot trauma
  - Patients should perform daily self foot examination
  - Provide early dedicated wound management for foot ulcers

DIAGNOSIS

Clinical Presentation

History
- Determine the duration of ulcer and history of prior episodes of foot osteomyelitis. Long-standing (>2 weeks) foot ulceration over bony prominence increases the likelihood of osteomyelitis.
- Ask about associated local (e.g., wound drainage, erythema, and tenderness) and systemic (e.g., fevers and chills) symptoms.
- Trauma may suggest fracture or presence of foreign body.

TABLE 8-4 LABORATORY MONITORING FOR OUTPATIENT ANTIBIOTIC THERAPY FOR COMMONLY USED ANTIBIOTICS

Antibiotic	Suggested labs/frequency
Vancomycin	CBC once weekly BMP twice weekly Vancomycin trough twice weekly (goal 15–20 mg/L)
Penicillin	CBC and BMP once weekly
Oxacillin or nafcillin	CBC and CMP once weekly
Cefazolin	CBC and BMP once weekly
Ceftriaxone	CBC and CMP once weekly
Carbapenems	CBC and CMP once weekly
Daptomycin	CBC, BMP, and CPK once weekly

BMP, basic metabolic profile; CBC, complete blood count; CMP, complete metabolic profile; CPK, creatine phosphokinase.

Physical Examination
- Measure size and depth of ulcer. Ulcers >2 cm^2 in size and >3 mm in depth increase the probability of underlying bone infection.[10]
- Check pedal pulses to assess vascular supply.
- Visible or probe-able bone indicates a presumptive diagnosis of osteomyelitis.

Differential Diagnosis

Infected diabetic foot ulcer without bone involvement and neuropathic changes (i.e., Charcot arthropathy) may mimic diabetic foot osteomyelitis in clinical presentation and imaging.

Diagnostic Testing

Laboratories
- Baseline testing, including a complete blood count and renal function and liver function tests, is indicated.
- WBC count may be normal or elevated.
- Elevated inflammatory markers such as ESR and CRP correlate with the presence of bone involvement, but are nonspecific. ESR elevation above 70 mm/h increases the likelihood of osteomyelitis by a factor of 11.[10]
- Blood cultures should be obtained if signs of systemic infection are present.

Imaging
- Plain films may demonstrate local osteopenia with bone lucencies or periosteal reactions, but may take 2 to 4 weeks to become positive.
- MRI is more useful than CT scan or nuclear tests and is the test of choice in most cases with a sensitivity of 90% to 100%.[11] Indium-111 scans can be useful in distinguishing between osteomyelitis and Charcot changes in selected patients.[11,12]

Diagnostic Procedures
- Superficial swab is not necessarily indicative of deeper pathogens, but can be used to identify resistant organisms, such as MRSA, which has the highest correlation between superficial and bone cultures (40%).[13]
- Transcutaneous bone biopsy can be useful to obtain bone samples for histology and culture.
- Vascular supply should be assessed (usually first by measuring ankle-brachial index) to determine need for revascularization procedures.

TREATMENT

Medications

- Cure via medical therapy without surgical intervention or with minimal debridement may be possible in cases without extensive gangrene, necrosis, or limb-threatening infection.[14]
- Antibiotics are generally administered for 4 to 6 weeks, which can be extended when chronically infected bone remains and shortened if all the infected tissue and bone is surgically removed.
- Oral antibiotics with high bioavailability (i.e., metronidazole and fluoroquinolones) can be used, but parenteral antibiotics are preferable in most cases.
- No single regimen has been shown superior and few head-to-head trials comparing antibiotic regimens exist to guide treatment.

- If deep culture results are available, therapy directed at isolated organisms should be used (Table 8-2).
- If deep culture results are not available, polymicrobial coverage should be included and considerations guiding therapeutic choice include the following:
  o Ease of outpatient administration
  o Risk factors for resistant gram-negative rods including *Pseudomonas* (prior antibiotic therapy, long-standing ulceration, and ulcer soaked in water) or MRSA infection
  o Superficial culture of resistant organisms
- Empiric regimens commonly used at our institution include the following:
  o Vancomycin 15 to 20 mg/kg intravenously every 12 hours **plus** ciprofloxacin 750 mg by mouth every 12 hours **plus** metronidazole 500 mg by mouth every 8 hours
  o Vancomycin 15 to 20 mg/kg intravenously every 12 hours **plus** ceftriaxone 2 g intravenously every 24 hours **plus** metronidazole 500 mg by mouth every 8 hours
  o Vancomycin 15 to 20 mg/kg intravenously every 12 hours **plus** cefepime 2 g intravenously every 8 to 12 hours **plus** metronidazole 500 mg by mouth every 8 hours
  o Vancomycin 15 to 20 mg/kg intravenously every 12 hours **plus** ertapenem 1 g intravenously every 24 hours

Other Nonpharmacologic Therapies

- Optimal glucose control is important for adequate healing in all diabetic patients.
- Local wound care with ongoing debridement of devitalized tissue is crucial.

Surgical Management

- Orthopedic surgery or podiatry consultation is usually indicated.
- Debridement and/or amputation is often necessary for cure, especially when chronically infected bone is present.
- Revascularization is needed for healing in cases of insufficient vascular supply.

SPECIAL CONSIDERATIONS

For dialysis patients, care should be taken to choose an antibiotic regimen that can be easily administered during dialysis (Table 8-3).

COMPLICATIONS

- Amputation of infected foot/limb carries high morbidity.
- Complications of long-term antibiotic therapy (e.g., line-related infections; hematological, renal, or liver toxicity; and other antibiotic-specific adverse events) can occur (see Table 8-4).

MONITORING/FOLLOW-UP

- Clinical reassessment for worsening of infection or poor wound healing should occur within the first 3 to 6 weeks of treatment.
- Concern for treatment failure is warranted if symptoms fail to improve and inflammatory markers (CRP and ESR) are persistently elevated.
- Reimaging is not routinely indicated.

OUTCOME/PROGNOSIS

More than one-third of patients require some level of amputation in the 1 to 3 years following treatment.[15]

OTHER CONTIGUOUS OSTEOMYELITIS

GENERAL PRINCIPLES

Epidemiology

There are three main types of contiguous osteomyelitis other than diabetic and peripheral vascular disease associated:
- Hardware or foreign body associated (except prosthetic joint infection that is discussed separately)
- Trauma associated, secondary to open fractures
- Osteomyelitis complicating decubitus ulcers

Etiology
- *S. aureus* is common in all types of contiguous osteomyelitis.
- Coagulase-negative staphylococci and *Propionibacterium* are associated with foreign body or hardware in subacute infection.
- Trauma-associated microbiology varies according to open fracture environment and can include unusual organisms.
- Decubitus ulcer–associated osteomyelitis is usually polymicrobial and fecal organisms are common.

Risk Factors
- Presence of hardware or foreign body
- Open fracture with gross contamination
- Nonhealing stage IV decubitus ulcer

DIAGNOSIS

Clinical Presentation

History
- Systemic symptoms, such as fever, are often absent in subacute or chronic osteomyelitis.
- Local symptoms such as increased pain, redness, or drainage are often found on examination.
- Query prior antibiotic use as this may impact organism recovery during culture.
- In the case of open fractures, the mechanism of injury and the degree and type of contamination may provide a clue as to causative organisms.
- Local signs of infection such as foul smelling, drainage, erythema, tenderness, poor wound healing, or exposed bone suggest infection.
- Increased pain may be the only symptom in patients with hardware-associated infection.

Physical Examination
- Inspect the wound for signs of infection (e.g., drainage, erythema, and swelling) in trauma- or hardware-associated infection.
- A draining sinus tract is often indicative of chronic osteomyelitis in trauma- or hardware-associated infection.
- Clinical diagnosis of osteomyelitis, even the presence of visible bone, is unreliable in decubitus ulcers.[16]

Differential Diagnosis

Osteomyelitis can be confused with soft tissue infection without bone involvement in all types of contiguous osteomyelitis and mechanical failure in hardware-associated osteomyelitis.

Diagnostic Testing

Laboratories
- Baseline testing, including a complete blood count and renal function and liver function tests, is indicated.
- WBC count may be normal or elevated
- Elevated inflammatory markers such as ESR and CRP correlate with the presence of bone involvement, but are nonspecific.
- Blood cultures should be obtained if signs of systemic infection are present.

Imaging
- Plain films may demonstrate soft tissue swelling, and bone destruction can be difficult to interpret in the background of abnormal bone from fractures, surgical changes, or pressure-related bone changes.[17] Hardware loosening (in hardware associated) or nonunion of fracture (in trauma) may also be seen.
- CT scan, MRI, or nuclear medicine studies can also be used to aid in diagnosis of decubitus ulcer–associated osteomyelitis.
- MRI has the best sensitivity (98%) and specificity (89%).[18]
- Practically, definitive diagnosis of trauma- or hardware-associated infection is often made surgically, rather than radiographically.

Diagnostic Procedures
- Superficial swab of decubitus ulcers indicates colonization and is generally not useful in defining causative organisms.[16]
- Deep operative specimens in trauma- or hardware-associated infection are often available and are invaluable for the choice of therapy.
- Bone biopsy with culture is useful in cases of suspected decubitus ulcer–associated osteomyelitis for both diagnostic purposes and therapeutic choices.

TREATMENT

A combined medical and surgical approach is almost always necessary for cure in these types of infections. Decubitus-associated chronic osteomyelitis may not require long-term antibiotics with the associated risk of adverse effects; instead, it may be reasonable to treat only clinically apparent "flares" in disease.

Medications

- Antibiotics are generally administered for 6 weeks, usually intravenously.
- If culture results are available, therapy directed at isolated organisms should be used (Table 8-2).
- Empiric therapy should be reserved for culture-negative hardware- or trauma-associated osteomyelitis.
- Empiric therapy for decubitus ulcer–associated osteomyelitis should cover gram-positive (including MRSA), gram-negative, and anaerobic organisms.
  - Gram-negative and gram-positive coverage (ciprofloxacin 750 mg PO twice daily **or** ceftriaxone 2 g intravenously once daily) **and** anaerobic coverage (metronidazole 500 mg PO three times daily) with the addition of parenteral vancomycin if MRSA is cultured or the patient is at high risk is a reasonable option.
  - Be aware of risk for resistant organisms in patients in long-term care facilities and those with prior antibiotic treatment and consider adding more extensive gram-negative coverage with a carbapenem, antipseudomonal penicillin, or fourth-generation cephalosporin.

Other Nonpharmacologic Therapies

Local wound care and ongoing debridement of devitalized tissue and unloading of pressure are useful in decubitus ulcers.

Surgical Management

- Debridement and hardware removal, if present, is often necessary for cure.
- Suppressive oral antibiotic therapy (discussed in the prosthetic joint infection section) is useful when hardware cannot be removed.
- Wound coverage through grafting or flaps may be necessary for complete wound closure.
- Diverting colostomy to prevent wound contamination in cases of decubitus ulcers may be useful in some cases.

SPECIAL CONSIDERATIONS

For dialysis patients, care should be taken to choose an antibiotic regimen that can be easily administered during dialysis (Table 8-3).

COMPLICATIONS

- Loss of functional limb (hardware- or trauma-associated osteomyelitis).
- Chronic osteomyelitis in decubitus ulcer–associated infection can result in difficult-to-cure infection.

MONITORING/FOLLOW-UP

- Clinical reassessment for worsening of infection or poor wound healing is indicated within the first 3 to 6 weeks of treatment.
- Concern for treatment failure is indicated if symptoms fail to improve and inflammatory markers (CRP and ESR) are persistently elevated.
- Reimaging is not routinely indicated.

OUTCOME/PROGNOSIS

- Prognosis is variable and depends on many factors including age, comorbidities, organism, and type of contiguous osteomyelitis.
- Bacteremia due to decubitus ulcers is associated with a high mortality rate in the elderly (up to 50%).[19]

SEPTIC ARTHRITIS OF THE NATIVE JOINTS

GONOCOCCAL ARTHRITIS

GENERAL PRINCIPLES

- Disseminated gonococcal infection (DGI) is the result of bacteremic spread of *Neisseria gonorrhoeae*.
- DGI presents in one of two ways:
  - Tenosynovitis, papulopustular dermatitis, and arthralgia (without obvious purulent arthritis)
  - Purulent arthritis without skin involvement
- *N. gonorrhoeae* produces many virulence factors that allow it to disseminate from mucosal colonization, and pili facilitate attachment to the synovium.[20]
- Gonococcal arthritis is the most common bacterial arthritis in young adults.
- Septic arthritis complicates DGI in one-half of cases and may be less likely to be associated with classic skin findings or tenosynovitis.
- Infection is due to occult bacteremia from usually asymptomatic mucosal infection (genitourinary, rectal, or oropharynx), which disseminates.
- Risk factors include young sexually active adults, female sex, menstruation, pregnancy and postpartum period in women, and complement deficiencies.[20]

DIAGNOSIS

Clinical Presentation

History
- The classic DGI triad of migratory polyarthralgias, tenosynovitis (mainly of the fingers, hands, and wrists) and dermatitis is less likely in the setting of septic arthritis.
- With septic arthritis, monoarthritis or oligoarthritis and fever may be the only clinical complaints.
- DGI has a predilection for the knee and wrist joints.

Physical Examination
- Examine the skin for characteristic, painless macules and papules on the arms, legs, or trunk
- Careful joint examination

Differential Diagnosis

Other causes of infectious and noninfectious arthritis (bacterial septic arthritis, gouty arthritis, and reactive arthritis [ReA]), meningococcemia, secondary syphilis, and connective tissue disease can be confused with DGI.

Diagnostic Testing

Diagnosis is usually based on clinical and epidemiological features due to the low yield of diagnostic procedures.

Laboratories

- WBC count and inflammatory markers (ESR and CRP) may be elevated, but are nonspecific.
- Skin cultures, synovial cultures, and blood cultures are rarely positive, but genitourinary cultures are positive in more than 80% of patients.[20]
- DNA probes and nucleic acid amplification tests are FDA-approved for urethral and endocervical specimens and are highly sensitive and specific.[21]
- Screening for other sexually transmitted diseases, including HIV, should be performed.

Imaging

- Plain films may demonstrate effusion.
- MRI or CT can be used to detect septic arthritis, effusions, abscesses, or tissue edema.

Diagnostic Procedures

- Arthrocentesis is the test of choice but has a low yield for positive cultures.
- Purulent effusion (>50,000 WBCs) should be present.
- Gram stain is positive in <25% of cases and culture in only 50%, but polymerase chain reaction can detect *N. gonorrhoeae* with a high degree of sensitivity.[22]

TREATMENT

Medications

- In the appropriate clinical setting (young adult who is sexually active), empiric treatment for DGI should be initiated:
  - Ceftriaxone 1 g intravenously every 24 hours or cefotaxime 1 g intravenously every 8 hours used for initial therapy
  - Can switch to oral therapy with cefixime 400 mg by mouth twice daily 24 to 48 hours after improvement[23]
- Treat for a total of 7 to 14 days.
- Patients should also receive treatment for chlamydial infection (doxycycline 100 mg PO twice daily for 7 days is one option).

Surgical Management

Drainage by repeated needle aspiration or arthroscopy is needed for purulent arthritis due to DGI.

SPECIAL CONSIDERATIONS

Sexual contacts should be treated for *Neisseria* and *Chlamydia* infection.

COMPLICATIONS

Complications are rare, but include joint damage, osteomyelitis, meningitis, and endocarditis.

MONITORING/FOLLOW-UP

Patients with recurrent *Neisseria* infection should be screened for complement deficiency.

OUTCOME/PROGNOSIS

Prognosis is good, with return to normal joint function in the vast majority of patients.

NONGONOCOCCAL ARTHRITIS

GENERAL PRINCIPLES

- Bacteria enter the joint space, triggering an acute inflammatory response with acute and chronic inflammatory cells. Cytokines and proteases degrade the cartilage and then progress to subchondral bone loss [24]
- Nongonococcal septic arthritis is the most rapidly destructive joint disease.
- There are 10 to 20 cases per 100,000 in the general population.[24]
- Large joints are affected more often than small joints and up to 60% of cases occur in the hip or knee.[25]
- Joint infection occurs most commonly from hematogenous seeding, which can be persistent with an identifiable source or transient, or less commonly from direct inoculation (joint surgery, arthrocentesis, and puncture wound).
- The most common cause of bacterial septic arthritis is *S. aureus*, including increasing incidence of MRSA.[26]
- Other common bacterial causes include group B streptococci in diabetics, gram-negative bacilli in elderly or debilitated patients, and coagulase-negative staphylococci following medical procedures.
- Risk factors include older age, rheumatoid arthritis, diabetes mellitus, malignancy, risk factors for bacteremia (e.g., vascular catheter and IVDA), and joint manipulation.

DIAGNOSIS

Clinical Presentation
- Patients present with acute onset of monoarticular arthritis consisting of pain, swelling, and limited motion of the affected joint, often accompanied by fever.
- Examination usually reveals a warm, tender joint with effusion and decreased active and passive range of motion; however, examination of the shoulder and hip joint may be difficult and unrevealing.

Differential Diagnosis
Nongonococcal septic arthritis must be differentiated from other causes of infectious and noninfectious arthritis (e.g., gonococcal arthritis, gout, pseudogout, and ReA), Lyme disease, and connective tissue disease.

Diagnostic Testing

Laboratories
- WBC count and inflammatory markers (ESR and CRP) may be elevated, but are nonspecific.
- Blood cultures should be performed.

Imaging
- Plain films may demonstrate effusion.
- MRI or CT can be used to detect septic arthritis, effusions, abscesses, or tissue edema.

Diagnostic Procedures
- **Arthrocentesis is the test of choice**.
- Fluoroscopic guidance may be necessary due to difficulty with access (hip joint).
- Fluid should be sent for examination for cell count and differential (>50,000 WBCs typical), crystal examination, Gram stain, and culture.
- Gram stain is positive in 50% of cases and cultures are positive in >80%.[27]

TREATMENT

Medications
- Empiric therapy should be based on the Gram stain and clinical scenario and may include treatment directed at *S. aureus* and streptococci.
  - Vancomycin 15 to 20 mg/kg intravenously every 8 to 12 hours **plus** ceftriaxone 2 g intravenously every 24 hours is one reasonable choice and can be continued for culture-negative cases.
- Targeted therapy is similar to that for other bone infections (Table 8-2).
- Treatment for 2 to 4 weeks is the standard of care.

Surgical Management
- Drainage by repeated needle aspiration (daily drainage may be required) or arthroscopy needed for purulent arthritis.
- If adequate drainage cannot be maintained by less invasive methods or the hip joint is involved, open surgical drainage is used.

SPECIAL CONSIDERATIONS

- Other causes of infectious septic arthritis include the following:
  - Mycobacterial and fungal arthritis, which present as a chronic arthritis
  - Lyme arthritis, which presents as a chronic monoarthritis, commonly of the knees
- For dialysis patients, care should be taken to choose an antibiotic regimen that can be easily administered during dialysis (Table 8-3).

COMPLICATIONS

- Complications include joint damage (50% of cases), osteomyelitis, and complications of prolonged bacteremia (endocarditis and seeding of other organs).
- Mortality rate is significant (5% to 15%).[28]

MONITORING/FOLLOW-UP

- Clinical reassessment for monitoring of infection is indicated within the first 4 weeks of treatment.
- Prompt repeat arthrocentesis or surgical drainage is indicated if symptoms worsen or fail to improve with appropriate therapy.

OUTCOME/PROGNOSIS

Prognosis is fair, but high rates of permanent joint damage (>40% of adults in one series had a poor joint outcome) and unchanged mortality rates are discouraging.[28]

PROSTHETIC JOINT INFECTIONS

GENERAL PRINCIPLES

- Microorganisms are introduced at the time of surgery or through transient or persistent bacteremia.
- Bacteria adhere to the prosthesis and biofilm formation protects organisms from the host immune response and limits antimicrobial penetration.[29]
- Prosthetic joint infections are mainly a disease of older adults due to the need for joint replacement surgery in advanced osteoarthritis.
- Infection rates are <1% in hip replacement and <2% in knee replacement, but hundreds of thousands of procedures are performed each year, resulting in a large number of infected prostheses.[29]
- **Early infection** (<3 months after surgery) and **delayed infection** (3 to 24 months after surgery) are mainly due to organisms introduced at the time of surgery.
- **Late infection** (>24 months after surgery) is usually due to hematogenous seeding from skin, respiratory tract, dental, or urinary tract infections.
- The most commonly isolated organisms are coagulase-negative staphylococci (30% to 43%), *S. aureus* (12% to 23%), mixed flora (10% to 11%), streptococci (9% to 10%), gram-negative bacilli (3% to 6%), enterococci (3% to 7%), and anaerobes (2% to 4%).[29]
- Risk factors include the following:
  - Older age
  - Comorbidities including rheumatoid arthritis, psoriasis, diabetes mellitus, immunocompromised state, malignancy, obesity, or poor nutritional status
  - Prior surgery at prosthesis site
  - First 2 years after joint replacement

DIAGNOSIS

Clinical Presentation

- Early infection often presents with acute onset of joint pain, effusion, erythema and warmth at prosthesis site, and fever.

- Delayed infection has a more insidious onset of symptoms such as loosening of the implant or pain with absence of systemic symptoms. Presentation of delayed infections depends on the virulence of the causative organism.
- Careful examination of the joint and incision site may reveal erythema and cellulitis, discharge, wound dehiscence, sinus tract formation, and pain with passive or active motion.

Differential Diagnosis

Aseptic mechanical problems (gout, pseudogout, hemarthrosis, or prosthesis loosening) can present similarly.

Diagnostic Testing

Differentiation of infection from mechanical problems is mainly accomplished through sampling of deep tissue or fluid by joint aspiration or surgical exploration.

Laboratories
- WBC count and inflammatory markers (ESR and CRP) may be elevated, but are nonspecific.
- Blood cultures should be performed, although yield is low.

Imaging
- Plain films may detect loosening of the prosthesis or osteomyelitis.
- MRI and CT scan are hindered by metal artifact.

Diagnostic Procedures
- Joint aspiration can demonstrate increased WBCs and organisms on Gram stain or culture consistent with infection, but often patients proceed directly to surgical exploration if suspicion of infection is high or prosthesis replacement or repair is required.
- Multiple specimens should be sent from all operative procedures to increase culture yield.

TREATMENT

Proven infection requires combined medical and surgical treatment.

Medications

- Empiric therapy should be based on the Gram stain and should be held until deep cultures are obtained if the patient is clinically stable.
- If empiric therapy is warranted, it should be targeted at most common organisms including *S. aureus*, coagulase-negative staphylococci, and gram-negative organisms.
- Targeted therapy is similar to that for other bone infections (Table 8-2), with an exception being the addition of rifampin with staphylococcal infection.
- **Rifampin 300 mg orally twice daily should be added to cases of retained hardware (i.e., early infection with retained hardware or late infection when hardware cannot be removed) in staphylococcal infections due to its activity against biofilms.**
- Treatment is recommended for 6 to 8 weeks.

Surgical Management

- Early infection (<3 months postsurgery) with <3 weeks of symptoms, stable prosthesis, and minimally damaged soft tissue can be treated with debridement and retention of the prosthesis with a >70% cure rate,[29] but infections with *S. aureus* may have a higher failure rate.[30]
- Late infections (>3 weeks) are optimally treated with a two-stage procedure where the implant is removed and antibiotic therapy is administered for 6 weeks followed by reimplantation of the prosthesis after an antibiotic-free window, which results in a >90% cure rate.[31]

SPECIAL CONSIDERATIONS

Dialysis Patients

Care should be taken to choose an antibiotic regimen that can be easily administered during dialysis (Table 8-3).

Retained Hardware When Removal Is Indicated

- In cases where prosthesis removal is not possible despite the presence of an indication for removal, acute therapy targeted at causative organisms plus rifampin if staphylococci are cultured followed by chronic oral antibiotic suppression therapy can be used following acute treatment.
- Chronic suppression is most successful with streptococci or coagulase-negative staphylococci, with higher failure rates for *S. aureus.*[32]
- An oral antibiotic should be chosen based on bacterial susceptibility, ease of administration, and least likelihood of adverse events.
- Commonly used antibiotics for chronic suppression include **trimethoprim–sulfamethoxazole or doxycycline**.

COMPLICATIONS

- Functional impairment of the joint is a feared complication.
- Severe systemic infection with systemic shock can occur with more virulent organisms.

MONITORING/FOLLOW-UP

- Clinical reassessment for worsening of infection or poor wound healing should occur within the first 3 to 6 weeks of treatment.
- Persistent or worsening symptoms or continued presence of elevated inflammatory markers should prompt further evaluation for continued infection.

OUTCOME/PROGNOSIS

Prognosis depends on the location, time since surgery, host factors, and infecting organism, but >90% of two-stage procedures and >70% of early infection treated with retained prosthesis result in a cure, generally with good prosthesis function.

SEPTIC BURSITIS

GENERAL PRINCIPLES

- Septic bursitis is bacterial infection of a bursa overlying a joint.
- Septic bursitis commonly affects subcutaneous olecranon, prepatellar, or infrapatellar bursae.
- Bacteria are introduced through trauma, percutaneously, or, rarely, hematogenous spread.
- Septic bursitis is due to *S. aureus* in >80% of cases.[33]
- Other causes include streptococci, gram-negative rods, mycobacteria, and fungi.
- The most significant risk factor is trauma to the bursa.

DIAGNOSIS

- Patients note pain, redness, and warmth over affected bursa, with or without systemic symptoms.
- Evidence of trauma or puncture wound is often evident over the affected bursa.
- Septic arthritis of the joint, gout, traumatic bursitis, and rheumatic bursitis can all present similarly.
- **Aspiration of the bursa is the test of choice**, with fluid sent for cell count and differential, crystals, Gram stain, and culture.
- Aspiration of joint space may be necessary to rule out septic arthritis.

TREATMENT

- Antibiotic therapy targeting the offending organism is indicated for a 10- to 14-day course (Table 8-2).
- Oral regimens are reasonable in mild cases in otherwise healthy patients.[33]
- Daily aspiration should be performed until sterile fluid is obtained.

OUTCOME/PROGNOSIS

- Prognosis is generally good, but bursitis can recur.
- Recurrent bursitis may require bursectomy.

VIRAL ARTHRITIS

GENERAL PRINCIPLES

- Viral arthritis is a syndrome of acute polyarthritis, fever, and rash due to viral infection.
- The pathophysiology of viral arthritis is poorly understood, but may result from direct infection of synovium or be due to host immune response.

- Complicates up to 60% of parvovirus infections,[34] and up to 20% of patients with acute hepatitis B or chronic hepatitis C viral infection have joint symptoms.[35]
- Parvovirus, hepatitis B and C, and rubella are the most common causes of viral arthritis. Rubella virus is a common cause of arthritis in the developing world.
- Other viruses that cause arthritis include HIV, Epstein-Barr virus, enterovirus, mumps, adenovirus, and alphaviruses.
- Risk of viral arthritis is dependent on risk factors for the individual viral infections.
- Women more likely than men experience arthritis following parvovirus infection (60% vs. 30%).[34]

DIAGNOSIS

Clinical Presentation

History
- Parvovirus infection often presents with symmetric polyarthritis of the hands, wrists, and ankles accompanied by facial erythema ("slapped cheek") and fever.
- A symmetric polyarthritis of the hands, wrists, knees, and ankles in acute hepatitis B infection often precedes the development of jaundice during the febrile prodrome.
- Chronic hepatitis C virus is often associated with arthralgias. Frank arthritis resembling rheumatoid arthritis develops in a smaller number of patients.[35]
- Rubella causes an arthritis most commonly in the small joints of the hands and is associated with onset of a rash.

Physical Examination
- Careful examination of the joints with attention to the hands, wrists, and ankles should demonstrate joint involvement.
- Skin examination may reveal a characteristic rash consistent with rubella or parvovirus.

Differential Diagnosis

Other causes of polyarthritis including rheumatoid arthritis, acute rheumatic fever, endocarditis, and DGI.

Diagnostic Testing

- Viral serology is generally most useful for diagnosis.
- Imaging is often unremarkable.
- Joint aspiration rarely is useful except to rule out other causes of arthritis as organisms are not generally recovered from the synovium.

TREATMENT

- Supportive care is the only treatment indicated for most cases of viral arthritis.
- Nonsteroidal antiinflammatory drugs (NSAIDs) are useful for symptom management.
- Treatment of hepatitis C or chronic hepatitis B may improve joint symptoms.

SPECIAL CONSIDERATIONS

Returning travelers with polyarthralgias should have a careful travel history performed to gauge risk for alphaviruses such as chikungunya virus or flaviviruses (e.g., dengue virus).

OUTCOME/PROGNOSIS

- Viral arthritis rarely presents significant long-term disability and most are self-limiting.
- Parvovirus may have a relapsing course in one-third of patients or chronic course lasting months in up to 20% of patients.[34]
- Joint symptoms with chronic hepatitis B or C may persist with the disease, but permanent joint damage is rare.

REACTIVE ARTHRITIS

GENERAL PRINCIPLES

- Reactive arthritis is defined as **sterile inflammation of joints** that may be related to a distant infection.
- ReA is hypothesized to be related to poor clearance of the organism and/or dysregulatory immune response.
- There is an association with other seronegative spondyloarthropathies and HLA-B27.[36] However, the relation to HLA-B27 is less strong than that of ankylosing spondylitis.
- ReA is an uncommon disease that mainly occurs in young adults. The male-to-female ratio is equal for ReA following gastroenteritis but much more common in males following genitourinary infection.
- ReA can occur in outbreaks from a single source of infection.
- Numerous microbial infections can cause ReA:
  ○ Enteric bacteria include *Yersinia*, *Salmonella*, *Shigella*, *Campylobacter*, and *C. difficile*.
  ○ *Chlamydia trachomatis* can cause ReA following urethritis.
  ○ *Chlamydophila pneumoniae* can cause ReA following a respiratory tract infection.

DIAGNOSIS

Clinical Presentation

- Antecedent respiratory, genitourinary, or gastrointestinal infection can often be elicited, but in other cases the initiating infection may be asymptomatic or not reported.
- There is usually a 1- to 2-week lag (up to 4 weeks with *Chlamydia*) between initial infection and joint symptoms.[36]
- It commonly presents as asymmetric oligoarthritis of the large joints of the lower extremities, along with extra-articular complaints. Back pain occurs in about half of

the cases. Enthesopathy (e.g., Achilles tendinitis, plantar fasciitis, and dactylitis) is not uncommon.

- Evidence of joint redness, swelling, and pain with range of motion is characteristic.
- Extra-articular symptoms including conjunctivitis, acute anterior uveitis, and skin findings (e.g., circinate balanitis, keratoderma blenorrhagicum, and erythema nodosum) may be seen.

Differential Diagnosis

ReA must be differentiated from other causes of acute poly- or oligoarthritis, including infectious and noninfectious causes.

Diagnostic Testing

- ReA is a rule-out diagnosis that should be considered in the appropriate clinical scenario when other causes of arthritis are ruled out.
- At the time of arthritis, cultures for triggering infection are often negative. An exception is *C. trachomatis*, which can often be identified in the urine via nucleic acid amplification tests or cultured from the urethra.[37]
- Serological tests, when available, may support the diagnosis.

TREATMENT

- Symptomatic treatment with NSAIDs and local steroid injections is useful.
- No significant evidence exists to favor antibiotic treatment for ReA per se, although culture-positive *C. trachomatis* should be treated.

OUTCOME/PROGNOSIS

Fifty percent of patients recover in the first 6 months of treatment, but a minority develop chronic or recurrent symptoms.[36]

REFERENCES

1. Foster TJ, Hook M. Surface protein adhesins of *Staphylococcus aureus*. *Trends Microbiol.* 1998;6:484-488.
2. Mylona E, Samarkos M, Kakalou E, et al. Pyogenic vertebral osteomyelitis: a systematic review of clinical characteristics. *Semin Arthritis Rheum.* 2009;39:10-17.
3. Bhavan K, Marschall J, Olsen M, et al. The epidemiology of hematogenous vertebral osteomyelitis: a cohort study in a tertiary care hospital. *BMC Infect Dis.* 2010;10:158.
4. Sapico FL, Montgomerie JZ. Pyogenic vertebral osteomyelitis: report of nine cases and review of the literature. *Rev Infect Dis.* 1979;1:754-776.
5. Pigrau C, Almirante B, Flores X, et al. Spontaneous pyogenic vertebral osteomyelitis and endocarditis: incidence, risk factors, and outcome. *Am J Med.* 2005;118:1287.
6. Modic MT, Feiglin DH, Piraino DW, et al. Vertebral osteomyelitis: assessment using MR. *Radiology.* 1985;157:157-166.
7. McHenry MC, Easley KA, Locker GA. Vertebral osteomyelitis: long-term outcome for 253 patients from 7 Cleveland-area hospitals. *Clin Infect Dis.* 2002;34:1342-1350.

8. Kowalski TJ, Berbari EF, Huddleston PM, et al. Do follow-up imaging examinations provide useful prognostic information in patients with spine infection? *Clin Infect Dis.* 2006;43:172-179.

9. Hartemann-Heurtier A, Senneville E. Diabetic foot osteomyelitis. *Diabetes Metab.* 2008;34:87-95.

10. Butalia S, Palda VA, Sargeant RJ, et al. Does this patient with diabetes have osteomyelitis of the lower extremity? *JAMA.* 2008;299:806-813.

11. Jeffcoate WJ, Lipsky BA. Controversies in diagnosing and managing osteomyelitis of the foot in diabetes. *Clin Infect Dis.* 2004;39:S115-S122.

12. Newman LG, Waller J, Palestro CJ, et al. Unsuspected osteomyelitis in diabetic foot ulcers. *JAMA.* 1991;266:1246-1251.

13. Senneville E, Melliez H, Beltrand E, et al. Culture of percutaneous bone biopsy specimens for diagnosis of diabetic foot osteomyelitis: concordance with ulcer swab cultures. *Clin Infect Dis.* 2006;42:57-62.

14. Shank CF, Feibel JB. Osteomyelitis in the diabetic foot: diagnosis and management. *Foot Ankle Clin.* 2006;11:775-789.

15. Apelqvist J, Larsson J, Agardh CD. Long-term prognosis for diabetic patients with foot ulcers. *J Intern Med.* 1993;233:485-491.

16. Darouiche RO, Landon GC, Klima M, et al. Osteomyelitis associated with pressure sores. *Arch Intern Med.* 1994;154:753-758.

17. Sugarman B. Pressure sores and underlying bone infection. *Arch Intern Med.* 1987;147:553-555.

18. Huang AB, Schweitzer ME, Hume E, et al. Osteomyelitis of the pelvis/hips in paralyzed patients: accuracy and clinical utility of MRI. *J Comput Assist Tomogr.* 1998;22:437-443.

19. Bryan CS, Dew CE, Reynolds KL. Bacteremia associated with decubitus ulcers. *Arch Intern Med.* 1983;143:2093-2095.

20. Cucurull E, Espinoza LR. Gonococcal arthritis. *Rheum Dis Clin North Am.* 1998;24:305-322.

21. Stary A, Ching SF, Teodorowicz L, Lee H. Comparison of ligase chain reaction and culture for detection of *Neisseria gonorrhoeae* in genital and extragenital specimens. *J Clin Microbiol.* 1997;35:239-242.

22. Liebling MR, Arkfeld DG, Michelini GA, et al. Identification of *Neisseria gonorrhoeae* in synovial fluid using the polymerase chain reaction. *Arthritis Rheum.* 1994;37:702-709.

23. Workowski KA, Berman S; Centers for Disease Control and Prevention (CDC). Sexually transmitted diseases treatment guidelines, 2010. *MMWR Recomm Rep.* 2010;59(RR-12):1-110.

24. Goldenberg DL. Septic arthritis. *Lancet.* 1998;351:197-202.

25. Mathews CJ, Coakley G. Septic arthritis: current diagnostic and therapeutic algorithm. *Curr Opin Rheumatol.* 2008;20:457-462.

26. Gupta MN, Sturrock RD, Field M. A prospective 2-year study of 75 patients with adult-onset septic arthritis. *Rheumatology.* 2001;40(1):24-30.

27. Weston VC, Jones AC, Bradbury N, et al. Clinical features and outcome of septic arthritis in a single UK Health District 1982–1991. *Ann Rheum Dis.* April 1999;58:214-219.

28. Kaandorp CJ, Krijnen P, Moens HJ, et al. The outcome of bacterial arthritis: a prospective community-based study. *Arthritis Rheum.* 1997;40:884-892.

29. Zimmerli W, Trampuz A, Ochsner PE. Prosthetic-joint infections. *N Engl J Med.* 2004;351:1645-1654.

30. Byren I, Bejon P, Atkins BL, et al. One hundred and twelve infected arthroplasties treated with "DAIR" (debridement, antibiotics and implant retention): antibiotic duration and outcome. *J Antimicrob Chemother.* 2009;63:1264-1271.

31. Trampuz A, Zimmerli W. Prosthetic joint infections: update in diagnosis and treatment. *Swiss Med Wkly.* 2005;135:243-251.

32. Segreti J, Nelson JA, Gordon MT. Prolonged suppressive antibiotic therapy for infected orthopedic prostheses. *Clin Infect Dis.* 1998;27:711-713.

33. Zimmermann B III, Mikolich DJ, Ho G Jr. Septic bursitis. *Semin Arthritis Rheum.* 1995;24:391-410.

34. Moore TL. Parvovirus-associated arthritis. *Curr Opin Rheumatol.* 2000;12:289-294.
35. Ohl C. Infectious arthritis of native joint. In: Mandell GL, Bennett JE, Dolin R, eds. *Mandell, Douglas, and Bennett's Principles and Practice of Infectious Diseases.* 7th ed. Philadelphia, PA: Churchill Livingstone, Elsevier; 2009:1443-1456.
36. Leirisalo-Repo M. Reactive arthritis. *Scand J Rheumatol.* 2005;34:251-259.
37. Galadari I, Galadari H. Nonspecific urethritis and reactive arthritis. *Clin Dermatol.* 2004;22:469-475.

Skin and Soft Tissue Infections

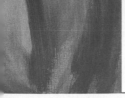

9

Molly F. Sarikonda and David J. Riddle

IMPETIGO

GENERAL PRINCIPLES

Definition

Impetigo is a contagious superficial infection of the epidermis caused by *Staphylococcus aureus* or β-hemolytic streptococci. It can be divided into bullous and nonbullous forms.

Epidemiology

- Nonbullous impetigo is more common.
- Impetigo usually affects young children (ages 2 to 5), but can occur in any age group.[1]
- Incidence is highest in tropical climates or during the summer months in temperate areas.[2]
- Infection is easily spread to others via contact with exposed skin.

Etiology

- ***S. aureus* is the most common cause of both forms of impetigo.**[2]
- β-hemolytic streptococci (primarily *Streptococcus pyogenes*) may cause nonbullous impetigo, either alone or as a coinfection with *S. aureus.*
- Bullous impetigo is caused by *S. aureus* strains that produce **exfoliative toxin A**.[3]
  - Cases caused by community-acquired methicillin-resistant *S. aureus* (CA-MRSA) are increasing, although the majority of cases are caused by methicillin-sensitive strains.[3]
  - Many CA-MRSA isolates do not possess the gene encoding for this virulence factor.[4]

Pathophysiology

- Streptococcal impetigo begins with skin colonization, followed by inoculation of the organisms via minor skin trauma. Staphylococcal impetigo is usually preceded by nasal colonization.
- *S. aureus* produces exfoliative toxin A, which causes disruption of the adhesive junctions in the superficial epidermis in bullous impetigo.

Risk Factors

- Poverty, poor hygiene, and crowded living conditions increase the likelihood of transmission.
- Minor trauma, insect bites, and inflammatory dermatosis also increase the risk of acquisition.[1]

DIAGNOSIS

Clinical Presentation

- Characteristic painful skin lesions are generally the only presenting complaint.
- Systemic symptoms are rare, but local lymphadenitis may be present.
- The lesions of nonbullous impetigo usually occur on the exposed areas of the face or extremities, whereas bullous impetigo is more commonly found on the trunk.
- Nonbullous impetigo begins with papules that develop into vesicles on a bed of erythema. These lesions enlarge to form pustules that rupture and become coated in the **characteristic thick golden crust** over the course of 4 to 6 days.
- Bullous impetigo begins with fragile vesicles that rapidly enlarge into flaccid fluid-filled bullae. These bullae frequently rupture and leave a thin brown crust.

Differential Diagnosis

The differential diagnosis includes contact dermatitis, bullous pemphigoid, and Stevens-Johnson syndrome.

Diagnostic Testing

- An appropriate history and clinical appearance are diagnostic.
- Lesions that fail to respond to appropriate therapy should be cultured and alternative diagnoses considered.

TREATMENT

- Topical therapy is as effective as oral systemic antibiotics in patients with few lesions.
  - ○ **Topical mupirocin** (2% applied three times daily) is the first-line topical agent.[1] Resistance to this agent among staphylococcal strains is increasing and treatment should be reassessed if there is no clinical improvement within 3 to 5 days.
  - ○ **Topical retapamulin** (1% applied twice daily) has been FDA approved for treatment and has comparable efficacy to mupirocin.[5]
- Oral systemic antibiotics should be used in cases of widespread disease or if lesions are present in an area where topical therapy is not practical.
  - ○ A penicillinase-resistant penicillin (dicloxacillin), β-lactam/β-lactamase inhibitor combination (amoxicillin/clavulanate), or first-generation cephalosporin (cephalexin) can be used since these agents are active against streptococci and β-lactamase-producing strains of *S. aureus* (see Table 9-1).[1]
  - ○ Clindamycin should be used when MRSA is suspected or in cases of serious β-lactam allergy. Linezolid should be considered if there is a high rate of inducible clindamycin resistance in the area (see Table 9-2).
- Duration of therapy should be based on clinical response, but is generally 7 to 10 days.[1]
- Hand washing should be promoted and patients and family members should be educated in ways to improve personal hygiene when applicable.

TABLE 9-1	ANTIBIOTIC DOSING AND ROUTES OF ADMINISTRATION FOR SELECTED ANTIBIOTICS COMMONLY USED IN SKIN AND SOFT TISSUE INFECTIONS

Oral options		
Antibiotic	**Dosage and administration**	
	Adults	**Children**
Penicillin V	500 mg four times daily	<12 y: 25–50 mg/kg/d divided three to four times daily (max 3 g/d)
		≥12 y: 500 mg four times daily
Dicloxacillin	500 mg four times daily	<40 kg: 25–50 mg/kg/d divided four times daily (max 2 g/d)
		≥40 kg: 500 mg four times daily
Cefalexin	500 mg four times daily	25–50 mg/kg/d divided four times daily (max 4 g/d)
Clindamycin	300–450 mg three to four times daily	30–40 mg/kg/d divided three to four times daily (max 1.8 g/d)
Amoxicillin–clavulanate	875 mg twice daily	<16 y and <40 kg: 25–45 mg amoxicillin component/kg/d divided every 12 h
		≥16 y or ≥40 kg: 875 mg twice daily
Intravenous options		
Penicillin G	3–4 million units intravenously every 4 h	100,000–400,000 units/kg/d divided every 4–6 h (max 24 million units/d)
Oxacillin	1–2 g every 4 h	100–200 mg/kg/d divided every 4–6 h (max 12 g/d)
Ampicillin–sulbactam	1.5–3 g every 6 h	100–200 mg ampicillin/kg/d divided every 6 h (max 12 g/d)
Cefazolin	1–1.5 g every 8 h	25–100 mg/kg/d divided every 6–8 h (max 6 g/d)
Cefepime	1 g every 12 h (increase to 2 g for treatment of *Pseudomonas aeruginosa*)	50 mg/kg/dose every 12 h (max 2 g/dose)
Piperacillin–tazobactam	4.5 g every 8 h (increase to every 6 h for treatment of *P. aeruginosa*)	240 mg piperacillin/kg/d divided every 8 h (increase to 300–400 mg piperacillin/kg/d divided every 6 h for treatment of *P. aeruginosa*, max 16 g/d)
Meropenem	500 mg every 8 h	10 mg/kg/dose every 8 h (max 500 mg/dose)
Clindamycin	600–900 mg every 8 h	25–40 mg/kg/d divided every 6–8 h (max 2.7 g/d)
Vancomycin	15–20 mg/kg every 12 h	15–20 mg/kg/dose every 6–8 h

TABLE 9-2	ANTIBIOTIC THERAPY FOR COMMUNITY-ACQUIRED METHICILLIN-RESISTANT *STAPHYLOCOCCUS AUERUS*	
Oral options		
Antibiotic name	**Dosage and administration**	
	Adults	**Children**
Trimethoprim–sulfamethoxazole	Two double-strength tablets twice daily	Age >2 mo: 8–12 mg TMP/kg/d divided twice daily (max 320 mg TMP/d)
Clindamycin	300–450 mg three to four times daily	30–40 mg/kg/d divided three to four times daily (max 1.8 g/d)
Doxycycline	100 mg twice daily	Avoid use in children <8 y of age 2–4 mg/kg/d divided twice daily (max 200 mg/d)
Linezolid	600 mg twice daily	<12 y: 30 mg/kg/d divided three times daily ≥12 y: 20 mg/kg/d divided twice daily (max 1200 mg/d)
Intravenous options		
Clindamycin	600–900 mg every 8 h	25–40 mg/kg/d divided every 6–8 h (max 2.7 g/d)
Vancomycin	15–20 mg/kg every 12 h	15–20 mg/kg/dose every 6–8 h
Daptomycin	6 mg/kg every 24 h	Not FDA approved in children 6 mg/kg every 24 h
Linezolid	600 mg every 12 h	<12 y: 30 mg/kg/d divided every 8 h ≥12 y: 20 mg/kg/d divided every 12 h (max 1200 mg/d)
Telavancin	10 mg/kg every 24 h	Not FDA approved, insufficient data
Tigecycline[a]	100 mg × 1 dose, then 50 mg every 12 h	Not FDA approved ≥12 y: 1.5 mg/kg × 1 dose (max 100 mg), then 1 mg/kg/dose every 12 h (max 50 mg)

[a]There may be an increased risk of mortality when using tigecycline in comparison with other antibiotics when treating serious infections.

COMPLICATIONS

Poststreptococcal glomerulonephritis may rarely follow streptococcal impetigo, but acute rheumatic fever has not been reported following streptococcal impetigo.

ABSCESSES, FURUNCLES, AND CARBUNCLES

GENERAL PRINCIPLES

Classification
- Skin abscesses are purulent infections that involve the dermis and deeper cutaneous tissue.
- Furuncles ("boils") are similar to skin abscesses but involve the hair follicles with small subcutaneous abscesses.
- A carbuncle is a collection of furuncles that form a single suppurative lesion that drains through multiple hair follicles.

Epidemiology
- Skin abscesses are very common and account for more than 3 million emergency center visits each year.[6] Furuncles and carbuncles are also common.
- Outbreaks of cutaneous abscesses and furunculosis, usually caused by *S. aureus*, can occur with close contact.[1]

Etiology
- **S. aureus is the predominant cause of skin abscesses, furuncles, and carbuncles.**
  - CA-MRSA causes up to 75% of these infections in some centers.[7]
- Other organisms less frequently cause these infections, depending on environmental and host factors.
  - Lesions adjacent to a mucous membrane (perioral, vulvovaginal, or perirectal) or associated with injection drug use may be polymicrobial.
  - Furuncles may also be caused by other organisms in skin flora, including *Candida* species.
  - *Pseudomonas aeruginosa* or atypical mycobacteria are seen with a history of water exposure.

Pathophysiology
- Inoculation of bacteria through nonintact skin is the most frequent cause of skin abscesses, although bacteremic seeding of the skin can occur.
- Furuncles can result as a progression of folliculitis. These infections may occur anywhere on hairy skin, but are usually found in areas exposed to friction or maceration (e.g., neck, axilla, and buttocks).
- Carbuncles are more likely to occur in the back of the neck and lower extremities.[1]
- Panton-Valentine leukocidin, a cytotoxin causing leukocyte destruction and tissue necrosis, is found in some strains of *S. aureus* and has been associated with necrotic skin lesions.[8]

Risk Factors

- Risk factors for cutaneous MRSA infections are presented in Table 9-3.
- Conditions leading to minor breaches in the skin (intravenous or subcutaneous drug use, dermatological conditions, and abrasions).

DIAGNOSIS

Clinical Presentation

- The presence of characteristic skin lesions is generally the only complaint.
- There may be a history of skin infections in close contacts or in the patient's past history.
- Skin abscesses appear as painful, erythematous, fluctuant nodules that often have an overlying pustule.
- Furuncles have a similar appearance, with a hair emerging through the pustule.
- Carbuncles present as a fluctuant mass with purulent drainage from multiple hair follicles.
- Scarring may occur, especially after multiple recurrences.

Differential Diagnosis

- Folliculitis is more superficial and without purulent drainage.
- Hidradenitis suppurativa is similar but has a more chronic course.
- Epidermoid cysts can be confused with skin abscesses.
- Skin lesions secondary to systemic infections with *Pseudomonas*, *Aspergillus*, *Nocardia*, or *Cryptococcus* can be seen in immunocompromised patients.

Diagnostic Testing

- Culture and Gram stain are helpful, especially with changing resistance profiles of CA-MRSA.
- In appropriate settings, stains and cultures for fungi and mycobacteria may be beneficial.

TABLE 9-3	**RISK FACTORS ASSOCIATED WITH COMMUNITY-ACQUIRED METHICILLIN-RESISTANT *STAPHYLOCOCCUS AUREUS* (CA-MRSA) SKIN AND SOFT TISSUE INFECTIONS**

Household or day-care contacts of a patient with proven community-associated MRSA infection

Children

Men who have sex with men

Military personnel

Incarcerated persons

Athletes, particularly in contact sports

Native Americans or Pacific Islanders

History of MRSA infection

Intravenous drug users

Hemodialysis

TREATMENT

- **Skin abscesses, large furuncles, and carbuncles should be incised and drained.**
- **Antibiotic therapy is often not necessary.** It should be considered in patients with extensive disease, surrounding cellulitis, systemic symptoms, abscesses in areas that are difficult to drain (i.e., face), and immunocompromise.
- Therapy should be directed against *S. aureus*, including MRSA. Oral antibiotics can be used for uncomplicated cases; patients that require hospital admission should receive intravenous antibiotics (see Table 9-2 for treatment options for CA-MRSA). Antibiotic duration is based on clinical response, typically 5 to 10 days.
- Small furuncles can be treated with warm compresses.
- Education on ways to improve personal hygiene and wound care when appropriate.

SPECIAL CONSIDERATIONS

- Antibiotic prophylaxis is given prior to incision and drainage of skin and soft tissue infections in patients with underlying cardiac conditions associated with the highest risk of adverse outcome from infective endocarditis. More than 20% of patients with *S. aureus* skin infection that require incision and drainage will suffer at least one recurrence.[9]
- Recurrent skin infections are associated with *S. aureus* colonization of the nares or skin and eradication of *S. aureus* in those with positive nasal swabs may decrease infection rates. **Decolonization may be considered if patients have recurrent infection despite appropriate hygiene interventions** (see Table 9-4 for decolonization regimen).

TABLE 9-4	OUTPATIENT REGIMEN FOR ERADICATION OF NASAL CARRIAGE OF *STAPHYLOCOCCUS AUREUS*

- Careful attention to personal hygiene.

- Avoid sharing personal items (i.e., razors, soaps, lotions, linens) and discard or launder all potentially contaminated personal items midway through decolonization regimen.

- Thoroughly clean household surfaces with cleaning solution active against MRSA (i.e., bleach solution).

- Mupirocin 2% ointment applied to nares twice daily for 5–10 d.

- 4% chlorhexidine whole-body wash once daily for 5–14 d. May substitute dilute bleach baths twice weekly for 3 mo.

- Oral regimens should be reserved for cases of recurrence despite the above measures and may include oral rifampin plus trimethoprim–sulfamethoxazole or clindamycin.

CELLULITIS AND ERYSIPELAS

GENERAL PRINCIPLES

Classification
- Cellulitis involves the deeper dermis and subcutaneous fat.
- Erysipelas is a more superficial infection that involves the upper layers of the dermis and superficial lymphatics.

Epidemiology
- Cellulitis is a relatively common condition with an estimated incidence rate of 25/1,000 person-years. The incidence is greatest in the middle-aged and elderly.
- The estimated incidence of erysipelas is about 0.1/1,000 person-years. Erysipelas has a bimodal age distribution.

Etiology
- Any breakdown in the cutaneous barrier allows the entry and spread of organisms colonizing the skin surface.
- The majority of cases are caused by gram-positive bacteria, with β-hemolytic streptococci, particularly *S. pyogenes*, **accounting for about 80%.**
- *S. aureus* (both methicillin-sensitive and methicillin-resistant strains) is a common cause of cellulitis in some regions of the United States.
- Other organisms can cause cellulitis depending on host and environmental factors (see Table 9-5).

TABLE 9-5	UNUSUAL ORGANISMS IN SKIN AND SOFT TISSUE INFECTIONS	
Organism	**Clues to diagnosis**	**Other considerations**
	Water exposure	
Vibrio vulnificus	Saltwater exposure	Treatment of choice for mild infections is doxycycline
Aeromonas hydrophila	Freshwater exposure	Treatment of choice for mild infections is ciprofloxacin
Mycobacterium marinum	Saltwater or freshwater exposure Lesion begins as papule	Treatment should include two active agents (clarithromycin plus either ethambutol or rifampin is preferred) Duration of therapy is typically 3–4 mo
Streptococcus iniae	Aquaculture workers Usually localized infection of the hands	Susceptible to penicillin

Occupational exposure

Erysipelothrix rhusiopathiae	Occupational animal exposure (fishermen, butchers, veterinarians) Usually localized infection of the hands	Susceptible to penicillin

Bites and injuries

Human oral flora (peptostreptococci, *Eikenella corrodens*, Viridans streptococci)	Human bite	Treatment of choice for mild infections is amoxicillin–clavulanate
Pasteurella multocida and Capnocytophaga canimorsus	Dog or cat bite	Cat bites warrant prophylactic antibiotics due to high rate of infection Treatment of choice is amoxicillin–clavulanate
Clostridium tetani	Devitalized tissue (e.g., crush injury) wound contamination with soil or rust	Can progress to generalized tetanus characterized most often by trismus ("lockjaw"). Age-appropriate tetanus vaccine should be given if ≥10 y since last vaccine in minor, clean wounds or if ≥5 y since last vaccine for all other wounds. Tetanus immunoglobulin should be given to patients with unknown or incomplete vaccination status in all but minor, clean wounds

Immunosuppression

Cryptococcus neoformans	Impairment of cell-mediated immunity	Represents disseminated disease, fluconazole is treatment of choice
Helicobacter cinaedi	HIV infection; multifocal cellulitis	Represents disseminated infection with bacteremia, treatment is not well defined

Risk Factors

- Surgical incisions, trauma, ulcerations, inflammatory dermatoses, and fissures secondary to tinea pedis are common predisposing skin disruptions.[10,11]
- Obesity, venous insufficiency, disruption of lymphatic drainage, and other conditions that cause chronic edema increase the risk of skin infection and may contribute to recurrent disease.
- Risk factors for CA-MRSA infections are outlined in Table 9-3.

DIAGNOSIS

Clinical Presentation

History

- Both cellulitis and erysipelas present as a **spreading area of cutaneous erythema, warmth, edema, and pain**.
- Systemic symptoms, such as fever and chills, are more common with erysipelas.
- Careful assessment of risk factors for unusual pathogens or CA-MRSA (see Tables 9-3 and 9-5) should be performed.

Physical Exam

- Both infections mainly occur on the lower extremities, although any body site may be affected. Erysipelas has been associated with a butterfly distribution on the face.
- They present as areas of skin warmth, edema, and erythema without an underlying focus of infection.
- Erysipelas appears as a raised lesion with clearly demarcated borders, while the borders in cellulitis are less distinct.[1]
- Skin may have an orange peel appearance (peau d'orange) due to superficial edema surrounding tethered hair follicles. There may be associated lymphangitis.
- Vesicles, bullae, petechiae, and ecchymoses may also occur.

Differential Diagnosis

- Differentiation from necrotizing fasciitis (NF) is essential (see Section "Necrotizing Fasciitis").
- Deeper foci of infection, such as osteomyelitis, septic arthritis, and bursitis, may present with overlying cutaneous inflammation.
- Herpes zoster, erythema migrans, and viral exanthems may present with erythema.
- Cutaneous malignancies, contact dermatitis, insect bites, gout, drug reactions, vasculitis, thrombophlebitis, and lipodermatosclerosis may mimic the appearance of cellulitis.

Diagnostic Testing

- Signs of inflammation such as elevated white blood cell (WBC) count or elevated erythrocyte sedimentation rate and C-reactive protein (CRP) may be present.
- Blood cultures are positive in <5% of cases and are usually performed only when signs of systemic toxicity are present.
- Cultures of intact skin are usually not helpful, but cultures of purulent discharge, unroofed vesicles, or bullae may be beneficial in cases where unusual or drug-resistant pathogens are suspected.

TREATMENT

Oral antibiotics are appropriate in mild infection, but intravenous administration should be used in patients with systemic symptoms or those that cannot tolerate oral intake (see Table 9-1 or Table 9-2).

Erysipelas

- If there is any uncertainty regarding the diagnosis, the patient should be treated as per the cellulitis recommendations.
- **Since the majority of cases of erysipelas are caused by streptococci, penicillin or amoxicillin remains the treatment of choice.**
  - ○ Patients with penicillin allergy may be treated with cephalosporins, in the absence of severe reactions, or clindamycin.
  - ○ If suspicion of *S. aureus* is high, an antistaphylococcal penicillin (i.e., dicloxacillin) or first-generation cephalosporin (i.e., cephalexin) should be used.

Cellulitis

- Empiric therapy should be directed toward β-hemolytic streptococci and *S. aureus*.
  - ○ Appropriate oral options include **dicloxacillin, amoxicillin/clavulanate, or cephalexin**. Clindamycin may be used in patients with severe β-lactam allergies.
  - ○ Parental antibiotic options include oxacillin or cefazolin. Clindamycin or vancomycin may be used in patients with severe β-lactam allergies.
- Patients with risk factors for MRSA infections (Table 9-3), from a community with a prevalence of MRSA >30%, with evidence of systemic toxicity, or with failure to respond to treatment should be treated with empiric antimicrobials effective against MRSA (see Table 9-2).
  - ○ Vancomycin is the most appropriate initial intravenous agent. Daptomycin, linezolid, and telavancin can be considered in patients unable to tolerate vancomycin or with a known history of vancomycin-intermediate or vancomycin-resistant *S. aureus*. Clindamycin may also be considered if the cellulitis is community acquired and the local resistance rates among CA-MRSA strains are low.
  - ○ Linezolid is an appropriate choice for oral therapy. Clindamycin may also be given orally if local resistance rates are low. Trimethoprim–sulfamethoxazole should be avoided unless it is certain that the infection is not due to streptococci.
- Treatment duration should be based on clinical response. Uncomplicated cases require only a 5-day course of antibiotic treatment[1]; however, longer treatment durations, usually 7 to 14 days, are necessary for complicated infections or those caused by drug-resistant pathogens such as MRSA.
- Patients with clinical presentations or risk factors for more unusual pathogens (Table 9-5) should be treated with empiric therapy directed toward these organisms.
- Elevation of the affected area reduces edema and may prevent lymphedema.[1]
- Treatment of underlying conditions (edema, ulcerations, dermatoses, and tinea infection) will reduce the risk of recurrence.[1]

COMPLICATIONS

- Acute complications include thrombophlebitis, NF, abscess formation, bacteremia, and toxic shock syndrome (TSS).
- Symptoms usually worsen in the first 24 hours of treatment due to exacerbation of inflammation.

OUTCOME/PROGNOSIS

- Most cases of cellulitis and erysipelas resolve with treatment.
- Recurrence is common, occurring in 15% to 30% of patients.
- Recurrent episodes of cellulitis can lead to cumulative lymphatic damage and lymphedema.

NECROTIZING FASCIITIS

GENERAL PRINCIPLES

Definition
NF is a life-threatening infection characterized by necrosis of the subcutaneous tissues with progression along superficial and deep fascia.[12]

Epidemiology
- NF is rare, occurring in less than 0.5 per 100,000 population.
- **NF type 1** is often associated with surgical wounds in immunocompromised patients.
- **NF type 2** is usually a spontaneous CA infection that may occur in healthy individuals.

Etiology
- **In NF type 1, an average of five organisms are involved**, including mixed obligate anaerobes (*Bacteroides* or *Peptostreptococcus*), facultative anaerobes (streptococcal species or *S. aureus*), and aerobic coliforms (*Escherichia coli* or *Klebsiella*).[1]
- **NF type 2 is usually due to *S. pyogenes***, but mixed infection with *S. pyogenes* and *S. aureus* has been reported. *S. aureus* (MRSA), *Vibrio vulnificus*, *Aeromonas hydrophila*, and other streptococci have also been reported in patients with risk factors for these organisms.[1]

Pathophysiology
- NF type 1 occurs following surgery, dental disease or oral trauma (cervical NF), urethral or lower gastrointestinal (GI) trauma (Fournier gangrene), or decubitus or lower extremity ulcerations.
- NF type 2 results from infection of a minor skin lesion, but 20% of cases have no apparent skin breakdown.
  - Once *S. pyogenes* gains access to deep tissues, secreted proteases degrade extracellular matrix.
  - Streptococcal virulence proteins prevent phagocytosis, inhibit neutrophil function, and cause neutrophil apoptosis.
  - Production of superantigens results in excessive immune response and triggers release of cytokines, leading to severe tissue damage, ischemia, and shock.
  - This necrotizing process spreads along superficial facial planes, causing a rapidly progressive and severe illness.

Risk Factors
- NF type 1 is most frequently associated with surgical procedure or trauma.
- NF type 2 may be associated with diabetes or peripheral vascular disease, but can occur as a sequelae of varicella or trauma.

DIAGNOSIS

Clinical Presentation
- NF is an infectious disease and surgical emergency, and early diagnosis is crucial.
- NF can be difficult to differentiate from cellulitis or other soft tissue infections, but several characteristic features should cause the clinician to consider the diagnosis.
  - Pain out of proportion to physical findings
  - Induration that extends beyond the area of visual skin involvement
  - Crepitus or subcutaneous gas
  - Rapid progression of skin findings
  - Systemic toxicity out of proportion to clinical findings
  - Failure to respond to appropriate medical therapy
- Patients may complain of exquisite pain early in the course of illness. This is followed by anesthesia as NF progresses.
- Findings may initially be quite subtle or indistinguishable from cellulitis. A dusky appearance to the skin, the presence of bullae, and/or crepitus are relatively specific findings for NF.

Differential Diagnosis
NF is most commonly mistaken for cellulitis, clostridial myonecrosis (CM), or pyomyositis.

Diagnostic Testing
- The Laboratory Risk Indicator for Necrotizing Fasciitis (LRINEC) includes several common laboratory findings. When severe skin infection is present, a score of ≥6 has a positive predictive value of 92% for NF.[13]
  - Elevated CRP >150 mg/L (4 points)
  - Leukocytosis with WBCs 15,000 to 25,000/mm³ (1 point) or >25,000/mm³ (2 points)
  - Anemia with hemoglobin 11 to 13.5 g/dL (1 point) or <11 g/dL (2 points)
  - Hyponatremia with Na <135 mmol/L (2 points)
  - Renal insufficiency with serum creatinine >1.6 mg/dL (2 points)
  - Serum glucose >180 mg/dL (1 point)
- Blood cultures are positive in 60% of cases of NF type 2, but are only positive in 20% of NF type 1 cases.
- Intraoperative cultures are most reliable and should be used to guide antibiotic therapy.
- Soft tissue plain radiographs, CT, or MRI may show subcutaneous gas or fascial edema.

TREATMENT

- **Treatment is both surgical and medical and should proceed rapidly**.
- Early surgical intervention with aggressive debridement is crucial and has been shown to decrease mortality.[1,14]
- Repeat evaluation in the operating room 24 to 36 hours after the initial debridement and daily thereafter until debridement is complete is usually required.[1]
- **Broad-spectrum antibiotics** should be initially directed at the likely causative organisms and modified as Gram stain and culture data are available.[1,14]

- NF type 1 should be treated with broad-spectrum antibiotics. These include carbapenems (meropenem), extended-spectrum penicillins with a β-lactamase inhibitor (piperacillin–tazobactam), or cefepime in combination with metronidazole (see Table 9-1).
- NF type 2 should be treated with vancomycin plus clindamycin (see Table 9-1 or Table 9-2). The clindamycin is used to inhibit toxin production. If the infection is due to *S. pyogenes*, therapy may be narrowed to penicillin and clindamycin.

OUTCOME/PROGNOSIS

- Mortality remains >20% and can approach 50% when associated with TSS.[15,16]
- Morbidity, including disfigurement and limb loss, is common even with appropriate intervention.

PYOMYOSITIS

GENERAL PRINCIPLES

- Pyomyositis is a suppurative infection of the skeletal muscle.
- In tropical regions, pyomyositis is most common in otherwise healthy young children and adults.
- Pyomyositis in temperate regions is generally a disease of immunocompromised young adults.[1]
- *S. aureus* is the most common cause, accounting for over 90% of tropical cases and 70% of temperate cases. MRSA is emerging as a common pathogen.[17]
  - *S. pyogenes* is second, followed by other streptococci, enteric gram-negative bacilli, or polymicrobial infections. *Bartonella*, mycobacteria, or anaerobes are rare causes.[17]
- Seeding of the skeletal muscle occurs during an episode of bacteremia.
- Muscle trauma, which may be clinically unapparent, forms a nidus for infection and abscess formation.
- **Around 50% of patients with pyomyositis in temperate areas have an underlying medical condition**, including HIV, diabetes mellitus, rheumatologic diseases, malignancies, or other immunocompromised states.[17]
- **About 50% of patients have a known history of trauma.** Strenuous exercise may lead to pyomyositis in young athletes.

DIAGNOSIS

Clinical Presentation
- Localized pain, swelling, and cramping in the involved muscle group.
- Systemic symptoms, such as fever and chills, are common.
- The lower extremity muscles, especially the thigh, are most commonly involved, but chest, abdominal, and gluteal muscle involvement has been reported.[17]

- Multiple muscle groups are infected in up to 20% of cases.
- Superficial signs of inflammation on exam may not be initially present.
- The overlying area is often indurated and has a woody or brawny appearance.

Differential Diagnosis

The differential diagnosis includes muscle hematoma, osteomyelitis, severe cellulitis, NF, neoplasms, deep vein thrombosis, and muscle strains.

Diagnostic Testing

Laboratories

- Although pyomyositis is an infection of skeletal muscle, creatine kinase levels are often normal or only mildly elevated.[17]
- Blood cultures are positive in up to 30% of cases.[1]
- *S. aureus* pyomyositis should prompt an evaluation for endocarditis.

Imaging

- Ultrasound (US) may show hyperechogenicity due to muscle edema and hypoechogenicity from muscle necrosis.
- CT can detect muscle edema and rim-enhancing fluid collections indicative of abscesses.
- MRI is most sensitive in early infections and helps localize and identify the extent of muscle damage.[18]

Diagnostic Procedures

- Cultures should be obtained under US or CT guidance prior to antibiotic administration when possible.
- Intraoperative specimens should also be sent for culture and antibiotic susceptibilities.

TREATMENT

- Drainage by interventional radiology, or surgical drainage and debridement, is essential.
- For immunocompetent patients, empiric antibiotic therapy with vancomycin (see Table 9-1) is an effective therapy for both MRSA and *S. pyogenes* (see Table 9-2 for alternative treatments of MRSA).
- Immunocompromised patients should receive vancomycin in combination with other broad-spectrum antibiotics such as meropenem or piperacillin–tazobactam (see Table 9-1).
- Antibiotic therapy should be adjusted as culture results become available.
- Duration of therapy should be guided by clinical response, but is generally 3 to 4 weeks in the absence of endocarditis or osteomyelitis.

COMPLICATIONS

- Endocarditis or osteomyelitis may be present secondary to bacteremia.
- Compartment syndrome requiring fasciotomy may occur.

CLOSTRIDIAL MYONECROSIS

GENERAL PRINCIPLES

Definition

- CM is a necrotizing infection of the skeletal muscle secondary to *Clostridium*. It is also commonly known as "gas gangrene."[1,19]
- It can be spontaneous or traumatic, including postsurgical.

Epidemiology

- Traumatic CM occurs in wounds complicated by compromised vascular supply.
- Spontaneous CM is usually seen in patients with neutropenia or GI malignancy.[1]

Etiology

- *Clostridium* species are anaerobic, gram-positive, spore-forming bacilli that are found in the soil and human GI tract.
- Traumatic CM is most frequently caused by *Clostridium perfringens.*
- Spontaneous CM is usually caused by *Clostridium septicum.*[1]

Pathophysiology

- Inoculation of *Clostridium* into deep tissue via crush injuries, knife lesions, or gunshot wounds that have created an anaerobic environment (caused by interruption of vascular supply) leads to traumatic CM.
- Spontaneous CM results when disruption in the GI mucosa allows *Clostridium* to spread hematogenously and seed the muscle.
- Once the muscle is seeded, infection proceeds very rapidly, sometimes in less than 24 hours.
- Clostridia cause this disease through the production of at least 10 different exotoxins, although the α-toxin is the most important. α-toxin hydrolyzes cell membranes and leads to tissue necrosis, hemolysis, platelet aggregation, and leukocyte inactivation. α-toxin also has a direct cardiodepressive effect that causes profound shock.[19,20]

Risk Factors

- Peripartum complications (i.e., abortion, retained placenta, prolonged rupture of membranes, and retained fetal tissue), subcutaneous drug injection ("skin popping"), surgery of the GI tract, and intramuscular injections are all risk factors.
- Spontaneous CM not only occurs with GI malignancy, but also occurs in immunocompromised patients (e.g., neutropenia and hematological malignancy).

DIAGNOSIS

Clinical Presentation

- Traumatic CM should be suspected in cases of severe pain at the site of the surgical incision or trauma within 24 hours of the event accompanied by signs of systemic toxicity.
- Spontaneous CM should be suspected in cases of abrupt onset of muscle pain and signs of systemic toxicity in the setting of known immunocompromise or GI disease, although these may not be immediately apparent.

- Overlying skin may initially appear pale, followed by a violaceous or erythematous discoloration and bullae.
- The area is extremely tender to palpation and underlying crepitus may be present.
- Patients may progress rapidly to severe shock.

Differential Diagnosis

- NF or pyomyositis can mimic CM.
- Spontaneous CM may be confused initially with muscle strain, injury, or other conditions leading to myalgia, such as influenza.

Diagnostic Testing

- Complete blood count and complete metabolic panel may show leukocytosis and signs of multiorgan failure including coagulopathy, hemolytic anemia, and renal and liver failure. The hemolytic anemia can be severe and recalcitrant to transfusion.
- Blood cultures are positive for *C. perfringens* in about 15% of cases of traumatic CM.
- Large, gram-variable rods may be recovered from wounds, bullae, and surgical samples.
- Plain films, CT scan, or MRI may demonstrate gas within tissue.

TREATMENT

- **Immediate surgical consultation should be sought when CM is suspected**.
- Early surgical debridement, antibiotics, and intensive supportive measures are required.
- Surgical intervention is often needed for definitive diagnosis and emergent treatment.
  - Necrotic, edematous, pale/gray muscle tissue that does not bleed or contract is often seen at the time of surgery.
  - There is usually an obvious release of gas upon surgically entering the infected muscle.
  - Pathology reveals gas, cell lysis, and absent inflammation.
- Multiple repeated debridements are often necessary.
- The recommended antibiotic regimen is **penicillin and clindamycin** (see Table 9-1). Infection due to *Clostridium tertium* is treated with vancomycin or metronidazole.
- Patients should be monitored in the intensive care unit with aggressive treatment of shock and multiorgan failure when indicated.
- The role of hyperbaric oxygen remains controversial.[1]

COMPLICATIONS

- Patients can progress quickly to septic shock and multiorgan failure.
- Intravascular hemolysis in the setting of CM can be severe and requires transfusion support.

OUTCOME/PROGNOSIS

- Mortality rates are extremely high for spontaneous CM (67% to 100%). Survivors should be evaluated for GI malignancy.[21,22]
- Mortality for traumatic CM is roughly 20%.[23]

SURGICAL SITE INFECTIONS

GENERAL PRINCLPLES

Definition
Surgical site infections (SSIs) are defined as the occurrence of infection at or near the site of a surgical procedure within 30 days or 1 year if a prosthesis is left in place.[17]

Classification
- SSIs are divided into categories based on the infected organ system, body space, or depth of tissue involvement.
- Superficial infections involve the skin or subcutaneous tissue and deep infections involve the deep soft tissues, muscle, or fascia.

Epidemiology
- SSIs account for 17% of all nosocomial infections.[24]
- Around 3% of patients undergoing surgery will develop an SSI.[1]
- SSIs increase the average cost of the hospital stay by $3,000 to $30,000 per case.[25]

Etiology
- *S. aureus*, including MRSA, coagulase-negative staphylococci, enterococci, enteric gram-negative bacilli, and *Pseudomonas* account for the majority of SSIs.[26]
- Multidrug-resistant organisms are common since infections are usually acquired in the hospital setting.[27]
- SSIs that are clinically evident within 48 hours after the procedure are usually due to *S. pyogenes* or *Clostridium* species.[1]
- Procedure site:
  - Genitourinary or GI tract SSIs are often caused by mixed aerobic and anaerobic organisms.
  - Axillary SSIs have a higher rate of gram-negative organisms.
  - Perineal SSIs are usually due to gram-negative organisms and anaerobes.
  - Head and neck SSIs are often caused by oral flora.

Pathophysiology
- SSIs can result from endogenous flora in proximity to the surgical incision, seeding from a distant focus of infection, or exogenous exposures (hands of medical personnel, surgical attire, operative equipment, or aerosolized via the ventilation system).
- Organisms gain access to deep tissues due to breach in the usual anatomic barriers, either through direct inoculation at the time of surgery or postoperatively.
- SSIs may lead to failure of wound healing, dehiscence, and increased scar formation.

Risk Factors
- Patient risk factors include older age, diabetes, poor nutritional status, smoking, obesity, preexisting infection at another body site, colonization with pathogens such as *S. aureus*, immunosuppression, and prolonged preoperative hospital stay.
- Procedure-related factors include longer procedure duration, presence of foreign bodies, contamination of the wound, and inappropriate preparatory measures (prophylactic antibiotic choice, skin preparation, sterilization of equipment, and scrub duration).
- The type of procedure also has a significant impact on the likelihood of SSI, with abdominal procedures carrying the greatest risk.

- The Center for Disease Control and Prevention's (CDC) National Healthcare Safety Network surgical patient risk index incorporates the anesthesiologist preoperative assessment score, cleanliness of the wound, and procedure duration to classify patients into different risk levels for SSIs.[28]

DIAGNOSIS

Clinical Presentation

- With the exception of infection due to *S. pyogenes* or *Clostridium* species, SSIs usually do not become clinically evident until at least 5 days after the operation, with 14 days being typical.[1]
- Exam of the incision usually shows tenderness, swelling, erythema, and purulent drainage.

Diagnostic Criteria

According to the CDC guidelines,[1] superficial SSIs must meet one of the following criteria:

- Purulent drainage from the surgical site
- Organisms isolated from an aseptically obtained culture of fluid or tissue from the incision site or spontaneous dehiscence of a deep incision
- Local signs of infection (pain, edema, erythema, or warmth) in superficial SSIs or the presence of an abscess in deep infections
- Diagnosis of the SSI by the surgeon or attending physician (although practically, the diagnosis is made by a wide variety of health care professionals)

Differential Diagnosis

Organ/space infection should be suspected if superficial SSIs fail to improve despite adequate treatment.

Diagnostic Testing

- Gram stain of drainage is helpful with suspected infection <48 hours after surgery in order to identify clostridial or streptococcal species.
- Infected surgical sites should be cultured.

TREATMENT

- Early surgical intervention to open the infected wound and to debride necrotic tissue is the hallmark of treatment.
- The role of antibiotics is controversial in patients with minimal signs of systemic toxicity and less impressive wound findings.
- In patients with superficial SSI and fever, tachycardia, >5 cm of erythema surrounding wound, or any wound necrosis, a short course of antibiotics is indicated.[1]
- In deep tissue or organ/space SSIs, choice of empiric therapy and duration of treatment should be guided by the location of the infection and adequacy of the surgical debridement/drainage.
  - Empiric therapy to cover MRSA and streptococcal species with vancomycin (see Table 9-1 or Table 9-2) is reasonable for cases where gram-negative and anaerobic organisms are not suspected.

- ○ Piperacillin–tazobactam, meropenem, or cefepime plus metronidazole may be used when gram-negative and anaerobic treatment is warranted.
- ○ Antibiotic choice should be modified as Gram stain and culture results become available.

OUTCOME/PROGNOSIS

- Significant morbidity can occur if incision does not heal promptly.
- Deep space and organ infections carry higher morbidity and mortality.

TOXIC SHOCK SYNDROME

GENERAL PRINCLPLES

Definition

TSS is a bacterial toxin–mediated illness characterized by acute onset of fever, hypotension, and multiorgan failure.[29]

Classification

TSS is classified based on the causal organism: staphylococcal TSS, which may be menstrual or nonmenstrual, and streptococcal TSS.

Epidemiology

- The overall incidence of staphylococcal TSS is estimated to be 1 to 3.4 per 100,000 women.
  - ○ 90% of staphylococcal TSS cases occur in women, with roughly half of these being associated with menstruation.
  - ○ The incidence of menstrual-associated staphylococcal TSS has significantly declined since the mid-1980s when most super-absorbency tampons were removed from the market.
- Invasive streptococcal diseases occur in an estimated 5 cases per 100,000 patients per year and up to 15% of these patients will develop streptococcal TSS.
- Half of the patients with NF will have associated TSS.

Etiology

- The majority of cases of staphylococcal TSS are caused by methicillin-sensitive strains of *S. aureus*. There are several case reports of TSS due to MRSA.
- Streptococcal TSS is caused by *S. pyogenes*.

Pathophysiology

- Bacterial superantigen production is a crucial component of the pathogenesis. Superantigens bind directly to MHC class II molecules and to T-cell receptors, which trigger excessive **unregulated T-cell activation** in which up to 30% of T cells begin releasing cytokines. This results in an **exaggerated systemic inflammatory response** that causes shock and multiorgan failure.[29]

○ Menstrual staphylococcal TSS occurs due to vaginal colonization with a toxin-producing strain of *S. aureus*. **TSS toxin 1** (TSST1) is the superantigen in these cases and is capable of crossing mucosal barriers.

○ Nonmenstrual staphylococcal TSS occurs when a toxin-producing *S. aureus* infects a wound or colonizes another mucosal surface. Only about 50% of non-menstrual cases are caused by organisms that produce TSST1. **Staphylococcal enterotoxin B** can act as an alternative superantigen in TSST1-negative strains.

○ Streptococcal TSS is usually associated with invasive diseases such as cellulitis, NF, or pyomyositis. *S. pyogenes* produces multiple virulence proteins that may function as superantigens, such as **streptococcal pyrogenic exotoxins** (SpeA, SpeB).

Risk Factors

- High-absorbency tampons for menstrual staphylococcal TSS
- Disruption of skin or mucous membranes (abscess, surgical procedures, and burns) in patients colonized or infected with the toxin-producing strains of *S. aureus*
- Trauma, surgery, older age, chronic illness, varicella infection, and nonsteroidal antiinflammatory use predispose patients to invasive streptococcal disease

DIAGNOSIS

Clinical Presentation

History
- Patients with TSS may present with an acute influenza-like illness that rapidly progresses to shock and multiorgan failure within 8 to 12 hours after symptom onset.
- A history of menstruation with tampon use suggests staphylococcal TSS.
- Patients may report a history of trauma or severe pain at the site of infection that can mimic peritonitis or myocardial infarction.

Physical Exam
- Tachycardia, respiratory distress, petechiae, ecchymoses, or jaundice may appear shortly after initial presentation.
- The rash associated with TSS is a **diffuse macular erythema** that may resemble sunburn. It often involves both the skin and mucous membranes, includes the palms and soles, and may be transitory.
- Female patients should undergo vaginal exam, which may reveal hyperemia. Tampons or other foreign bodies should be removed.
- Patients with streptococcal TSS will often have an identifiable focus on exam.

Diagnostic Criteria
- Diagnostic criteria for staphylococcal TSS are presented in Table 9-6.
- Diagnostic criteria for streptococcal TSS are presented in Table 9-7.

TABLE 9-6	DIAGNOSTIC CRITERIA FOR STAPHYLOCOCCAL TOXIC SHOCK SYNDROME

1. Fever: ≥38.9°C (°F)

2. Rash: diffuse macular erythroderma

3. Desquamation: occurs 1–2 wk after onset of illness, especially palms and soles

4. Hypotension: systolic blood pressure (BP) ≤90 mm Hg, orthostatic decrease in diastolic BP ≥15 mmHg

5. Multisystem involvement (≥3 systems):

   a. Gastrointestinal: vomiting or diarrhea

   b. Muscular: severe myalgia or creatine kinase >2× normal

   c. Mucous membranes: vaginal, oropharyngeal, conjunctival hyperemia

   d. Renal: BUN or creatinine >2× normal, pyuria

   e. Hepatic: total bilirubin >2× normal

   f. Hematological: platelets ≤100,000/μL

   g. CNS: disorientation or alteration of consciousness without focal neurological signs

6. Negative results of blood, throat, or CSF cultures (blood cultures may be *Staphylococcus aureus* positive) and no rise in antibody titers against *Rickettsia rickettsii, Leptospira* spp., and rubeola

Confirmed case satisfies all six criteria.

Probable case satisfies five of six criteria.

BUN, blood urea nitrogen; CNS, central nervous system; CSF, cerebrospinal fluid.

TABLE 9-7	DIAGNOSTIC CRITERIA FOR STREPTOCOCCAL TOXIC SHOCK SYNDROME

1. Hypotension: systolic blood pressure ≤90 mm Hg

2. Two or more of the following:

   a. Renal impairment: creatinine ≥2 mg/dL

   b. Coagulopathy: platelets ≤100,000/μL or disseminated intravascular coagulation

   c. Hepatic involvement: transaminases or bilirubin >2× normal

   d. Generalized, erythematous, macular rash that may desquamate

   e. Adult respiratory distress syndrome

   f. Soft tissue necrosis (necrotizing fasciitis, pyomyositis)

Confirmed case includes isolation of *Streptococcus pyogenes* from a normally sterile site (blood, cerebrospinal fluid, peritoneal fluid, and tissue biopsy) in addition to satisfying both criteria.

Probable case includes isolation of *S. pyogenes* from a nonsterile site (throat, skin, and vagina) in addition to satisfying both criteria.

Differential Diagnosis

The differential for TSS is broad and includes systemic infections such as gram-negative sepsis (including meningococcemia), Rocky Mountain spotted fever, and leptospirosis in previously healthy individuals.

Diagnostic Testing

- Blood cultures are positive in <5% of cases of staphylococcal TSS, but are positive in roughly 60% of cases of streptococcal TSS.
- Mucosal or wound cultures are positive in up to 90% of patients with staphylococcal TSS.
- Laboratory studies will show signs of multiorgan failure (see Tables 9-6 and 9-7).

TREATMENT

- Staphylococcal and streptococcal TSS should be treated with an appropriate **cell wall–acting antibiotic in combination with clindamycin**.
- Empiric choice of cell wall–acting antibiotic for staphylococcal TSS should include an agent that is effective against MRSA.
  - **Vancomycin** is the typical first-line choice, but linezolid, daptomycin, and telavancin are possible alternatives (see Table 9-2).
  - If *S. aureus* is found to be methicillin sensitive, the patient should be treated with **oxacillin or nafcillin**.
  - **Penicillin** is the most appropriate cell wall–acting antibiotic for the treatment of streptococcal TSS (see Table 9-1).
- Since clindamycin binds to the 50S ribosomal subunits and prevents peptide bond formation, it is used to halt toxin production and arrest disease progression. In cases where clindamycin cannot be used, linezolid is an alternative that also arrests toxin production in vitro.
- **Intravenous immunoglobulin** (IVIG) may be considered for the treatment of both streptococcal and staphylococcal TSS with consideration of the following:
  - IVIG contains neutralizing antibodies against many of the superantigens implicated in causing both syndromes.
  - Studies have failed to show statistically significant improvement in patients treated with IVIG due to small samples sizes, but it is generally used, especially if patients are not responding to therapy.[29-31]
- Duration of antibiotic treatment is usually at least 14 days, but depends on clinical response, the presence or absence of a focus of infection, and associated bacteremia.
- **Extensive fluid resuscitation is often required**.
- Vasopressors and mechanical ventilation may also be necessary.
- Aggressive debridement of any focus of infection, including SSIs, is important.
- Multiorgan failure is common (see Tables 9-6 and 9-7).

OUTCOME/PROGNOSIS

- Menstrual staphylococcal TSS has the best prognosis with a mortality rate of less than 2%.[32]
- Nonmenstrual staphylococcal TSS has a mortality rate of up to 5%.[32]
- The mortality rate for streptococcal TSS remains high, approximately 40% to 60%.[16,33,34]
- Recurrences of TSS are possible and can occur in one-third of patients with menstrual TSS. Recurrent episodes tend to be less severe.

REFERENCES

1. Stevens DL, Bisno AL, Chambers HF, et al. Practice guidelines for the diagnosis and management of skin and soft tissue infections. *Clin Infect Dis.* 2005;41:1373-1406.
2. Rørtveit S, Rørtveit G. Impetigo in epidemic and nonepidemic phases: an incidence study over 4(½) years in a general population. *Br J Dermatol.* 2007;157:100-105.
3. Durupt F, Mayor L, Bes M, et al. Prevalence of *Staphylococcus aureus* toxins and nasal carriage in furuncles and impetigo. *Br J Dermatol.* 2007;157:1161-1167.
4. Tristan A, Bes M, Meugnier H, et al. Global distribution of Panton-Valentine leukocidin-positive methicillin-resistant *Staphylococcus aureus,* 2006. *Emerg Infect Dis.* 2007;13:594-600.
5. Oranje AP, Chosidow O, Sacchidanand S, et al. Topical retapamulin ointment, 1%, versus sodium fusidate ointment, 2%, for impetigo: a randomized, observer-blinded, noninferiority study. *Dermatology.* 2007;215:331-340.
6. Taira BR, Singer AJ, Thode HC Jr, Lee CC. National epidemiology of cutaneous abscesses: 1996 to 2005. *Am J Emerg Med.* 2009;27:289-292.
7. Moran GJ, Krishnadasan A, Gorwitz RJ, et al. Methicillin-resistant *S. aureus* infections among patients in the emergency department. *N Engl J Med.* 2006;355:666-674.
8. Lina G, Piémont Y, Godail-Gamot F, et al. Involvement of Panton-Valentine leukocidin-producing *Staphylococcus aureus* in primary skin infections and pneumonia. *Clin Infect Dis.* 1999;29:1128-1132.
9. Liu C, Bayer A, Cosgrove SE, et al. Clinical practice guidelines by the Infectious Diseases Society of America for the treatment of methicillin-resistant *Staphylococcus aureus* infections in adults and children: executive summary. *Clin Infect Dis.* 2011;52:285-292.
10. Björnsdóttir S, Gottfredsson M, Thórisdóttir AS, et al. Risk factors for acute cellulitis of the lower limb: a prospective case-control study. *Clin Infect Dis.* 2005;41:1416-1422.
11. Dupuy A, Benchikhi H, Roujeau J-C, et al. Risk factors for erysipelas of the leg (cellulitis): case-control study. *Br Med J.* 1999;318:1591-1594.
12. Brook I, Frazier EH. Clinical and microbiological features of necrotizing fasciitis. *J Clin Microbiol.* 1995;33:2382-2387.
13. Wong CH, Khin LW. Clinical relevance of the LRINEC (Laboratory Risk Indicator for Necrotizing Fasciitis) score for assessment of early necrotizing fasciitis. *Crit Care Med.* 2005;33:1677.
14. Anaya DA, Dellinger EP. Clinical practices: necrotizing soft-tissue infection: diagnosis and management. *Clin Infect Dis.* 2007;44:705-710.
15. Wong CH, Chang HC, Pasupathy S, et al. Necrotizing fasciitis: clinical presentation, microbiology, and determinants of mortality. *J Bone Joint Surg Am.* 2003:85-A:1454-1460.
16. Darenberg J, Luca-Harari G, Jasir A, et al. Molecular and clinical characteristics of invasive group A streptococcal infection in Sweden. *Clin Infect Dis.* 2007;45:450-488.
17. Crum NF. Bacterial pyomyositis in the United States. *Am J Med.* 2004;117:420-428.
18. Turecki MB, Taljanovic MS, Stubbs AY, et al. Imaging of musculoskeletal soft tissue infections. *Skeletal Radiol.* 2010;39:957-971.
19. Stevens DL, Bryant AE. The role of clostridial toxins in the pathogenesis of gas gangrene. *Clin Infect Dis.* 2002;35:S93-S100.
20. Sakurai J, Nagahama M, Oda M. *Clostridium perfringens* alpha-toxin: characterization and mode of action. *J Biochem.* 2004;136:569-574.
21. Nordkild P, Crone P. Spontaneous clostridial myonecrosis. A collective review and report of a case. *Ann Chir Gynaecol.* 1986;75:274-279.
22. Bodey GP, Rodriquez S, Fainstein V, Elting LS. *Cancer.* 1991;67:1928-1942.
23. Hart GB, Lamb RC, Strauss MB. Gas gangrene. *J Trauma.* 1983;23:991-1000.
24. Perencevich EN, Sands KE, Cosgrove SE, et al. Health and economic impact of surgical site infections diagnosed after hospital discharge. *Emerg Infect Dis.* 2003;9:196-203.
25. Urban JA. Cost analysis of surgical site infections. *Surg Infect.* 2006;7:S19-S22.

26. Mangram AJ, Horan TC, Pearson ML, et al. Guideline for prevention of surgical site infection, 1999. Hospital Practice Advisory Committee. *Infect Control Hosp Epidemiol.* 1999;20:250-278.

27. Hidron AI, Edwards JR, Patel J, et al. NHSN annual update: antimicrobial-resistant pathogens associated with healthcare-associated infections: annual summary of data reported to the Nation Healthcare Safety Network at the Centers for Disease Control and Prevention, 2006–2007. *Infect Control Hosp Epidemiol.* 2008;29:996-1011.

28. Haley R, Culver DH, Morgan WM, et al. Identifying patients at high risk of surgical wound infection. A simple multivariate index of patient susceptibility and wound contamination. *Am J Epidemiol.* 1985;121:206-215.

29. Lappin E, Ferguson AJ. Gram-positive toxic shock syndromes. *Lancet Infect Dis.* 2009;9:281-290.

30. Darenberg J, Ihendyane N, Sjölin J, et al. Intravenous immunoglobulin G therapy in streptococcal toxic shock syndrome: a European randomized, double-blind, placebo-controlled trial. *Clin Infect Dis.* 2003;37:333-340.

31. Shah SS, Hall M, Srivastava R, et al. Intravenous immunoglobulin in children with streptococcal toxic shock syndrome. *Clin Infect Dis.* 2009;49:1369-1376.

32. Hajjeh RA, Reingold A, Weil A, et al. Toxic shock syndrome in the United States: surveillance update, 1979–1996. *Emerg Infect Dis.* 1999;5:807-810.

33. Hasegawa T, Hashikawa SN, Nakamura T, et al. Factors determining prognosis in streptococcal toxic shock-like syndrome: results of a nationwide investigation in Japan. *Microbes Infect.* 2004;6:1073-1077.

34. Ekelund K, Skinhøj P, Madsen J, Konradsen HB. Reemergence of emm1 and a changed superantigen profile for group A streptococci causing invasive infections: results from a nationwide study. *J Clin Microbiol.* 2005;43:1789-1796.

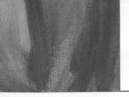

Central Nervous System Infections

10

Susana Lazarte and Robyn S. Klein

- Central nervous system (CNS) infections can be associated with high morbidity and mortality. A high level of suspicion is necessary to diagnose and treat them as soon as possible.
- The clinical presentation depends on the CNS compartment involved and the pathogen. Infection should be suspected whenever a patient presents with fever, headache, and a change in mental status or focal neurologic involvement.

MENINGITIS

- Inflammation of the meninges, which usually presents with headache, fever, meningismus, and an elevated number of white blood cells (pleocytosis) in the cerebrospinal fluid (CSF).
- It can be **acute** (hours to days) or **chronic** (symptoms lasting over 4 weeks).[1]
- It is classified as bacterial, fungal, parasitic, or aseptic, the latter of which can be infectious (usually viral) or noninfectious, such as drug induced.
- Possible complications of meningitis include brain abscess, hydrocephalus, seizures, respiratory failure, coma, brain stem herniation due to intracranial hypertension, cortical vein phlebitis, sagittal sinus thrombosis, deafness, blindness, and developmental delay.

ACUTE MENINGITIS

GENERAL PRINCIPLES

Etiology

- Etiologies vary according to age group and risk factor (Table 10-1), and empiric therapy is based on these. The cause can be inferred from the cell count and characteristics of the CSF.
  - If there are >1,000 neutrophils/mL, the predominant therapy should be directed against bacteria.
  - Lymphocytic pleocytosis, with <100 lymphocytes, would suggest an alternative etiology (Table 10-2).
- **Bacterial**. The most common organism causing acute meningitis in adults in developed countries is **_Streptococcus pneumoniae_**, followed by _Neisseria meningitidis_. Type B _Haemophilus influenzae_ in industrialized countries has decreased with the introduction of immunization, but it is still an important cause in developing countries. Other etiologies include group B streptococci, enterococci, and gram-negative rods.

TABLE 10-1	MOST COMMON ETIOLOGIES OF ACUTE BACTERIAL MENINGITIS BY AGE AND RISK FACTOR
Age/risk factor	**Common bacterial pathogens**
<1 mo	*Streptococcus agalactiae, Escherichia coli, Listeria monocytogenes, Klebsiella* spp.
1–23 mo	*Streptococcus pneumoniae, S. agalactiae, Haemophilus influenzae, E. coli, Neisseria meningitidis*
2–50 y	*N. meningitidis, S. pneumoniae*
>50 y	*S. pneumoniae, N. meningitidis, L. monocytogenes,* gram-negative bacilli
Immunocompromised	*S. pneumoniae, N. meningitidis, L. monocytogenes,* gram-negative bacilli
Penetrating head trauma	*Staphylococcus aureus,* coagulase-negative *Staphylococcus,* gram-negative bacilli (including *Pseudomonas aeruginosa*)
Basilar skull fracture	*S. pneumoniae, H. influenzae,* group A β-hemolytic streptococci
Postneurosurgery	*S. aureus,* coagulase-negative staphylococci, gram-negative bacilli (incl. *P. aeruginosa*)
Cerebrospinal fluid shunt	*Staphylococcus epidermidis* (coagulase-negative staphylococci), *S. aureus,* gram-negative bacilli, *Propionibacterium acnes*

Adapted from Tunkel AR, Hartman BJ, Kaplan SL, et al. Practice guidelines for the management of bacterial meningitis. *Clin Infect Dis.* 2004;39:1267-1284; Tunkel A, van de Beek D, Scheld WM. Acute meningitis. In: Dolin R, Mandell GL, Bennett JE, eds. *Mandell, Douglas and, Bennett's Principles and Practice of Infectious Diseases.* 7th ed. Philadelphia, PA: Elsevier Churchill Livingston; 2010:1189-1230.

○ *Listeria monocytogenes* is an important pathogen in the elderly and immunosuppressed.
○ Coagulase-negative staphylococci and other skin flora are more common in patients with intraventricular shunts.
○ *Treponema pallidum* (syphilis) can present as acute meningitis in primary syphilis.
- **Viral. Enteroviruses** account for >85% of viral meningitis. Other viruses include West Nile virus (WNV), mumps, herpes simplex virus (HSV)-2 (Mollaret meningitis), HSV-1, lymphocytic choriomeningitis virus, St. Louis encephalitis virus, and HIV.
- **Fungal.** Usually chronic. In the immunosuppressed, *Histoplasma, Aspergillus,* and *Cryptococcus* can present as acute meningitis.
- **Parasitic.** *Naegleria fowleri, Acanthamoeba* spp., and *Balamuthia mandrillaris* are free living amebas causing meningoencephalitis, usually fatal. In the United States, *B. mandrillaris* is more prevalent in individuals of Hispanic origin.[2] *Angiostrongylus cantonensis* is the cause of eosinophilic meningitis, predominantly in Southeast Asia, Pacific Islands, and the Caribbean.

TABLE 10-2	TYPICAL CEREBROSPINAL FLUID FINDING IN MENINGITIS IN ADULTS				
	Opening pressure (mm H_2O)	White cells/ mm^3	Glucose (mg/dL)	Protein (mg/dL)	Laboratory diagnosis
Normal	<180	0–5	50–75	15–40	None
Bacterial meningitis	⇑	100–5,000 neutrophils	<40	100–500	Gram stain, culture
Tuberculous meningitis	⇑	<500 lymphocytes	<50	100–200	Acid-fast bacilli (AFB) smear, culture, PCR (*M. tuberculosis*)
Crypto-coccal meningitis	⇑	10–200 lymphocytes	<40	50–200	Cryptococcal antigen, India ink stain, fungal culture
Viral meningitis	⇑	10–1,000 lymphocytes	Normal	50–100	Virus-specific PCR (polymerase chain reaction)

- **Noninfectious. Drugs** (e.g., nonsteroidal antiinflammatory drugs [NSAIDs], trimethoprim–sulfamethoxazole, OKT3 monoclonal antibodies, and carbamazepine) are the most common noninfectious causes of aseptic meningitis.
- **Posttrauma or surgery.** Skin flora, especially staphylococci and streptococci, are the most common cause of acute meningitis following trauma or manipulation of CNS, followed by oropharyngeal bacteria and gram-negative rods.

Pathophysiology

- Bacteremia from nasopharyngeal source precedes CNS invasion and replication in subarachnoid space. Blood cultures may be helpful in diagnosis.
- The polysaccharide capsules of *S. pneumoniae* and *H. influenzae* are important virulence factors; patients with hypocomplementemia or splenectomy are at increased risk (due to decreased opsonization).
- Viral invasion may follow viremia, but may also occur via the olfactory nerve and afferent nerve axons (e.g., HSV).
- Enteroviruses are transmitted via the fecal–oral route and systemic invasion occurs via lymphoid tissues in the gut.

Risk Factors

- Age, lack of vaccination, immunosuppression, splenectomy, disruption of the blood–brain barrier, history of trauma, and presence of intraventricular shunt are major risk factors.
- Enteroviral meningitis is more common in summer.
- Travel and water-related activities are relevant if fungal or parasitic etiologies are considered.
- *L. monocytogenes* can be transmitted via unpasteurized dairy products, deli, or any raw food item.

Prevention

Vaccination

- Vaccines are available for *H. influenzae* type B, most strains of meningococcus, and pneumococcus.
- **H. influenzae**
  - Vaccination against *H. influenzae* type B has led to >90% decreased incidence in developed countries; decreased rates of nasopharyngeal colonization has contributed to herd immunity.
  - Current recommendations by the Advisory Committee on Immunization Practices (ACIP) include doses at 2, 4, and 6 months of age, with a booster at 12 to 15 months of age.[3]
- **N. meningitidis**
  - The current meningococcal conjugated vaccine covers serogroups A, C, W135, and Y, but **not serogroup B**.
  - The ACIP recommends one dose for all those within ages 11 to 18, as transmission is highest in high schools and colleges.[3]
  - Children between ages 2 and 10 with risk factors such as asplenia or hypocomplementemia, adults who are splenectomized, and military recruits or travelers to endemic areas, such as sub-Saharan Africa and Saudi Arabia, should also be vaccinated.
- **S. pneumoniae**
  Conjugate pneumococcal vaccines have decreased the rates of invasive pneumococcal disease in children and adults. Recently, invasive disease by serogroups not covered by vaccine has increased.

Chemoprophylaxis

- **H. influenzae.** Controversial. Some experts recommend rifampin for close contacts aged <2, such as day care settings.
- **N. meningitidis**
  - **Prophylaxis is recommended for close contacts of a patient with meningococcal meningitis.**
  - Close contact is defined as exposure to oral secretions (e.g., kissing, mouth-to-mouth resuscitations, and endotracheal intubation) or prolonged contact within 3 feet or less, within 1 week before the onset of symptoms until 24 hours after initiation of appropriate antibiotic therapy.
  - **Household contacts, day care contacts, and health care personnel who were exposed to the patient's oral secretions need prophylaxis**, but NOT all health care personnel who are exposed to the patient.
  - The current recommendations for prophylaxis include the following[4]:
    - **Ciprofloxacin**. Only in adults, 500 mg orally once.

- **Rifampin**. 600 mg PO q12h for 2 days for adults; 10 mg/kg PO q12h for 2 days for children >1 month of age; 5 mg/kg PO q12h for 2 days for infants <1 month of age.
- **Ceftriaxone**. 250 mg IM once in adults and 125 mg IM once in children.
- ○ Chemoprophylaxis is indicated **even in individuals who received meningococcal vaccination in the past**, since it does not protect against serotype B.

DIAGNOSIS

Clinical Presentation

History
- Age, risk factors, exposures, vaccinations, and seasonality should be elicited.
- The patient may complain of acute onset of headache, neck stiffness/pain, and fever.

Physical Examination
- Fever is usually present in all forms of meningitis.
- Meningeal signs include nuchal rigidity and Kernig and Brudzinski signs. However, the absence of these findings does not exclude the diagnosis of meningitis.
- Evidence of intracranial hypertension such as anisocoria, papilledema, nausea, vomiting, or cranial nerve paralysis provides information regarding severity and following diagnostic steps.
- Altered mental status or even coma can be present in patients with prolonged course of symptoms and patients.

Differential Diagnosis
- Noninfectious causes of similar symptoms include subarachnoid hemorrhage; tumors; cysts; illicit drug or alcohol intoxications; aseptic meningitis, such as that from trimethoprim/sulfamethoxazole, NSAIDs, OKT3 monoclonal antibodies, intravenous immunoglobulins, and carbamazepine; seizures; and migraine headache.
- HSV-2 can present as recurrent meningitis (Mollaret meningitis), which is self-limited and usually resolves spontaneously and needs no treatment.

Diagnostic Testing

Laboratories
- Peripheral blood should be obtained for cell count with differential looking for leukocytosis as well as a complete metabolic panel.
- Blood cultures may provide the etiology, especially important if the lumbar puncture (LP) cannot be performed.
- CSF studies are discussed under the section "Diagnostic Procedures."

Imaging
Computed tomography or magnetic resonance is indicated in patients with suspected mass lesion or risk of herniation, as indicated by the presence of focal signs or papilledema.

Diagnostic Procedures
- Analysis of the CSF is essential. **An LP should be performed promptly unless clearly contraindicated.**
- **Signs of increased intracranial pressure should prompt studies to rule out a mass before an LP.**

- CSF should be sent for cell count with differential, protein, glucose, Gram stain, and culture in all patients. Specific tests such as enterovirus polymerase chain reaction (PCR) or WNV IgM will depend on risk factors, initial CSF analysis, and seasonality.
- Opening pressure should be obtained when performing LP (normal 50 to 195 mm H_2O).
- Bacterial meningitis presents with higher pleocytosis (up to the range of several thousand), with neutrophil predominance, low glucose (<40 mg/dL, CSF/serum ratio <0.5), and elevated protein. Gram stain is positive in 60% to 90% of patients with bacterial meningitis with pleocytosis.
- A management algorithm is presented in Figure 10-1.

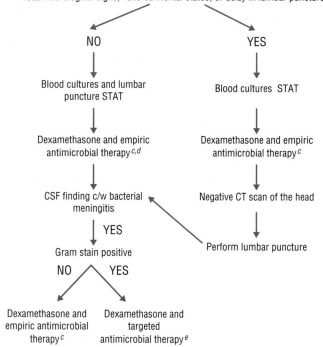

FIGURE 10-1 Algorithm for the management of acute bacterial meningitis in adults, from the guidelines of the Infectious Diseases Society of America.

[a]Mass lesion, stroke, or abscess; [b]dilated nonreactive pupil, gaze palsy, abnormal visual fields or ocular mobility, leg or arm drift; [c]see Table 10-3; [d]administer immediately after lumbar puncture; [e]see Table 10-4.

Adapted from Tunkel AR, Hartman BJ, Kaplan SL, et al. Practice guidelines for the management of bacterial meningitis. *Clin Infect Dis.* 2004;39:1267-1284.

TREATMENT

- **Bacterial meningitis is a medical emergency, and treatment should not be delayed** (Figure 10-1).
- Administration of systemic antibiotics does not affect CSF findings for 24 hours. Recommendations for empiric treatment are given according to age groups and identified risk factors (Table 10-3).

Medications

Corticosteroids
- In adults, evidence supports the use of adjunctive steroids for suspected acute bacterial meningitis due to pneumococcus.[1,5]
- In children, the use of concomitant steroids is indicated for meningitis due to *H. influenzae* type B.
- Dexamethasone at 0.15 mg/kg q6h should be started **with the first dose of antibiotics.**
- In adults, steroids should be discontinued if further studies do not support the diagnosis of bacterial meningitis, specifically if no evidence of pneumococcal infection is found.[1,5]
- The use of dexamethasone prior or with the first dose of antimicrobials has decreased the rates of hearing loss and short-term mortality in high-income countries.

TABLE 10-3	EMPIRIC ANTIBIOTIC RECOMMENDATIONS FOR ACUTE BACTERIAL MENINGITIS
Age/risk factor	**Empiric antimicrobial therapy**
<1 mo	Ampicillin plus cefotaxime or ampicillin plus aminoglycoside
1–23 mo	Vancomycin plus third-generation cephalosporin (ceftriaxone or cefotaxime)
2–50 y	Vancomycin plus ceftriaxone
>50 y	Vancomycin plus ceftriaxone (or cefotaxime) plus ampicillin
Immunocompromised	Vancomycin plus ampicillin plus cefepime or meropenem
Penetrating head trauma	Vancomycin plus ceftazidime, cefepime, or meropenem
Basilar skull fracture	Vancomycin plus ceftriaxone or cefotaxime
Postneurosurgery	Vancomycin plus ceftazidime, cefepime, or meropenem
Cerebrospinal fluid shunt	Vancomycin plus ceftazidime, cefepime, or meropenem

Adapted from Tunkel AR, Hartman BJ, Kaplan SL, et al. Practice guidelines for the management of bacterial meningitis. *Clin Infect Dis.* 2004;39:1267-1284.

TABLE 10-4	SPECIFIC ANTIMICROBIAL THERAPY FOR ACUTE BACTERIAL MENINGITIS IN ADULTS ONCE PRESUMPTIVE ORGANISM IDENTIFIED	
Microorganism	**Recommended therapy**	**Alternative therapies**
Streptococcus pneumoniae	Vancomycin (30–45 mg/kg/d in 2–3 doses) plus third-generation cephalosporin (cefotaxime or ceftriaxone)	Cefepime, meropenem, fluoroquinolone Vancomycin continued only if MIC >1 µg/mL Penicillin or ampicillin if MIC <0.1 µg/mL
Neisseria meningitidis	Ceftriaxone (2 g q12h)	Chloramphenicol, meropenem
Haemophilus influenzae type B	Third-generation cephalosporin	Cefepime, chloramphenicol, fluoroquinolone
Listeria monocytogenes	Ampicillin or penicillin G	Meropenem, trimethoprim–sulfamethoxazole
Streptococcus agalactiae	Ampicillin or penicillin G	Third-generation cephalosporin
Pseudomonas aeruginosa	Cefepime or ceftazidime	Carbapenem (except ertapenem)

Adapted from Tunkel AR, Hartman BJ, Kaplan SL, et al. Practice guidelines for the management of bacterial meningitis. *Clin Infect Dis*. 2004;39:1267-1284.

Antimicrobials

Antimicrobial treatment for acute meningitis is presented in Table 10-4.

PROGNOSIS/OUTCOME

- Delay in treatment is a strong predictor for death.
- Deafness, blindness, mental retardation, and paralysis are the most common sequelae among survivors.

CHRONIC MENINGITIS

GENERAL PRINCIPLES

Definition

Chronic meningitis is defined as signs and symptoms suggestive of meningeal disease with CSF pleocytosis lasting 4 weeks or more.

Etiology

- **The most common infectious cause of chronic meningitis worldwide is tuberculosis**, especially in the developing world.

- **Fungi are the second most common causes**, including *Cryptococcus neoformans*, *Coccidioides immitis, Histoplasma capsulatum, Blastomyces hominis*, and *Candida* spp.
- Parasitic causes include *Acanthamoeba* spp. and neurocysticercosis (*Taenia solium*).
- Other bacterial causes include *T. pallidum, Borrelia burgdorferi, Brucella* spp., and *Tropheryma whippelii.*
- Potential noninfectious causes include meningeal carcinomatosis, collagen vascular disease (e.g., lupus and other forms of vasculitis), sarcoidosis, and toxin/drug induced.
- A significant minority of cases are idiopathic.

Pathophysiology

Depending on the infectious agent, the manifestations can be due to granuloma formation irritating the meninges, perivascular inflammation, or rupture of a parameningeal site, including an abscess or cyst with leakage into the meningeal space.[6]

Risk Factors

- Travel (for even short periods) to the Southwest United States and Mexico should raise the suspicion of coccidioidomycosis.
- Tuberculous meningitis should be suspected in immigrants from tropical or developing countries and if immunosuppressed patients travel to an endemic country.
- Histoplasmosis and blastomycosis should be suspected in patients from endemic areas.
- Immunosuppression. HIV infected patients, transplant recipients, and patients on immunosuppressive drugs are at increased risk of cryptococcal meningitis, *Mycobacterium tuberculosis*, and Whipple disease.
- Exposures: Sexual behavior (neurosyphilis) and unpasteurized cheese from endemic countries (*Brucella*).

DIAGNOSIS

Clinical Presentation

History

- Symptoms can wax and wane over a period of time, making the diagnosis difficult.
- Headaches, nausea, memory loss, and confusion are the most common symptoms.
- Fever may be absent.
- With progression of disease and possible development of hydrocephalus, other symptoms such as diplopia, ataxia, and dementia may occur.
- History of exposures, travel and immunosuppression, and occupational activities should be obtained.
- Associated symptoms such as weight loss, night sweats, tumors, or skin lesions may lead toward a certain etiology such as tuberculosis, malignancy, or fungal infection.
- History of sexually transmitted diseases and genital lesions suggests neurosyphilis as a possibility.
- Presence of oral ulcers, visual problems, and uveitis is suggestive of noninfectious causes such as Behçet disease.

Physical Examination

- Skin lesions may be present in fungal infections such as blastomycosis or cryptococcosis.
- Lymphadenopathy should raise suspicion of hematologic malignancy, sarcoidosis, or tuberculosis.

- A detailed neurological examination is essential.
- Cranial nerve abnormalities can be seen due to chronic meningeal inflammation, without intracranial hypertension.

Differential Diagnosis

Other causes of headache, focal neurologic signs, dementia, and delirium should be considered when appropriate.

Diagnostic Testing

Laboratories
- Peripheral blood should be obtained for cell count with differential looking for leukocytosis as well as a complete metabolic panel.
- Serologies may be useful for coccidioidomycosis (serum complement fixation), Lyme disease, syphilis, and brucellosis.
- CSF studies are discussed under the section "Diagnostic Procedures."

Imaging
- MRI is the imaging method of choice. It may show blunting of sulci as evidence of edema, hydrocephalus, and meningeal enhancement.
- Granulomas may be seen in tuberculosis or cryptococcosis, especially if disseminated hematogenously (miliary tuberculosis).
- Intraparenchymal or intraventricular lesions may be seen in neurocysticercosis.

Diagnostic Procedures
- **CSF evaluation is essential**.
- Cell count with differential, glucose, protein, Gram stain, aerobic, mycobacterial, and fungal cultures should be sent. Larger volumes are needed for mycobacterial and fungal cultures.
- Pleocytosis is usually lymphocytic.
- Low-glucose concentrations are more typical of tuberculosis and fungal infections.
- If lymphocytic carcinomatosis is suspected, flow cytometry should be ordered.
- For the most common specific etiologies, the following CSF tests should be ordered:
  - *M. tuberculosis*. Acid-fast stains are not sensitive. At least 3 to 5 mL should be sent for culture. Nucleic acid amplification tests have varied sensitivity and specificity depending on the laboratory. Adenosine deaminase is not routinely ordered but if high can aid in the diagnosis of tuberculosis.[7,8]
  - **Cryptococcal meningitis**. The organism may be seen with India ink stain. CSF cryptococcal antigen has very high sensitivity but can remain positive even in treated patients. If unable to obtain CSF, a positive serum cryptococcal antigen correlates well in immunosuppressed patients.
  - *C. immitis*. CSF complement fixation antibody.
  - *H. capsulatum*. *Histoplasma* antigen in CSF. Urine *Histoplasma* antigen not useful unless the patient has evidence of disseminated infection.
  - **Syphilis**. CSF VDRL or RPR. Indicate high suspicion for neurosyphilis on laboratory requisition.
  - Lyme disease and Whipple disease: PCR for the specific antigen.
- Opening pressure should always be checked when LP is performed.
- A lumbar drain may be required in cases with very high intracranial pressure, such as with cryptococcal meningitis.

- Meningeal biopsy may be required in cases when the diagnosis is unclear. The presence of granulomas or the evidence of malignancy or vascular inflammation can help establish the diagnosis.
- Tuberculosis skin test (PPD) should be placed in all patients, although it may be negative in immunosuppressed patients. In patients with known history of negative PPD, **a new positive test should prompt treatment even if CSF studies are negative**.

TREATMENT

May need to treat empirically if suspicion is high for an etiologic agent (e.g., *M. tuberculosis*), in immunosuppressed patients, or if patient decompensates quickly and action is required.[7]

Medications

- **M. tuberculosis**. Four-drug therapy is recommended (i.e., isoniazid, rifampin, ethambutol, and pyrazinamide) for 2 months followed by consolidation with isoniazid and rifampin for 9 to 12 months, although the length has not been determined well by any clinical trial.[9]
  - ○ If the organism is susceptible, ethambutol can be discontinued.[9]
  - ○ Corticosteroids (dexamethasone or prednisone) have been shown to improve outcomes, especially in HIV-negative patients. Taper steroids over 3 weeks.
- **Cryptococcal meningitis**
  - ○ See Chapter 13.
  - ○ In immunocompetent patients, use amphotericin B deoxycholate (0.7 to 1 mg/kg/d) or liposomal amphotericin B (3 to 7 mg/kg/d) IV with or without flucytosine orally (100 mg/d) followed by 8 weeks of fluconazole 800 mg orally per day.
- **Coccidioidomycosis**. Fluconazole is the mainstay of treatment for *C. immitis* meningitis.
- Amphotericin B should be started in patients with suspected fungal meningitis. Switch to fluconazole or itraconazole, once a specific fungus is diagnosed. Therapy should be given over several months.

Other Nonpharmacologic Therapies

Persistent intracranial hypertension in cryptococcal meningitis may require serial LPs, lumbar drain, or CSF shunts if there is hydrocephalus.

COMPLICATIONS

- Hydrocephalus, especially in cryptococcal meningitis.
- Tuberculous meningitis may result in cerebral ischemia/infarction, growth of a tuberculoma, seizures, hyponatremia, and death.

PROGNOSIS/OUTCOME

- Prognosis depends on the specific etiology, age, immunocompromised status and severity of disease at presentation, and time to initiation of treatment.

- Tuberculous meningitis is associated with 50% mortality, even with treatment.[8,9] Sequelae include cranial nerve palsies, blindness, deafness, psychiatric disorders, and seizures.
- Similar sequelae can occur in all forms of fungal meningitis.

ENCEPHALITIS

GENERAL PRINCIPLES

Definition
- Encephalitis is an inflammation of the brain parenchyma, which usually presents as altered mental status or personality changes.[10,11]
- It can be associated with meningitis and is referred to as meningoencephalitis.

Etiology
- Most infectious encephalitis is of viral origin, but the etiology is unknown in many patients.[10,11]
- **The most common cause of sporadic encephalitis is HSV**, which has a high morbidity and mortality if untreated.
- Viral etiologies depend on the epidemiology, geography, time of the year, and exposures. In the United States, WNV has emerged as a common cause, followed by **enteroviruses**. Rabies is a fatal yet preventable cause of encephalitis.
- Nonviral causes include *M. tuberculosis*, *Mycoplasma pneumoniae*, *Bartonella* spp., syphilis, fungi, and parasitic infections such as free living amebas (Table 10-5).[10]

TABLE 10-5	CAUSES OF ENCEPHALITIS
Agent	**Exposure or risk factor**
Viruses	
Adenovirus	Children, immunosuppressed, previous respiratory disease
California encephalitis group	Mosquito-borne; camping in California, Midwest, and US East Coast; exposure to squirrels and chipmunks
Colorado tick fever virus	Tick exposure, Rocky Mountains, gastrointestinal disease
Chikungunya virus	Travel to India, area of outbreak, mosquito-borne, severe arthralgias
Cytomegalovirus	HIV/AIDS, solid organ transplant patients, blood transfusions
Eastern equine encephalitis	Mosquito-borne, Eastern US, Caribbean
Epstein-Barr virus	History of mononucleosis, organ transplant, blood transfusions, exposure to infected saliva

Enterovirus	Summer, swimming
Human herpes virus 6	Immunosuppressed, transplant recipients
HIV	Sexual risk factors, intravenous drug use, health care workers
Herpes simplex virus-1	Previous gingivostomatitis, recurrent oral infection, immunosuppression
Herpes simplex virus-2	Perinatal transmission, recurrent infection
Influenza virus	Winter months, lack of vaccination
Japanese encephalitis virus	Mosquito-borne, travel to Southeast Asia, China, India
JC virus	HIV, solid organ transplant, steroids, tumor necrosis factor inhibitors, sarcoidosis, natalizumab
Lymphocytic choriomeningitis virus	Exposure to rodent urine, feces, secretions
Measles virus	Lack of vaccination, developing countries, mostly postinfectious
Mumps virus	Lack of vaccination, previous parotitis
Murray Valley encephalitis virus	Mosquito-borne, travel to Australia
Poliovirus	Lack of vaccination, travel to countries with no immunization program, oral vaccine
Rabies virus	Unvaccinated dog or cat bites, wild foxes, raccoons, skunks, human contact with bats
Rift Valley fever virus	Mosquito vector, travel to sub-Saharan Africa, Egypt
Rubella virus	Lack of vaccination, exposure to infected patients
St. Louis encephalitis virus	Mosquito-borne, Mississippi river basin, summer months, elderly
Tick-borne encephalitis virus	Travel to Russia, Western Europe, China
Vaccinia virus	Postinfectious
Varicella zoster virus	Primary infection, disseminated zoster, immunosuppressed
West Nile virus	Summer months, mosquito-borne, throughout US, organ transplantation, blood transfusion, older age
Western equine encephalitis virus	Mosquito-borne, warm months, Western US

(continued)

TABLE 10-5 (CONTINUED)

Bacteria

Bartonella bacilliformis	Sand fly vector, patients or travelers from Andean mountains
Bartonella henselae	Children, cat, dog, or rodent exposure
Listeria monocytogenes	Elderly, exposure to unpasteurized dairy products, deli, immunosuppressed
Mycoplasma pneumoniae	Children, young adults, preceding respiratory symptoms, probably postinfectious
Anaplasma phagocytophilum	Tick-borne, warm months, Europe, Northern US
Coxiella burnetii	Exposure to goats, sheep, ingestion of unpasteurized dairy products
Ehrlichia chaffeensis	Tick-borne, Midwestern, Southeastern US, warm months
Rickettsia rickettsii	Tick vector, camping in the US between Oklahoma and North Carolina
Borrelia burgdorferi	Tick vector, endemic areas in the US, Europe
Treponema pallidum	Sexual contact, primary or tertiary syphilis

Fungi

Coccidioides spp.	Travel or resident in Southwestern US, Mexico, Central America
Histoplasma capsulatum	Immunocompromised, Ohio and Mississippi River valleys

Protozoa

Acanthamoeba spp.	Immunocompromised
Balamuthia mandrillaris	Endemic countries, swimming in freshwater
Naegleria fowleri	Swimming in lakes, brackish water
Plasmodium falciparum	Travel to tropical and subtropical endemic countries, lack of prophylaxis
Toxoplasma gondii	Perinatal transmission, ingestion of raw meat, immunocompromised, HIV/AIDS
Trypanosoma brucei	Tsetse fly vector, travel to West or East Africa

Helminths

Baylisascaris procyonis	Raccoon or raccoon feces exposure
Gnathostoma spp.	Southeast Asia, Latin America, ingestion of undercooked fish

- Encephalitis may also be postinfectious, such as postimmunization or acute demyelinating encephalomyelitis (ADEM). *M. pneumoniae* and streptococcal disease may be associated with ADEM.
- JC virus causes progressive multiple leukoencephalopathy, seen in immunosuppressed patients, HIV infection, sarcoidosis, and patients on steroids and other immunosuppressed medications.
- Whipple's disease is caused by *T. whippelii*.
- Varicella zoster virus (VZV) as a complication of chicken pox (primary infection) or disseminated herpes zoster, particularly in the immunosuppressed.
- Cytomegalovirus (CMV), particularly in HIV and solid organ or bone marrow transplant patients.
- Epstein-Barr virus (EBV) and adenovirus are less common etiologies of encephalitis.

Pathophysiology

- The cardinal pathological feature is inflammation of the brain parenchyma. Damage may be caused by direct pathogen invasion or by an immune-mediated mechanism causing demyelination and vasculitis.
- Herpes simplex encephalitis
  - **The most common herpes encephalitis in adults is HSV 1.**
  - Direct invasion from the trigeminal or olfactory nerve may occur.[12]
  - This may follow an acute oropharyngeal infection, reactivation, or recurrent HSV-1. In approximately one-third of patients, it can reactivate within the CNS without a known primary or recurrent HSV-1 infection.
- Arboviral encephalitis
  - In the United States, the most common arboviral infection is **WNV**, which has emerged in the last 20 years.
  - Worldwide, other arboviral infections include Japanese encephalitis virus (JEV) (Southeast Asia and China), chikungunya virus (India, sub Saharan Africa, Pakistan, and Italy), and tick-borne encephalitis (Western Europe, Russia, and China).
  - After a mosquito (*Aedes* spp. or *Culex* spp.) or tick bite (*Ixodes*), there is virus replication, which results in viremia and subsequent dissemination to the CNS.
- Rabies
  - Rabies is transmitted to humans through the saliva of an infected animal following a bite. It can be transmitted by bats, raccoons, foxes, and dogs.
  - The incubation period can be long, up to 7 years, with a median of 2 months.
- Table 10-5 presents more details regarding etiologies and exposures.

Risk Factors

- Travel to endemic areas: China (JEV), United States and Europe (WNV in summer months), and the East coast (eastern equine encephalitis)
- Mosquito or tick exposure
- Exposure to wild animals: dogs, raccoons, and bats (rabies)
- Seasonality: Summer months for WNV and ehrlichiosis/anaplasmosis
- Activities: Camping (insect exposure), swimming (free living amebas and enterovirus), and sexual contact (HIV)
- Immunocompromised: VZV, CMV, and JC virus
- Recent vaccination: ADEM
- Primary HSV infection in those <18 years old
- Ingestion of unpasteurized milk or other dairy products (*Listeria*) and raw meat (*Toxoplasma*)

Prevention
- Avoid exposures as above.
- Rabies vaccine as well as rabies immunoglobulin should be administered to anyone who has been bitten by a wild animal or unimmunized dog or bats (even without clear evidence of bite) (www.cdc.gov/rabies/exposure, last accessed May 1, 2012).
- A JEV vaccine is approved for travelers to endemic areas (www.cdc.gov/travel, last accessed May 1, 2012).

DIAGNOSIS

Clinical Presentation
History
- Risk factors should be assessed.
- **Altered mental status is the hallmark of encephalitis** and may precede other symptoms.
- HSV-1 should always be considered in patients with meningoencephalitis, even without a recent outbreak of herpes.
- Personality change and auditory hallucinations suggestive of temporal involvement should raise suspicion of HSV-1 infection.
- The patient may not be able to provide a history; so if unable to obtain any information, immediate action should be taken for diagnosis and management.
- Prodromal symptoms and exposures to sick people (e.g., *Mycoplasma*).
- Fever, altered consciousness, behavioral changes, headache, seizures, and/or focal neurological signs may occur.
- Meningeal signs and symptoms may be present in cases of meningoencephalitis.

Physical Examination
- Fever and altered mental status are the most common findings.
- Meningismus is usually absent.
- Focal neurologic signs, including aphasia and personality changes, ataxia, and cranial nerve palsies (tuberculosis and syphilis), may be seen.
- Generalized or focal seizures may be present.
- Movement disorders may suggest a flavivirus infection, such as WNV or JEV, or a postinfectious syndrome, such as ADEM or poststreptococcal chorea.
- Various rashes and animal/arthropod bites may provide useful clues.

Differential Diagnosis
- Possibilities include glioblastoma or meningioma, brain abscesses, meningitis, sarcoidosis, systemic lupus erythematosus, vasculitis, drugs, alcohol or other toxic encephalopathies, and delirium.
- In children with a history of recent immunization or recent viral infection, ADEM should be considered.

Diagnostic Testing
Imaging
- MRI is the most sensitive neuroimaging study.
- If MRI is unavailable or contraindicated, then a CT (with and without contrast) should be obtained.

- Findings may include temporal involvement (HSV-1), white matter lesions (demyelinating diseases), hemorrhages (VZV), lack of enhancement (JC virus), periventricular lesions, or mass lesions including tuberculomas and free living amebiasis.

Diagnostic Procedures
- **All patients with a suspicion of encephalitis should undergo an LP unless clearly contraindicated.**
- The most common finding is a mild-to-moderate pleocytosis with lymphocytic predominance; glucose is usually normal and protein elevated.
- **A normal CSF in a patient with a history suggestive of HSV encephalitis should not delay treatment and specific testing.**
- Nucleic acid amplification tests (e.g., PCR):
  ○ **HSV PCR should be sent in all patients with encephalitis.**
  ○ The sensitivity of HSV PCR is 98% and specificity 96%, although this varies according to the laboratory
  ○ Note that HSV PCR may be negative on day 1 or day 2 of the disease, so if the clinical picture and imaging suggest HSV, a PCR should be repeated later.[12,13]
  ○ Other PCRs are available for enterovirus, adenovirus, influenza, JC, EBV, CMV, VZV, rabies, *Ehrlichia*, *Bartonella*, and *Mycoplasma*.
- Antibodies:
  ○ The diagnosis of WNV is made by the presence of IgM antibodies in the CSF or serum.[12] There is cross-reactivity with other flaviviruses, such as St. Louis encephalitis virus or JEV.
  ○ CSF and serum antibodies should be sent if rabies is suspected.
- If rabies is suspected, a skin biopsy from the nape of the neck can be done; fluorescent antibody staining may reveal rabies antigen in cutaneous nerve fibers. PCR testing can also be done on saliva.
- For Whipple's disease, small bowel biopsy with PAS staining is required.

TREATMENT

- The treatment of HSV encephalitis is intravenous acyclovir at 10 mg/kg every 8 hours for 14 to 21 days.
- **Acyclovir should be started empirically on every patient who presents with a picture consistent with encephalitis.**
- For other viral etiologies, the treatment is mainly supportive.
- A humanized monoclonal antibody is currently in clinical trials for WNV.

PROGNOSIS/OUTCOME

- If untreated, mortality due to herpes simplex encephalitis can be as high as 70%; morbidity is high (>28%), and most survivors have some type of sequelae including severe cognitive impairment and disability.[12,13]
- WNV encephalitis can be severe in patients aged >50. Residual neurologic findings may include a poliomyelitis-like syndrome, persistent headaches and fatigue, and focal signs that can persist for months.

BRAIN ABSCESS

GENERAL PRINCIPLES

Etiology

The etiologic agent is usually determined by the location of the abscess or the predisposing factor (Table 10-6). Most are caused by bacteria; fungi and parasites are less common causes.

Pathophysiology

There are four distinct phases of development in a brain abscess[14]
- Early cerebritis with focal inflammation and edema (first few days)
- Late cerebritis with increasing size and development of a necrotic center
- Early capsular stage when a ring-enhancing capsule develops (1 to 2 weeks)
- In the late capsular phase, a well-formed collagenous capsule develops and walls off the abscess (after about 2 weeks)

Risk Factors

- **Pyogenic brain abscess**
  - ○ **Contiguous source. This is the most common source** including chronic otitis media, mastoiditis, cholesteatoma, chronic sinusitis, odontogenic fistulas/caries/abscesses, and cavernous sinus thrombosis.[14]
  - ○ **Hematogenous**: dissemination of infectious agent from an intrathoracic or intraperitoneal source to the brain including endocarditis, pulmonary arteriovenous malformation (e.g., as in hereditary hemorrhagic telangiectasia [HHT]), ventricular septal defects, and persistent ductus arteriosus
  - ○ **Trauma**: gunshot wounds, patients in combat
  - ○ **Open brain surgery**
- **Fungal**. Fungal brain abscesses occur in immunocompromised patients, such as bone marrow and solid organ transplant patients, patients on corticosteroids, uncontrolled diabetics with ketoacidosis (mucormycosis), and HIV
- **Parasitic**. Toxoplasmosis occurs in HIV-infected patients; neurocysticercosis in immigrants from endemic areas.

DIAGNOSIS

Clinical Presentation

History
- Presentation is usually indolent, especially if there is a contiguous source focus.
- Presentation varies according to location and if there are single or multiple abscesses.
- Most common symptom is headache, followed by fever and focal neurologic deficits.[14,15]
- Fever, hemiparesis, and symptoms of increased intracranial pressure should heighten suspicion for brain abscess.
- Seizures can be the only presenting symptom.
- If localized to the frontal lobe, headache and altered mental status may be presenting features.
- Look for predisposing conditions, immunosuppressed status, previous surgeries, or dental procedures.
- Family history of arteriovenous malformations or HHT may be helpful.

TABLE 10-6   BRAIN ABSCESS: SOURCE, LOCATION, AND PATHOGENS

Underlying condition	Probable site of abscess	Probable pathogens
Paranasal sinus disease	Frontal lobe	*Streptococci* (especially *S. milleri* group), *S. aureus*, *Haemophilus* spp., *Bacteroides* spp., *Fusobacterium* spp.
Otogenic source	Temporal lobe, cerebellum	Enterobacteriaceae, *Pseudomonas* spp., *Streptococcus* spp., *Bacteroides* spp., *S. aureus*
Odontogenic source	Frontal lobe	Streptococci, *Actinomyces* sp, *Bacteroides* sp, *Fusobacterium* sp
Pulmonary infection	Any lobe, possible multiple lobe involvement	*Streptococcus* spp., methicillin-resistant *S. aureus*, *Bacteroides*, *Fusobacterium* spp., Enterobacteriaceae, *Actinomyces* spp.
Bacterial endocarditis	Multiple lobe involvement, usually multiple abscesses in vascularized areas	*S. aureus*, *S. viridians*
Penetrating head trauma	Depends on site of wound	*S. aureus* (methicillin sensitive and resistant), *Staphylococcus epidermidis*, *Streptococci* spp., Enterobacteriaceae, *Clostridium* spp.
Postneurosurgery	Depends on site of wound	*S. aureus*, *S. epidermidis*, *Pseudomonas* spp., Enterobacteriaceae
Right-to-left shunt (congenital cyanotic heart disease, pulmonary arteriovenous malformations)	Multiple abscesses, multiple lobes	*Streptococcus* spp., *Staphylococcus* spp., *Peptostreptococcus* spp., *Haemophilus* spp.
Immunosuppressed patients (transplant recipients, immunosuppressant drugs)	Multiple abscesses, multiple lobes	*Aspergillus* spp., *Nocardia* spp., *Candida* spp., *Toxoplasma gondii*, *Listeria monocytogenes*, mucormycosis, *Mycobacterium* spp., *Cryptococcus* spp.
HIV infection	Multiple abscesses, any lobe	*T. gondii*, *Mycobacterium* spp., *Cryptococcus neoformans*, *Aspergillus* spp., *Nocardia* spp.

Adapted from Kastenbauer S, Pfister HW, Wispelwey B, Scheld WM. Brain abscess. In: Scheld SM, Whitley RJ, Marra C, eds. *Infections of the Central Nervous System.* 3rd ed. Philadelphia, PA: Lippincott Williams & Wilkins; 2004:479-508.

Physical Examination
- Fever may not be present.
- Focal signs and deficits and signs of increased intracranial pressure may be present.

Differential Diagnosis

The differential diagnosis is broad and includes brain tumors (primary or metastatic), epidural or subdural empyema, subdural hematoma, CNS lymphoma (difficult to distinguish from toxoplasmosis), cerebrovascular accident, venous sinus thrombosis (which may present with associated abscess), and sarcoidosis.

Diagnostic Testing

Laboratories
- The absence of leukocytosis does not rule out a brain abscess.
- Blood cultures should be obtained before administration of antibiotics.

Imaging
- Both CT with contrast and MRI with gadolinium can be used for diagnosis. MRI is more sensitive.[15]
- CT scan findings include the following:
  ○ Early cerebritis. Hypodense irregular area without enhancement
  ○ Abscess. Hypodense lesion with ring enhancement. Edema can be seen around lesion
  ○ A contiguous focus of infection may be identified
- MRI findings include the following:
  ○ T1: Hypointense lesion with ring enhancement
  ○ T2: Hyperintense central area with hypointense surrounding capsule and surrounding hyperintense edema
  ○ Diffusion-weighted imaging may be helpful in differentiating from malignancies

Diagnostic Procedures
- LP is generally contraindicated due to the risk of herniation.
- The only way to obtain definitive diagnosis is through examination of the contents of abscess.[14,15]
- Stereotactic biopsy with needle aspiration is the method of choice (CT guided) if the abscess is accessible.
- If the abscess is in a deep part of the brain, then surgical excision may be needed.
- Aspirate should be sent for histopathology, Gram stain, aerobic and anaerobic cultures, and for fungal or mycobacterial cultures if indicated.
- To identify a potential source, other diagnostic tests may include echocardiography, panorex, chest plain radiograph, and CT pulmonary angiography.

TREATMENT

Medications

- Empiric **antibiotic treatment** should be initiated if abscesses are small (<2.5 cm), when diagnostic sample cannot be obtained, while awaiting results, or if studies fail to identify etiology.[14,15]
  ○ Empiric therapy should include an antibiotic with activity against anaerobes (e.g., metronidazole) until a specific etiology is found.

TABLE 10-7	RECOMMENDED EMPIRIC ANTIMICROBIAL TREATMENT BASED ON PRESUMED SOURCE OF ABSCESS
Source of abscess	**Empiric antimicrobial treatment**
Paranasal sinus	Metronidazole plus either third-generation cephalosporin (plus vancomycin if methicillin-resistant *S. aureus* suspected)
Otogenic infection	Metronidazole plus ceftazidime or cefepime
Dental infection	Penicillin plus metronidazole
Bacterial endocarditis	Vancomycin plus/minus gentamicin plus metronidazole plus third-generation cephalosporin
Pulmonary infection	Penicillin plus metronidazole plus trimethoprim–sulfamethoxazole (if *Nocardia* is suspected)
Penetrating trauma	Vancomycin plus third-generation cephalosporin (may use fourth generation if *Pseudomonas* suspected)
Postoperative	Vancomycin plus cefepime or ceftazidime
Unknown	Vancomycin plus metronidazole plus third-generation cephalosporin

Doses: Vancomycin IV 30–45 mg/kg/d divided into 2–3 doses/d; metronidazole 500 mg IV q6-8h; ceftriaxone 2 g q12h, cefotaxime 2 g IV q4-6h.

- ○ Recommendations are given based on presumed source of the abscess (Table 10-7).
- ○ Intravenous antibiotic treatment should be prolonged (6 to 8 weeks) and tailored to the specific etiology if possible.
- **Corticosteroids**. Dexamethasone 10 mg every 6 hours is recommended if there is significant edema and life-threatening mass effect.[15]

Surgical Treatment

- Drainage, either via burr hole aspiration or surgical excision, should be performed on all abscesses >2.5 cm.[14,15]
- Open craniotomy with excision is indicated if abscesses fail to respond to antibiotics, for fungal abscesses, and if a foreign body is present.

COMPLICATIONS

Complications include seizures, obstructive hydrocephalus, and intraventricular rupture.

PROGNOSIS/OUTCOME

- Mortality used to be up to 80% in the preantibiotic and pre-CT era.
- With the advent of CT and combined treatment, mortality averages 13% in developed countries.[15]
- Long-term sequelae (20% to 70%) include seizures and focal deficits such as aphasia, ataxia, and cranial nerve palsies.
- There may be up to a 25% rate of recurrence.[15]

REFERENCES

1. Tunkel AR, Hartman BJ, Kaplan SL, et al. Practice guidelines for the management of bacterial meningitis. *Clin Infect Dis.* 2004;39:1267-1284.
2. Bravo F, Alvarez P, Gotuzzo E. *Balamuthia mandrillaris* infection of the skin and central nervous system: an emerging disease of concern to many specialties in medicine. *Curr Opin Infect Dis.* 2011;24:112-117.
3. Centers for Disease Control and Prevention. Recommended adult immunization schedule. *MMWR Morbid Mortal Wkly Rep.* 2011;60:1-4.
4. Gardner P. Prevention of meningococcal disease. *N Engl J Med.* 2006;355:1466-1473.
5. Brouwer MC, McIntyre P, de Gans J, et al. Corticosteroids for acute bacterial meningitis. *Cochrane Database Syst Rev.* 2010;9:CD004405.
6. Helbok R, Broessner G, Pfausler B, Schutzhard E. Chronic meningitis. *J Neurol.* 2009;256:168-175.
7. Christie LJ, Loeffler AM, Honarmand S, et al. Diagnostic challenges of central nervous system tuberculosis. *Emerg Infect Dis.* 2008;14:1473-1475.
8. Thwaites G, Fisher M, Hemingway C, et al. British Infection Society guidelines for the diagnosis and treatment of tuberculosis of the central nervous system in adults and children. *J Infect.* 2009;59:167-187.
9. Centers for Disease Control and Prevention. Treatment of tuberculosis. American Thoracic Society, CDC and Infectious Diseases Society of America. *MMWR Morbid Mortal Wkly Rep.* 2003;52:1-74.
10. Glaser CA, Gilliam S, Schnurr D, et al. In search of encephalitis etiologies: diagnostic challenges of the California Encephalitis Project, 1998–2000. *Clin Infect Dis.* 2003;36:731-742.
11. Glaser CA, Honarmand S, Anderson LJ, et al. Beyond viruses: clinical profiles and etiologies associated with encephalitis. *Clin Infect Dis.* 2006;43:1565-1577.
12. Tunkel AR, Glaser CA, Block KC, et al. The management of encephalitis: clinical practice guidelines by the Infectious Diseases Society of America. *Clin Infect Dis.* 2008;47:303-327.
13. Whitley RJ. Herpes simplex encephalitis: adolescents and adults. *Antiviral Res.* 2006;71:141-148.
14. Mathisen G, Johnson JP. Brain abscess. *Clin Infect Dis.* 1997;25:763-781.
15. Mamelak AN, Mampalam TJ, Obana WG, et al. Improved management of multiple brain abscesses: a combined surgical and medical approach. *Neurosurgery.* 1995;36:76-86.

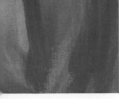

Sexually Transmitted Infections

11

Amelia M. Kasper and Hilary Reno

Sexually transmitted infections (STIs) are a significant cause of morbidity worldwide, with 19 million cases diagnosed annually in the United States alone. The standard clinical approach toward a patient at risk for STI is to match the clinical picture (a syndrome of typical symptoms in the setting of a corresponding history) with a diagnosis and then to also develop a complete differential diagnosis list to insure consideration of other infections presenting atypically.

A thorough sexual history should be elicited, including the number and gender of partners, frequency of sexual contact, types of activity, consistency of correct condom use, and history of prior STIs. It is vital to ask these questions in a direct, nonjudgmental way, even though it may be uncomfortable to the interviewer and the patient. Studies have shown that primary care providers do not adequately assess their patients' risk for STIs.

Physical exam should focus on a detailed survey of the skin, oropharynx, external genitalia, lymph nodes, and anus; for women, a speculum and bimanual exam should be included. HIV screening and pretest counseling is warranted for all patients who present for STI evaluation.

Prompt treatment of sex partners is a key component in controlling STIs. Local health departments can provide assistance in confidentially informing contacts, but traditionally, the responsibility has been placed on the patient to inform their sex partners of exposure.

Another option that is gradually gaining acceptance is allowing patients to provide their partners with proper medications or a prescription, also known as **expedited partner therapy** (EPT).[1,2] This has been shown to be particularly effective in treating male partners of women with chlamydia or gonorrhea. Providers need to be aware of the laws specific to their jurisdiction concerning EPT, because it is only legislated in some states. Providers should also be aware of state-specific reporting guidelines and how to report to local health authorities. **Syphilis, gonorrhea, chlamydia, chancroid, and HIV/AIDS are reportable diseases in all states**.

PAINFUL GENITAL ULCER DISEASES

- STIs that cause genital ulcers can be categorized by the presence of painful and painless ulcers.
- Lesions caused by genital herpes and chancroid tend to be painful, while those caused by syphilis, lymphogranuloma venereum (LGV), and granuloma inguinale tend to be painless.
- Genital ulcers may also be caused by noninfectious causes, such as Beçhet's disease, malignancy, and trauma.

GENITAL HERPES

GENERAL PRINCIPLES

Epidemiology

- Painful ulceration is most likely caused by herpes simplex virus (HSV).
- Traditionally, type 1 HSV (HSV-1) has been associated with oral lesions and type 2 HSV (HSV-2) with genital lesions; however, **either subtype may occur in either distribution**.
- One in six people in the United States aged 14 to 49 have genital HSV-2 infection, and it is estimated that 80% to 90% of people with HSV-2 are unaware that they are infected.
- Seroprevalence increases with age, and more women are affected than men.
- Genital HSV is especially a concern because it increases the risk of both acquiring and transmitting HIV.

Pathophysiology

- HSV is a double-stranded DNA virus that is spread by direct contact. Abraded skin or mucous membranes are more susceptible than intact skin.
- HSV-2 is typically transmitted through sexual contact and HSV-1 through non-sexual contact, though this rule is not absolute. Transmission of either HSV-1 or HSV-2 can occur perinatally.
- **Transmission can occur even without active lesions**, since viral shedding continues even during asymptomatic periods.
- After entering the skin, the virus is transported along peripheral nerves to sensory and autonomic ganglia. Infection may spread by direct cell-to-cell invasion or by sensory nerve pathways. As replication involves nerve endings, the retrograde transport of virions occurs, which allows for infection to appear at other sites (e.g., thighs or buttocks). Central nervous system (CNS) disease may also occur as a result.
- **The virus can remain latent in ganglia indefinitely**, with periodic recurrences due to reactivation of latent virus. Viral latency and reactivation are not well understood, but often occur in the setting of recent trauma, illness, or emotional stress.

DIAGNOSIS

Diagnosis is suggested by recognizing the clinical syndrome on history and physical exam. **All genital ulcers atypical for genital herpes should be evaluated for syphilis**.

Clinical Presentation

- If symptoms develop, the incubation period is 2 to 12 days after infection.
- Virtually any genital lesion may be herpetic regardless of clinical characteristics.
- Lesions are typically **small, painful grouped vesicles** in the genital and perianal regions, which rapidly ulcerate and form shallow, tender lesions.
- Lesions are usually present for 2 to 3 weeks; viral shedding decreases with crusting.
- The first episode is usually the most severe and may be associated with inguinal adenopathy, fever, headache, myalgias, and aseptic meningitis.
- Cervicitis, proctitis, and urethritis may also occur.

- Less common manifestations include ocular disease, stomatitis, esophagitis, fulminant hepatitis, autonomic dysfunction, encephalitis, myelitis, and neuropathy.
- Symptoms are usually less severe if antibodies to either HSV-1 or HSV-2 are already present.
- Recurrent episodes are commonly preceded by prodromal tingling or pain and are typically less severe and of shorter duration (4 to 6 days). Patients with a prolonged primary episode are more likely to experience a recurrence. In general, patients with HSV-1 genital infection have fewer recurrences and less asymptomatic viral shedding.
- Patients with immunocompromising conditions such as HIV, cancer, or organ transplants may experience prolonged or extensive outbreaks.

Diagnostic Testing

- Viral culture is the preferred method for making a diagnosis of genital HSV infection, but is only sensitive during the vesicular stage of the initial outbreak. Sensitivity declines rapidly as lesions heal. Vesicular fluid from an unroofed lesion should be placed in viral culture media and brought to the laboratory as soon as possible.
- Direct fluorescent antibody (DFA) staining of a scraped lesion or unroofed vesicle is another option, but is less sensitive than culture.
- Type-specific HSV antibodies appear weeks after infection. Assays are available and may be useful in determining seroprevalence for epidemiologic studies as well as counseling.
- HSV polymerase chain reaction (PCR) is more sensitive and is the preferred test at some centers, but commercial kits are neither readily available nor approved for genital HSV. PCR of the CSF with viral culture and typing are the tests of choice for suspected CNS infections.

TREATMENT

- Patients presenting with an initial episode of genital HSV should be treated. It is important to remember that **treatment decreases but does not eliminate viral shedding**. Recommended treatment regimens appear in Table 11-1.[3]
- All patients need to be counseled on the importance of informing their partners of their HSV status, avoiding sexual contact when lesions are present, using barrier methods even when lesions are not present, and the risk of vertical neonatal transmission.

CHANCROID

GENERAL PRINCIPLES

- Chancroid is highly infectious and is caused by *Haemophilus ducreyi*, a fastidious gram-negative bacillus.
- The reported incidence of chancroid is low but the true incidence is likely much higher, as testing for *H. ducreyi* is infrequent and difficult.
- Some parts of Africa and the Caribbean probably have a higher incidence but epidemiologic data are sparse.
- Like HSV, infection with chancroid **increases the risk of HIV transmission and acquisition**.

TABLE 11-1	TREATMENT FOR HSV INFECTIONS	

		Regimen
First episode		• **Acyclovir** 400 mg PO tid × 7–10 d OR 200 mg PO 5× a day for 7–10 d **OR** • **Famciclovir** 250 mg PO tid for 7–10 d **OR** • **Valacyclovir** 1 g PO bid for 7–10 d
Recurrent episodes	HIV positive	• **Acyclovir** 400 mg PO tid × 5–10 d **OR** • **Famciclovir** 500 mg PO bid × 5–10 d **OR** • **Valacyclovir** 1 g PO **qd** × 5–10 d
	HIV negative	• **Acyclovir** 400 mg PO tid × 5 d, 800 mg PO bid × 5 d, or 800 mg tid × 2 d **OR** • **Famciclovir** 125 mg PO bid × 5 d, 1 g PO bid × 1 d, 500 mg PO once then 250 mg PO bid × 2 d, or 500 mg PO × 3 d **OR** • **Valacyclovir** 1 g PO bid × 5–10 d
Suppressive therapy (patients with >6 episodes/year)	HIV positive	• **Acyclovir** 400–800 mg PO bid or tid **OR** • **Famciclovir** 500 mg PO bid **OR** • **Valacyclovir** 500 mg PO bid
	HIV negative	• **Acyclovir** 400 mg PO bid **OR** • **Famciclovir** 250 mg PO bid **OR** • **Valacyclovir** 500 mg PO qd[a] **OR** 1 g PO qd

HSV, herpes simplex virus.
[a]May be less effective for patients with very frequent outbreaks (>10/year).

DIAGNOSIS

Clinical Presentation

• Consider chancroid if the patient presents with typical manifestations, especially if there is a history of traveling to an endemic area (Africa, Asia, and the Caribbean).

- The lesion is a **painful, nonindurated genital ulcer with a yellow-gray base, undermined edges, and a surrounding ring of erythema**. Multiple ulcers may be present.
- It is often associated with **inguinal lymphadenopathy**, which is tender and may suppurate.
- Suppurative lymph nodes commonly develop secondary bacterial infections.

Diagnostic Testing

- **All ulcers suspicious for chancroid should be evaluated for HSV and syphilis**.
  - Perform a dark-field exam for *Treponema pallidum* if ulcers have been present for <7 days.
  - If ulcers have been present for >7 days, perform a serum rapid plasma reagent (RPR).
- Isolating the organism on culture requires special media that are not widely available. Sensitivity is <80% even when cultured appropriately.[3]
- PCR testing is rarely available.

TREATMENT

- **Azithromycin 1 g PO × 1 OR ceftriaxone 250 mg IM × 1** OR ciprofloxacin 500 mg PO bid × 3 days OR erythromycin base 500 mg PO tid × 7 days.[3]
- Lesions should be reexamined in 3 to 7 days and then weekly until healed (as long as 2 weeks).
- Treatment failures have been reported and are more common in patients with HIV. Longer regimens may be more appropriate for patients who have HIV or are unable to follow-up.
- Large ulcers may not heal for several weeks and may result in permanent scarring.
- Inguinal buboes may require needle aspiration or incision and drainage.
- Partners should be treated if they had sexual contact with the patient up to 10 days prior to symptom onset.

PAINLESS GENITAL ULCER DISEASES

In the United States, the most common STI-related cause of painless genital ulcers is syphilis. **The presence of any genital ulceration should prompt evaluation for syphilis**.

SYPHILIS

GENERAL PRINCIPLES

- Syphilis is a disease caused by a spirochete, *Treponema pallidum*.
- It follows a complex but predictable staged course of clinical manifestations interspersed with periods of latency.
- The systemic symptoms of syphilis are often nonspecific, thus earning its moniker "The Great Imitator."
- Treponemes enter the body through abrasions on skin or mucous membranes during sexual contact.

- Within hours, the organism spreads through the lymphatic system, to local lymph nodes, and into the blood stream.
- The organism can also be spread vertically through transplacental transmission.

DIAGNOSIS

Clinical Presentation

- See Table 11-2 for more detailed descriptions of the stages of syphilis.
- The incubation period between initial infection and the primary chancre is 10 to 90 days (average 21 days).
- Primary lesions in the vagina or anus are often overlooked.
- The chancre usually lasts 1 to 6 weeks and resolves spontaneously with no scarring even without treatment.
- Secondary syphilis develops 4 to 10 weeks after the chancre resolves.
- Tertiary (symptomatic late latent) syphilis follows between 1 and 30 years after infection.
- These stages may overlap or present atypically in the setting of HIV coinfection.

Diagnostic Testing

- *T. pallidum* cannot be cultured in vitro, and the diagnosis relies on either **direct visualization of the organism or serologic testing**.
- In **primary syphilis**, the chancre should be evaluated for spirochetes with **darkfield microscopy or DFA testing**. Both are highly dependent on adequate sample collection and operator skill.
- Serologic testing and treatment for presumptive primary syphilis should be performed if a suspicious lesion is present.
- **Nontreponemal diagnostic tests** (e.g., RPR, Venereal Disease Research Laboratory [VDRL]) are **sensitive in immunocompetent patients, but are not specific**.
  - They may give a false-positive result during pregnancy, in IV drug users, or in the presence of other diseases, such as other spirochete infections, tuberculosis, and autoimmune disorders.
  - False-negative results may occur very early in infection.
  - In advanced HIV disease, false-negative results or delayed appearance of seropositivity may be seen due to late antibody production.[3,4]
  - Very high antibody concentrations may interfere with RPR/VDRL testing and result in a false-negative test (prozone effect). The prozone effect is more common in patients with HIV.[5]
  - Titers tend to correspond to disease activity.
  - Patients with a history of treated syphilis may have low titers indefinitely. A fourfold increase in titer is indicative of reinfection.[3]
- **A positive RPR or VDRL should be followed by a confirmatory treponemal-specific test**, such as fluorescent treponemal antibody absorption (FTA-ABS), *T. pallidum* particle agglutination assay (TP-PA), or enzyme immunoassay (EIA).
- Some laboratories are conducting EIA for initial screening. A positive EIA should be followed with RPR with titer.
- **All patients with syphilis should be tested for HIV.**

TABLE 11-2	CLINICAL MANIFESTATIONS, DIAGNOSTIC TESTS, AND TREATMENT FOR SYPHILIS			
Stage	Symptoms	Laboratory diagnosis	Treatment	Alternative regimen
Early—primary	Painless ulcer at inoculum site, local lymphadenopathy	DFA (if available) AND serologic testing	**Benzathine PCN G** 2.4 million units IM × 1	If PCN-allergic: **Doxycycline** 100 mg PO bid × 14 d **OR** **Tetracycline** 500 mg PO four times daily × 14 d
Early—secondary	Macular or papular rash (palmar/plantar or generalized), mucous membrane lesions, constitutional symptoms (malaise, fever, headache, myalgias, arthralgias), generalized lymphadenopathy, patchy hair loss, condyloma lata, neurosyphilis (rare)	Nontreponemal serologic test (e.g., RPR), followed by treponemal-specific test for confirmation (e.g., TP-PA)	same	same
Early—latent (<1 y)	Generally asymptomatic		same	same
Late latent (>1 y or unknown)	Usually asymptomatic	Nontreponemal serologic test followed by treponemal-specific test for confirmation\n\nCSF VDRL if patient has HIV with low CD4, higher RPR, or neurologic symptoms; or in patients without HIV with symptoms of tertiary syphilis, or if evidence of neurologic/ophthalmic disease present	**Benzathine PCN G** 2.4 mu IM × 3 doses at 1-wk intervals	If PCN-allergic: **Doxycycline** 100 mg PO bid × 28 d **OR** **Tetracycline** 500 mg PO four times daily × 28 d

(continued)

TABLE 11-2 (CONTINUED)

Tertiary	Cardiovascular involvement (aortic aneurysm, aortic insufficiency, coronary ostial stenosis) or gummatous disease	**Benzathine PCN G** 2.4 mu IM × 3 doses at 1-wk intervals. Some experts recommend treating cardiovascular syphilis with **IV PCN** (see Neurosyphilis)	If PCN-allergic: **Doxycycline** 100 mg PO bid × 28 d
Neurosyphilis	Often asymptomatic; involvement may be divided into categories: *Ophthalmologic involvement*—early or late *Early*—Cranial nerve palsies, CVA, seizures *Late*—Tabes dorsalis (ataxia, lightning pains, pupillary abnormalities, wide-based gait) or general paresis (dementia, personality changes, tremor, reflex abnormalities)	**Aqueous crystalline PCN G** 3–4 mu IV q4h × 10–14 d	If compliance ensured: **Procaine PCN** 2.4 mu IM qd + **probenecid** 500 mg PO four times daily × 10–14 d
Pregnancy	Same as for patients who are not pregnant	**PCN is the only recommended treatment—desensitize if necessary**	

DFA, Direct fluorescent antibody; RPR, rapid plasma reagent; TP-PA, *T. pallidum* particle agglutination assay; PCN, penicillin; CVA, cerebrovascular accident.

TREATMENT

- Recommended treatment regimes are listed in Table 11-2.[3]
- Partners should be treated if they had sexual contact with the patient up to 3 months prior to symptom onset.
- **Jarisch-Herxheimer reaction (i.e., fevers, headaches, and myalgias) is common** within 24 hours posttreatment, affecting up to 90% of patients treated with penicillin for early syphilis and up to 25% during later stages. Antipyretics can be used to alleviate symptoms. This reaction may precipitate early labor in pregnant women, but should not bar timely and appropriate treatment.

LYMPHOGRANULOMA VENEREUM

GENERAL PRINCIPLES

- Lymphogranuloma venereum is caused by invasive *Chlamydia trachomatis* serovars L_1, L_2, and L_3.
- There are reports of increasing incidence in the United States, especially among men who have sex with men.

DIAGNOSIS

Clinical Presentation
- LGV is usually diagnosed clinically due to the lack of widespread serovar-specific testing.
- LGV initially manifests as a **painless, self-limited ulcer or papule at the inoculation site** 3 to 30 days after exposure. The ulcer is often missed and heals without scarring.
- The second stage is the development of **tender inguinal or femoral lymphadenopathy**. The enlarged nodes are usually unilateral and may become fluctuant and spontaneously drain. Constitutional symptoms and urethritis may also develop.
- The "groove sign" may be visible when the inguinal ligament forms a depression between enlarged inguinal and femoral lymph nodes. Its presence is suggestive of LGV, but is not frequently seen.
- Exposure through receptive anal intercourse can lead to proctocolitis, which may progress to colorectal fistulas and strictures. Symptoms include anal discharge, rectal bleeding, and tenesmus.
- The third stage of the disease, which may not occur until years after exposure, is **hypertrophic granulomatous enlargement and ulceration of the external genitalia**. Elephantiasis of the genitalia may also occur by lymphatic obstruction.

Diagnostic Testing
- A swab of a lesion or a bubo aspirate may be sent for culture, but this is not a sensitive method.
- **Nucleic acid amplification testing (NAAT) is the test of choice** for detecting all chlamydial serovars, but is not approved for rectal testing.
- Genotyping to identify serovars is not widely available; if a patient has symptoms suspicious for LGV proctocolitis, a rectal swab should be sent to the state laboratory or the CDC for evaluation.

TREATMENT

- **Doxycycline 100 mg PO bid for 3 weeks OR erythromycin base 500 mg PO qid for 3 weeks.**[3]
- Pregnant women should be treated with erythromycin.
- Prolonged courses of azithromycin have been reportedly effective, but this has not been well-studied. A recent case of LGV with doxycycline failure was reportedly cured with moxifloxacin.[6]
- Patients should be reexamined to ensure response to treatment.
- Large, fluctuant buboes should be drained to speed resolution and prevent complications.
- Anyone who had sexual contact with the patient during the 2 months prior to developing symptoms should be examined and treated prophylactically with azithromycin 1 g PO × 1 dose or doxycycline 100 mg PO bid × 7 days.

GRANULOMA INGUINALE (DONOVANOSIS)

GENERAL PRINCIPLES

- Granuloma inguinale is caused by the intracellular gram-negative organism *Klebsiella granulomatis* (formerly *Calymmatobacterium granulomatis*).
- It is locally endemic in parts of the developing world and is relatively uncommon in the United States.

DIAGNOSIS

Clinical Presentation

- The characteristic lesion is a **painless, beefy red vascular ulcerative lesion that tends to bleed when mechanically irritated**. Multiple lesions may be seen. There is typically no associated lymphadenopathy.
- The incubation period is thought to be 1 to 3 weeks.
- Rarely, extragenital infection can occur.

Diagnostic Testing

- *K. granulomatis* cannot be directly cultured.
- Tissue crush preparation or biopsy may show intracytoplasmic, bipolar-staining Donovan bodies. Tissue should also be evaluated for LGV, chancroid, and syphilis.
- Coinfection with other STIs is common.

TREATMENT

- **Doxycycline 100 mg PO bid × 3 weeks** OR azithromycin 1 g PO weekly × 3 weeks OR ciprofloxacin 750 mg PO bid × 3 weeks OR erythromycin base 500 mg PO qid × 3 weeks OR trimethoprim–sulfamethoxazole DS one tab PO bid for 3 weeks.[3]
- Longer treatment courses may be necessary, especially in immunocompromised patients, and adding on an aminoglycoside may speed resolution.

GONORRHEA, MUCOPURULENT CERVICITIS, AND NONGONOCOCCAL URETHRITIS

GENERAL PRINCIPLES

- **Cervicitis** presents as a symptom complex of mucopurulent vaginal discharge, abnormal vaginal bleeding, and/or dysuria. *Chlamydia*, gonorrhea, HSV, *Trichomonas vaginalis*, and human papilloma virus (HPV) can cause mucopurulent cervicitis.
- **Urethritis** is the corresponding symptom complex in men, causing mucopurulent penile discharge and dysuria. Urethritis is caused by gonorrhea or "nongonococcal urethritis" (NGU); the most common cause of NGU is *Chlamydia*, but it can also be caused by *T. vaginalis*, *Ureaplasma urealyticum*, *Mycoplasma hominis*, HSV, and adenovirus.
- All patients presenting with cervicitis or urethritis should receive appropriate antibiotic treatment and safer sex counseling. Partners should also be tested and treated.

Epidemiology

- **Chlamydia is the most common reportable STI in the United States, with 1 million cases reported annually.**
- **Gonorrhea is the second most common reportable bacterial STI in the United States.** It is estimated that only half of the cases are reported.
- Adolescents and young adults have the highest incidence of chlamydia and gonorrhea.

Pathophysiology

- *Neisseria gonorrhoeae* is a gram-negative intracellular diplococcus, visible within neutrophils on Gram stain.
- *C. trachomatis* is a gram-negative, obligate intracellular bacterium.
- *C. trachomatis* and *N. gonorrhoeae* infect columnar epithelial cells in the oropharynx, cervix, urethra, and rectum.
- Adolescent females are predisposed to chlamydia and gonorrhea because of the continued presence of columnar epithelium in the exocervix.

Risk Factors

Age ≤25, people with a history of sexual contact with new or multiple partners, forgoing barrier protection, drug use, or exchanging sex for drugs or money are high-risk groups for chlamydia and gonorrhea.

DIAGNOSIS

- **All sexually active women aged 25 or younger should be screened for chlamydia and gonorrhea annually.**
- Pregnant women should be screened during the first prenatal visit and again in the third trimester if any risk factors are present.
- Older women with multiple or new sex partners should also be screened.
- **In high-prevalence settings, all sexually active men should be tested for chlamydia and gonorrhea.**
- Annual screening for urethral and rectal chlamydia and gonorrhea, as well as pharyngeal gonorrhea, is recommended for men who have sex with men.

Clinical Presentation

- Asymptomatic chlamydial infection is common in both men and women. If symptoms of urethritis or cervicitis do develop, they will generally appear 7 to 21 days after exposure.
- Anorectal chlamydial infection may present as proctitis with anal irritation or itching, mucopurulent discharge, or tenesmus.
- Chlamydial conjunctivitis is associated with conjunctival hyperemia and eye discomfort; a mucoid discharge may be present.
- Among men with urethral gonorrhea, 90% will develop mucopurulent discharge and dysuria 2 to 14 days after exposure.
- It is estimated that 50% of women with gonorrhea are asymptomatic, but nonspecific cervicitis symptoms may start in 1 to 2 weeks after exposure.
- Anorectal gonococcal infection may present as proctitis.
- Pharyngeal gonococcal infection is usually asymptomatic, but patients might develop a mild pharyngitis.
- Purulent ocular drainage can result from gonococcal conjunctivitis; gonococcal and chlamydial conjunctivitis in adults is usually a result of auto-inoculation.

Diagnostic Testing

- Mucopurulent urethral drainage in men should be evaluated with a Gram stain and urinalysis.
  - Gram stain of secretions will show ≥5 leukocytes per high-power field (HPF) and, if gonorrhea is present, gram-negative intracellular diplococci.
  - A negative microscopic exam does not exclude infection in asymptomatic men.
- Gram staining of endocervical, anorectal, or pharyngeal secretion specimens for diagnostic purposes is not recommended.
- Patients with a history of multiple routes of exposure (i.e., vaginal, oral, and anal) should have all sites tested.
- Urinalysis may be positive for leukocyte esterase or show ≥10 leukocytes per HPF. Urine culture should be sent to evaluate for typical urinary tract infections.
- Culture has good specificity for both chlamydia and gonorrhea, but is less sensitive than other methods and time consuming.
  - For gonorrhea, the swabbed specimen should be used to directly inoculate Thayer-Martin media and sent to the laboratory as soon as possible.
  - Diagnostic cultures are usually reserved for cases with an unclear diagnosis or in the case of gonorrhea, unknown antibiotic susceptibility.
  - Culture is the legal standard for testing following suspected sexual assault.
- NAAT is routinely used to test urine, vaginal, penile, and ocular discharge. While more sensitive than culture for pharyngeal and rectal specimens, NAAT is not yet approved for this purpose and is only available at certain laboratories.

TREATMENT

- **Because of the high coincidence of chlamydial infection and gonorrhea, treatment for both is recommended when there is suspicion for either**.
- Treatment for both can be accomplished with a **one-time, directly observed dose of azithromycin and ceftriaxone**. This is generally the best option, especially if follow-up is a concern.

- Sex partners within the last 60 days should be evaluated and treated.
- Reinfection is very common. Partners need to be treated, and the patient should avoid all sexual contact until treatment is completed or 7 days following single-dose treatment.
- Test of cure is only indicated for pregnant women, if symptoms persist, or if there are concerns about antibiotic resistance or proper completion of therapy. All other patients should be encouraged to return for repeat testing in 3 to 4 months because of high rates of reinfection.
- See Table 11-3 for more details.

COMPLICATIONS

- In women, bacterial cervicitis may progress to pelvic inflammatory disease (PID; see section "Pelvic Inflammatory Disease").
- Bartholin or Skene gland infection may result in abscesses requiring drainage.
- Chlamydial urethritis can lead to epididymitis, prostatitis, or reactive arthritis in men.
- Gonorrhea can lead to epididymo-orchitis, prostatitis, and rarely urethral strictures.
- Disseminated gonococcal infection presents in one of two ways:
  - Tenosynovitis, papulopustular dermatitis, and arthralgia (without obvious purulent arthritis).
  - Purulent arthritis without skin involvement
  - Gonococcal arthritis is the most common bacterial arthritis in young adults.
- Women who are within 7 days after the onset of menses are at higher risk of developing disseminated infection.

PELVIC INFLAMMATORY DISEASE

GENERAL PRINCIPLES

- Pelvic inflammatory disease is an ascending infection causing endometritis, salpingitis, tubo-ovarian abscess (TOA), and pelvic peritonitis.
- It is a known complication of chlamydial infection and gonorrhea, but other vaginal flora can also cause PID.
- If left untreated, 10% of women develop infertility. Other complications are ectopic pregnancy and chronic pelvic pain.

DIAGNOSIS

Clinical Presentation

History
- There is a wide range of clinical severity of PID, from asymptomatic infection to frank septic shock.
- Patients may have symptoms of cervicitis plus dyspareunia.
- Lower abdominal or pelvic pain suggests PID in a patient with cervicitis.

TABLE 11-3	DIAGNOSIS AND TREATMENT OF SEXUALLY TRANSMITTED INFECTIONS ASSOCIATED WITH URETHRITIS OR CERVICITIS			
Disease	Diagnostic testing	Treatment	Alternative treatment	Notes
CT (Chlamydia trachomatis)	(1) History and exam (2) Urinalysis and urine culture (3) NAAT of endocervical or urethral secretions (4) Culture if indicated and NAAT not available	Azithromycin 1 g PO × 1 OR Doxycycline 100 mg PO bid × 7 d	Erythromycin base 500 mg PO q6h × 7 d OR Erythromycin ethylsuccinate 800 mg PO q6h × 7 d OR Ofloxacin 300 mg PO bid × 7 d OR Levofloxacin 500 mg PO qd × 7 d	Doxycycline, erythromycin estolate, and FQs should be avoided during pregnancy
Uncomplicated GC ("the clap")	(1) History and exam (2) Urinalysis and urine culture (3) Gram stain of urethral exudate, if present (4) NAAT of endocervical or urethral secretions (5) Culture if indicated and NAAT not available	Ceftriaxone 250 mg IM × 1 OR Cefixime 400 mg PO × 1 Plus concurrent treatment for CT Gonococcal conjunctivitis: Ceftriaxone 1 g IM × 1	History of severe cephalosporin allergy: best to desensitize, then treat with ceftriaxone OR Azithromycin 2 g PO × 1 (resistance reported, use only when no other option available) OR Spectinomycin 2 g IM × 1 (not available in the US)	High levels of circulating FQ resistance now preclude the use of any FQ to treat any GC infections in the US. Emerging macrolide resistance is also a concern
Disseminated gonococcal infection	(1) History and exam (2) Culture and/or NAAT of all potential mucosal sites of infection	Ceftriaxone 1 g IV or IM q24h OR Cefotaxime 1 g IV q8h × 7 days OR Ceftizoxime 1 g IV q8h	Can switch to cefixime 400 mg PO bid × 24–48 h after clinical improvement	If diagnosis is unclear, a trial of antibiotic therapy is warranted. If DGI, will usually improve rapidly.

	(3) Blood cultures (often negative) (4) Arthrocentesis for cell count and culture in joints suspicious for septic arthritis	Plus concurrent treatment for CT	Higher doses and prolonged therapy are needed for meningitis or endocarditis
Trichomonas vaginalis ("trich")	In women: wet mount exam of vaginal secretion; rapid EIA and nucleic acid probe are also available. In men: culture only approved test	Metronidazole 2 g PO × 1 OR tinidazole 2 g PO × 1 Metronidazole 500 mg PO bid × 7 d	If pregnant, advise patient on risks and benefits of treatment. Some providers wait until after 37 wk gestation to treat
NGU or MPC	(1) History and exam (2) Test for CT and GC (3) In women: test for BV and trichomoniasis	Azithromycin 1 g PO × 1 OR Doxycycline 100 mg PO bid × 7 d Treat empirically for GC if local prevalence high or if patient is of high risk	If NGU persists after initial treatment: Metronidazole 2 g PO × 1 OR Tinidazole 2 g PO × 1
PID	(1) History and exam (2) Test for CT and GC (3) Wet prep exam for WBCs, clue cells, and trichomonads	*IV Regimen A:* Doxycycline 100 mg PO or IV q12h AND Cefotetan 2 g IV q12h OR cefoxitin 2 g IV q6h IV: Ampicillin/sulbactam 3 g IV q6h PLUS Doxycycline 100 mg PO or IV q12h	Can switch to PO therapy after 24 h of improvement. If no improvement after 72 h of PO regimen, reevaluate and switch to IV regimen

(continued)

TABLE 11-3 (CONTINUED)

(4) Transvaginal ultrasound, laparoscopy, or endometrial biopsy reserved for difficult to diagnose cases	*IV Regimen B:* Clindamycin 900 mg IV q8h PLUS Gentamicin 2 mg/kg IV loading dose, with 1.5 mg/kg IV q8h for maintenance	*PO:* If unable to tolerate cephalosporins, consider treatment with levofloxacin 500 mg PO qd OR Ofloxacin 400 mg PO bid × 14 d if risk for GC is low. Test for GC prior to treatment. If NAAT positive, will need to treat for GC as above. If culture positive, treatment based on susceptibilities
	PO Regimen A: Ceftriaxone 250 mg IM × 1 AND Doxycycline 100 mg PO bid q14d and/or Metronidazole 500 mg PO bid × 14 d	
	PO Regimen B: Cefoxitin 2 g IM × 1 with probenecid 1 g PO × 1 AND Doxycycline 100 mg PO bid × 14 d and/or Metronidazole 500 mg PO bid × 14 d	
	PO Regimen C: IV third-generation cephalosporin AND Doxycycline 100 mg PO bid × 14 d and/or Metronidazole 500 mg PO bid × 14 d	

CT, *Chlamydia trachomatis*; NAAT, Nucleic acid amplification testing; FQ, fluoroquinolone; GC, *Neisseria gonorrhoeae*; DGI, disseminated gonococcal infection; EIA, enzyme immunoassay; NGU, nongonococcal urethritis; MPC, mucopurulent cervicitis; BV, bacterial vaginosis; PID, pelvic inflammatory disease; WBC, white blood cells.

Physical Exam
- The diagnosis of PID is supported by fever >38.3°C (100.9°F).[3]
- Cervicitis may be noted on a speculum exam.
- Bimanual exam will usually reveal uterine, adnexal, and/or cervical motion tenderness.
- Right upper quadrant pain and transaminitis suggest perihepatitis, or Fitz-Hugh-Curtis syndrome. Severe pain is caused by inflammation of Glisson capsule and the surrounding peritoneum.
- Consider another diagnosis (e.g., appendicitis and ectopic pregnancy) if mucopurulent discharge is not present and there are no leukocytes on wet prep exam.

Diagnostic Testing
- All women with PID should be tested for chlamydia, gonorrhea, and HIV.
- Diagnosis of PID is supported by elevated erythrocyte sedimentation rate and/or C-reactive protein (CRP), documented infection with *C. trachomatis* and/or *N. gonorrhoeae*, and fever >38.3°C (100.9°F).[3]
- More invasive studies, such as transvaginal ultrasonography, MRI, laparoscopy, or endometrial biopsy, are more specific tests for PID.

TREATMENT

- Antibiotic regimens are presented in Table 11-3.[3]
- Hospitalize patients who are acutely ill or have symptoms of an acute abdomen, are pregnant, are not tolerating or responding to outpatient antibiotics, or have a TOA.
- For women with mild or moderate PID, hospitalization is usually not necessary, and PO antibiotics provide effective treatment.
- If clinical improvement is seen on IV antibiotics, continue monitoring for another 24 hours before transitioning to PO antibiotics.
- If no improvement is seen within 72 hours, diagnostic laparoscopy may be necessary to further evaluate. If there has been no improvement after 72 hours of an outpatient PO regimen, reevaluate the patient and consider hospitalization with parenteral antibiotics.

VULVOVAGINITIS AND VAGINOSIS

GENERAL PRINCIPLES

- Symptoms of vulvar or vaginal infection include abnormal vaginal discharge or odor, as well as vulvar itching and irritation.
- Trichomoniasis, bacterial vaginosis (BV), and candidiasis can cause these symptoms.
- BV represents shifting in the normal genital flora (especially *Lactobacillus*) to anaerobes, *Gardnerella vaginalis*, and Mycoplasma species.
- Candidiasis is not generally sexually transmitted. Patients who are immunosuppressed are at higher risk of developing recurrent or severe vulvovaginal candidiasis and may benefit from longer courses of therapy.
- **Trichomoniasis is sexually transmitted. Men are almost always asymptomatic, but may have mild urethritis.**

DIAGNOSIS

- Trichomoniasis may cause diffuse cervical and vaginal erythema ("strawberry cervix") and a malodorous, frothy discharge with a pH ≥4.5.
  - Wet mount exam will often show mobile trichomonads.
  - Culture is available in some locations.
  - Point-of-care EIA and nucleic acid testing are now available, which are more sensitive than microscopic exam.
- A wet mount exam should be performed on patients with suspected BV, which will show clue cells (i.e., vaginal epithelial cells with a stippled appearance due to adherent coccobacilli). A homogenous white vaginal discharge with pH ≥ 4.5 and positive whiff test are suggestive of BV.
- Vulvovaginal candidiasis is diagnosed by a characteristic thick, curd-like vaginal discharge with intense vulvar inflammation, which will show fungal elements on 10% KOH preparation.

TREATMENT

- See Table 11-3 for treatment regimens for trichomoniasis.[3] Instruct patients to abstain from sexual activity until all partners are treated. Reinfection is very common.
- Treat BV with metronidazole 500 mg PO bid × 7 days OR metronidazole gel 0.75%, 5 g (1 applicator) intravaginally qHS × 5 days OR clindamycin cream 2%, 5 g (1 applicator) intravaginally qHS × 7 days.
  - BV is associated with adverse pregnancy outcomes; symptomatic pregnant women should be tested and treated.
  - Clindamycin cream is associated with adverse outcomes in the second half of pregnancy and should be avoided.
  - Sex partners do not need to be treated.
- Vulvovaginal candidiasis is treated with over-the-counter intravaginal azole creams and suppositories or fluconazole 150 mg PO × 1 dose.

GENITAL WARTS

GENERAL PRINCIPLES

- Genital warts are caused by HPV. Multiple subtypes exist; **types 6 and 11** are associated with genital warts, while types 16, 18, 31, 33, and 35 are associated with cervical or anorectal neoplasias.
- Genital HPV is a very common infection, with an estimated 6.2 million new cases annually in the United States. It is thought that 50% of sexually active adults will acquire genital HPV over their lifetimes.
- **Most cases are asymptomatic.**
- **Viral shedding occurs during and between symptomatic periods.** The incubation period is thought to be weeks to months.
- **Young adults should receive the HPV vaccine** to protect against certain high-risk subtypes of HPV.

DIAGNOSIS

- The appearance can vary considerably; usually, they are verrucous papules approximately 1 cm in diameter, which can spontaneously remit and recur.
- **Visual inspection is usually sufficient for diagnosis.** Biopsy is only indicated if the diagnosis is uncertain, if the patient is immunocompromised, or if the lesions do not respond to treatment, have an unusual appearance (pigmented, fixed, or indurated), or persistently ulcerate or bleed.

TREATMENT

- Treatment is focused on the removal of visible warts and to induce as long a wart-free interval as possible.
- Treatment options are as follows[3]:
  - Podofilox 0.5% solution or gel. Patients should be instructed to apply bid for 3 days, followed by 4 days of no therapy. This cycle may be repeated up to four times to treat visible warts. The total area treated should not exceed 10 cm^2.
  - Imiquimod 5% cream. Patients apply the cream to warts qHS, three times a week for up to 16 weeks; 6 to 10 hours after application, the affected areas should be washed with soap and water.
  - Cryotherapy. Treatment can be repeated every 1 to 2 weeks.
  - Podophyllin resin 10% to 20%, a small amount is applied weekly as needed. Application should be limited to <0.5 mL of resin per treatment, and the treatment area should be washed with soap and water 1 to 4 hours after treatment.
  - Trichloroacetic acid (TCA), a small amount is applied weekly as needed.
  - Surgical removal.
  - Podofilox, imiquimod, and podophyllin are cytotoxins and should not be used during pregnancy.

MOLLUSCUM CONTAGIOSUM

GENERAL PRINCIPLES

- Molluscum contagiosum is a superficial skin infection caused by the poxvirus molluscum contagiosum virus (MCV).
- The incubation period ranges from 2 weeks to 6 months. Transmission is through direct skin contact or fomites, including sexual contact, shared clothes or towels, and contact sports.
- Patients with atopic dermatitis are at particular risk of auto-inoculation and refractory infection.

DIAGNOSIS

- The diagnosis is usually made based on the appearance of the lesions. They are usually 2 to 5 mm, **waxy, painless, and umbilicated**. The central core of the lesion contains infectious viral particles.

- Patients who are immunocompromised may develop giant molluscum (≥15 mm). Biopsy may be required to exclude fungal infections or malignancy.

TREATMENT

- Most cases resolve spontaneously within 6 to 12 months. Lesions may persist for years in patients who are immunocompromised. The lesions rarely scar but may become secondarily infected.
- No single treatment has been proven to be more effective than others in treating MCV.
  - In adults, lesions may be treated by **curettage or cryotherapy in the office setting, followed by patient-applied topical imiquimod**.
  - Imiquimod should be started three times weekly; if no irritation develops, applications should be increased to once daily.
  - Other treatments include salicylic acid, TCA, KOH, cantharidin, electrocauterization, and photodynamic therapy.
- Patients should be advised to keep lesions covered whenever possible and to avoid shaving over affected areas.
- Giant molluscum is very resistant to treatment. Lesions should be treated before they coalesce into giant lesions.
- In patients with HIV, lesions usually improve with antiretroviral therapy.

ECTOPARASITES

GENERAL PRINCIPLES

- Pediculosis pubis ("crabs") is caused by a lice, *Phthirus pubis.* Infestation causes intense itching and inflammation. Lice and nits may be visible.
- *Sarcoptes scabiei* infestation is frequently sexually associated in adults.
- See Chapter 16 for further information.

DIAGNOSIS

Diagnosis is direct visualization of lice or nits.

TREATMENT

- Treatment for *P. pubis* is permethrin 1% cream applied for 10 minutes OR pyrethrins plus piperonyl butoxide applied for 10 minutes OR malathion 0.5% lotion applied for 8 to 12 hours OR ivermectin 250 µg/kg PO once, repeated in 2 weeks.
- Switch treatments if initial treatment fails.
- Bedsheets, towels, and clothes should be machine-laundered in hot water and machine-dried using heat.
- Treatment for scabies is permethrin cream 5% applied from the neck down and rinsed off in 8 to 14 hours OR ivermectin 200 µg/kg PO once then repeated in 2 weeks.

REFERENCES

1. Shiely F, Hayes K, Thomas KK, et al. Expedited partner therapy: a robust intervention. *Sex Transm Dis.* 2010;37:602-607.
2. Golden MR, Whittington WL, Handsfield HH, et al. Effect of expedited treatment of sex partners on recurrent or persistent gonorrhea or chlamydial infection. *N Engl J Med.* 2005;352:676-685.
3. Workowski KA, Berman S; Centers for Disease Control and Prevention (CDC). Sexually transmitted diseases treatment guidelines, 2010. *MMWR Recomm Rep.* 2010;59(RR-12):1-110.
4. Kingston AA, Vujevich J, Shapiro M, et al. Seronegative secondary syphilis in 2 patients coinfected with human immunodeficiency virus. *Arch Dermatol.* 2005;141:431-433.
5. Jurado RL, Campbell J, Martin PD. Prozone phenomenon in secondary syphilis. Has its time arrived? *Arch Intern Med.* 1993;153:2496-2498.
6. Méchaï F, de Barbeyrac B, Aoun O, et al. Doxycycline failure in lymphogranuloma venereum. *Sex Transm Infect.* 2010;86:278-278.

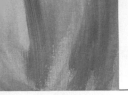

Human Immunodeficiency Virus Infection

12

Toshibumi Taniguchi and Diana Nurutdinova

GENERAL PRINCIPLES

- The first reports of cases of acquired human immunodeficiency syndrome (AIDS) were reported in the early 1980s and the virus that causes AIDS was discovered in 1983.
- HIV is no longer a "deadly" diagnosis; it has been transformed into a chronic disease requiring complex multidisciplinary care. Better understanding of pathogenesis of HIV and wide use of effective combination antiretroviral therapy (cART) led to dramatic declines in morbidity and mortality.

Definition

The unique feature of this virus is the preference for the cells that bear CD4 receptor (primarily T lymphocytes) resulting in depletion of the lymphocytes and impairment of cell-mediated immune response.

Classification

- CDC classification is widely used for public health surveillance purposes. The classification utilizes clinical conditions (Table 12-1) and CD4+ cell count to group patients.
- Details are available at http://www.cdc.gov/hiv/resources/guidelines/ (last accessed May 7, 2012).

Epidemiology

- HIV affects more than 33 million people worldwide, with the highest disease burden in sub-Saharan Africa.
- In the United States, more than a million people are living with HIV.
- Men who have sex with men account for more than a half of all new HIV infections in the United States each year and are the only risk group in which new infections have been on the rise.
- African Americans are disproportionately affected by HIV, accounting for almost half of people living with HIV, and new infections each year.

Etiology

- HIV is a lentivirus that is part of the retrovirus family.
- HIV most likely originated from simian immunodeficiency virus.
- Different HIV-1 subtypes dominate various regions worldwide.
  - HIV-1 infection in the United States is predominantly caused by subtype B.
  - HIV-2 is the virus that closely resembles HIV-1 but is characterized by a much slower progression to AIDS. It is predominant in West Africa and quite rare in the United States.

TABLE 12-1	AIDS-DEFINING CONDITIONS (ADULTS AND ADOLESCENTS AGE ≥13)

Candidiasis of bronchi, trachea, or lungs

Candidiasis of esophagus

Cervical cancer, invasive

Coccidioidomycosis, disseminated or extrapulmonary

Cryptococcosis, extrapulmonary

Cryptosporidiosis, chronic intestinal (>1 mo duration)

Cytomegalovirus disease (other than liver, spleen, or nodes)

Cytomegalovirus retinitis (with loss of vision)

Encephalopathy, HIV related

Herpes simplex: chronic ulcers (>1 mo duration) or bronchitis, pneumonitis, or esophagitis

Histoplasmosis, disseminated or extrapulmonary

Isosporiasis, chronic intestinal (>1 mo duration)

Kaposi sarcoma

Lymphoma, Burkitt (or equivalent term)

Lymphoma, immunoblastic (or equivalent term)

Lymphoma, primary, of brain

Mycobacterium avium complex or *Mycobacterium kansasii*, disseminated or extrapulmonary

Mycobacterium tuberculosis of any site, pulmonary, disseminated, or extrapulmonary

Mycobacterium, other species or unidentified species, disseminated or extrapulmonary

Pneumocystis jiroveci pneumonia

Pneumonia, recurrent

Progressive multifocal leukoencephalopathy

Salmonella septicemia, recurrent

Toxoplasmosis of brain

Wasting syndrome attributed to HIV

Pathophysiology

- Understanding of the HIV life cycle and its structure plays a critical role in appreciating the mechanism of action of antiretrovirals.
- During the early stages of infection, there is massive replication of the virus in the gut lymphatic tissue accompanied by cytokine production. Subsequently chronic

immune system activation determines the course of the illness. Specific T-cell response is generated as a result of the infection early but antibodies cannot effectively neutralize the virus.

- Permanent viral reservoirs containing proviral DNA are established in latent T cells or macrophages, making HIV infection nearly impossible to eradicate.
- The HIV viral envelope consists of a lipid bilayer with embedded gp120/gp41 complex. The viral capsid is made of p24; the core contains two single strands of RNA packaged with structural proteins and surrounded by the p17 matrix.
- The first step in the HIV replication cycle is the binding of the viral gp120 surface protein to CD4 receptor–containing cells (T cells, macrophages, and microglial cells).
- In order for viral entry to occur, coreceptor binding is necessary. HIV can bind to two chemokine receptors: CCR5 or CXCR4. Strains of HIV can express tropism for either of the coreceptors or have a dual tropism. Upon binding to the chemokine coreceptor, gp120/gp41 undergoes a conformational change, resulting in a hairpin-like structure that promotes fusion between the cell membrane and the virion.
  - ○ **Fusion inhibitor**. Enfuvirtide (T-20) binds to gp41, preventing the fusion of the virion with the cell
  - ○ **Chemokine receptor inhibitor**. Maraviroc (MVC) blocks the CCR5 receptor. An antagonist for a CXCR4 receptor is not clinically available.
- Once inside the cytoplasm, the virion undergoes reverse transcription. Viral RNA becomes double-stranded DNA that is later transported to the nucleus.
  - ○ **Nucleoside reverse transcriptase inhibitors** (NRTIs) are structural analogs of normal nucleosides or nucleotides, which target the reverse transcriptase and terminate HIV DNA synthesis.
  - ○ **Nonnucleoside reverse transcriptase inhibitors** (NNRTIs) bind to the reverse transcriptase and block polymerization of the viral DNA.
- After entering the nucleus, the double-stranded DNA integrates into the host chromosomal DNA, which is mediated by the HIV integrase. This process is referred to as DNA strand transfer.
  - ○ **Integrase strand transfer inhibitors** (INSTIs). Raltegravir (RAL) binds to HIV integrase and prevents DNA strand transfer.
- As viral RNA is produced, it gets packaged in a new virion with structural proteins and enzymes and then buds into the extracellular environment. Trimming of the structural proteins by HIV protease is necessary.
  - ○ **Protease inhibitors** (PIs). Bind to HIV protease preventing the packaging of virion. The majority of PIs require combination with low-dose ritonavir to boost blood levels.

Risk Factors

- HIV transmission can occur via blood, semen, vaginal fluid, or breast milk that may contain cell-bound or free viral particles.
- Transmission occurs via unprotected sexual intercourse, contaminated blood (sharing needles or equipment for illicit drugs or occupational exposure), and perinatally from mother to child.
- Unprotected anal receptive intercourse carries the highest risk of HIV acquisition.
- The presence of genital ulcer disease also increases the risk of transmission.

Prevention

- Prevention strategies are based on each specific mode of transmission.
- **Preexposure prophylaxis** is a strategy to prevent HIV by using antiretroviral medications **prior to a potential exposure to HIV**.

○ Using antiretrovirals before a potential high-risk HIV exposure is under investigation.

○ Use of microbicides or antiretroviral topical formulations to prevent HIV transmission is in clinical trials.

• **Treatment as prevention** (universal test and treat) is an emerging concept, which is based on the hypothesis that enhanced identification of HIV patients followed by rapid initiation of cART regardless of CD4 cell count or disease stage would reduce transmission and thus HIV infection rates at the population level.

• **Postexposure prophylaxis** can be divided into two categories: occupational and nonoccupational exposures.

○ **Occupational exposure**

■ Assess the source, volume of fluid, type, and timing of the exposure. HIV and hepatitis B (HBV) and C (HCV) testing is required.

■ Testing for exposed person: at baseline, 6 weeks, 12 weeks, and 6 months.

■ Offer 28 days of antiretrovirals for exposures with increased transmission risk. Table 12-2 summarizes the recommendations based on exposure types. However, with better tolerated antiretrovirals, three-drug regimens are usually used (Table 12-3).

○ **Nonoccupational exposure**

■ Nonoccupational postexposure prophylaxis (nPEP) is offered **for high-risk exposures (sexual or needle sharing) from a known HIV-positive source, presenting within 72 hours**. For nPEP, three-drug antiretroviral regimen is provided for 28 days.

■ nPEP for a high-risk exposure from a source with an unknown HIV status has to be individualized.

■ nPEP is not recommended if the exposed person presents after 72 hours.

DIAGNOSIS

• **HIV screening tests**

○ **The CDC recommends routine HIV screening for all adolescents and adults (aged 13 to 64) in health care settings, as a part of routine medical care.** Separate consent is not required but the patient should be informed of the HIV testing. Educational materials on HIV testing should be provided.

○ **HIV screening of all pregnant women is recommended, using an opt-out approach.** Repeat testing should be performed in the third trimester in women who tested negative at the initial screening.

○ Screening for HIV infection can be performed with a conventional enzyme-linked immunosorbent assay (ELISA) or a rapid HIV test that detects both HIV-1 and 2.

○ Newer assays that combine both antigen (p24) and antibody have high sensitivity and specificity.

○ Rapid HIV tests are utilized in the settings where the advantage of providing quick results is imperative (e.g., emergency rooms, urgent care, labor, and delivery).

○ **ELISA may be false negative during the interval between HIV infection and antibody detection** (serological window period). This window period is about 2 to 8 weeks depending on an assay utilized.

○ Confirmatory testing should follow any positive screening test.

TABLE 12-2	CDC RECOMMENDATIONS FOR HIV OCCUPATIONAL POSTEXPOSURE PROPHYLAXIS		
Exposure type	Infection status of the source		
	HIV positive, class 1[a]	HIV positive, class 2[b]	Source of unknown HIV status
Percutaneous			
Less severe[c]	Basic two-drug PEP recommended	Expanded three-drug PEP recommended	PEP generally not warranted; may consider basic two-drug PEP[d] when exposure to HIV is likely
More severe[e]	Expanded three-drug PEP recommended	Expanded three-drug PEP recommended	PEP generally not warranted; may consider basic two-drug PEP[d] when exposure to HIV is likely
Mucous membrane or nonintact skin			
Small volume[f]	Consider basic two-drug PEP	Basic two-drug PEP recommended	PEP generally not warranted
Large volume[g]	Basic two-drug PEP recommended	Expanded three-drug PEP recommended	PEP generally not warranted; may consider basic two-drug PEP[d] when exposure to HIV is likely

PEP, postexposure prophylaxis.

[a]HIV positive, class 1—asymptomatic HIV infection or known low viral load (e.g., <1,500 RNA copies/mL).

[b]HIV positive, class 2—symptomatic HIV infection, acquired immunodeficiency syndrome, acute seroconversion, or known high viral load.

[c]Solid needle or superficial injury.

[d]The designation "consider PEP" indicates that PEP is optional; a decision to initiate PEP should be based on a discussion between the exposed person and the treating clinician of the risks vs. benefits of PEP.

[e]Large-bore hollow needle, deep puncture, visible blood on device, or needle used in patient's artery or vein.

[f]A few drops.

[g]A major blood splash.

- **Confirmatory tests**
  - HIV Western blot (or indirect immunofluorescence assay) is used to confirm the HIV screening test. Western blot is positive in the presence of two of the following bands: p24, gp41, and gp160/120. When there are no bands present, the test result is interpreted as negative. Indeterminate test result is the presence of any other bands that do not meet the positive criteria.

TABLE 12-3	ANTIRETROVIRAL THERAPY FOR POSTEXPOSURE PROPHYLAXIS

Occupational exposures

- Basic two-drug regimen: (ZDV or TDF) plus (3TC or FTC)
- Expanded three-drug regimen: Basic two-drug regimen plus LPV/r
  ATV/r can be the third agent as well
- If drug resistance of the source is known, adjust the regimen accordingly

Nonoccupational exposures

- (ZDV or TDF) plus (3TC or FTC) plus EFV **OR**
- (ZDV or TDF) plus (3TC or FTC) plus LPV/r
  o ATV/r can be the third agent as well
  o We recommend use of **PIs** instead of NNRTIs due to high transmission prevalence of NNRTI-resistant HIV.

ZDV, zidovudine; TDF, tenofovir; 3TC, lamivudine; FTC, emtricitabine; LPV, lopinavir; ATV, atazanavir; EFV, efavirenz; PI, protease inhibitor; NNRTI, nonnucleoside reverse transcriptase inhibitor.

- o If the HIV Western blot test result is indeterminate, follow-up testing should be performed 4 weeks after the initial test. **Western blot may be false negative if the patient is in the serological window period**. In this case, HIV RNA assay should be considered.
- o HIV-2 infection is confirmed by HIV-2 Western blot, in patients with high suspicion for this infection but with negative or indeterminate HIV-1 Western blot result and negative HIV-1 RNA level.

Clinical Presentation

- **Acute HIV infection**
  - o The symptoms of acute HIV infection resemble infectious mononucleosis with fever, pharyngitis, adenopathy, rash, myalgia or arthralgia, headaches, and fatigue. Oral ulcers and gastrointestinal symptoms (diarrhea, odynophagia, anorexia, abdominal pain, and vomiting) may also occur.
  - o The severity of illness may impact the long-term outcome, predicting the progression of disease.
  - o The time from exposure to clinical manifestations of the acute HIV is typically 2 to 4 weeks and lasts for about 3 weeks.
  - o Massive depletion of CD4 cells and rapid increase in HIV RNA is seen as the initial response to the infection. With evolution of HIV-specific immunity (primarily from HIV-specific CD8+ cytotoxic T lymphocytes), HIV RNA level falls by 2 to 3 logs and the symptoms of acute retroviral syndrome resolve. CD4 cell count rebounds but remains below the baseline. Initiation of HIV therapy at this stage remains controversial.
- **Chronic HIV infection**
  - o The length of time from initial infection to the clinical disease varies.
  - o During the asymptomatic, chronic phase of HIV infection, active virus replication is ongoing and progressive. Persons with high levels of HIV RNA may progress to symptomatic disease faster than those with low HIV RNA levels.

○ Patients in this stage have chronic inflammation evidenced by increase in various inflammatory markers, likely from chronic immune activation caused by HIV infection. This increases the risk of non–AIDS-related comorbidities, such as cardiovascular disease, renal dysfunction, and non–AIDS-related malignancies. ART is known to reduce chronic immune activation; therefore, some experts recommend starting cART earlier (CD4 cell count >500 cells/mm^3) in the asymptomatic, chronic HIV infection stage.

○ The spectrum of disease changes as the CD4 cell depletion continues. **Life-threatening opportunistic infections occur when the CD4 cell count drops to <200 cells/mm^3.**

○ There are several unique subsets of patients with different disease progression patterns compared with an average HIV-infected person.

■ **Long-term progressors**. These patients show little or no decline in CD4 cell count over an extended period of time and usually have only low-level viremia.

■ **Elite controllers**. Show slight or no decline in CD4 cell counts over an extended period of time and usually have extremely low HIV RNA, often <50 copies/mL.

■ **Rapid progressors**. Progress to AIDS rapidly. The mechanism of rapid progression is still unknown, but infection with CXCR4 tropic virus seems to accelerate the HIV disease.

History

Initial evaluation of persons with HIV infection (either newly diagnosed or care transferred from another physician) should include the following:

• **History of present illness**. Date of diagnosis of HIV infection and approximate onset of infection, mode of acquisition, occurrence of symptoms suggestive of acute HIV infection, history of opportunistic infections, prior negative HIV test result if available, detailed medication history (including exposure to antiretrovirals), and knowledge of initial and most recent CD4 cell counts and HIV RNA level (viral load).

• **Past medical history**. Particular emphasis should be placed on viral hepatitis coinfection, cardiovascular risk factors, tuberculosis, malignancies, HIV-associated complications, and opportunistic infections. Inquire about immunization history.

• **Social and family history**

○ Substance use history: Obtain detailed information on tobacco, alcohol, and illicit substance use.

○ Sexual history: prior history of sexually transmitted infections and current sexual activity including safe sex practices and birth control

○ Family history: As HIV-infected patients are living longer, they should be asked about family history of conditions that may predispose them to medical illness (e.g., hypertension, diabetes, hyperlipidemia, malignancies, neurologic diseases, and heart disease).

• **Medications and allergies**. Over-the-counter medication use, including supplements, natural remedies, and vitamins, should be elicited as many have interactions with ART.

• **Employment and travel history**. Social support is key for successful management of HIV-infected patients. Employment, housing, and insurance status should be discussed. Travel history and residence in certain endemic areas is essential due to the risk of reactivation of some infections (e.g., histoplasmosis, coccidioidomycosis, penicilliosis, and tuberculosis).

• **Review of systems**. Comprehensive review of systems should be completed including common HIV-related symptoms such as fever, night sweats, weight loss, headaches, visual changes, oral thrush or ulceration, swallowing difficulties, respiratory and gastrointestinal symptoms, skin rashes or lesions, and changes in neurological function or mental status.

- **Depression and domestic violence screening**. Depression is prevalent in HIV-infected patients; routine screening should be done. Patients should also be assessed for domestic violence and sexual abuse.

Physical Examination

A complete physical examination should be performed on initial presentation.

- **Skin**. Skin conditions associated with HIV infection (e.g., seborrheic dermatitis, eosinophilic folliculitis, psoriasis, superficial fungal disease, molluscum contagiosum, and Kaposi sarcoma) should be assessed.
- **Body habitus**. Assess for the presence of fat redistribution (increased dorsocervical fat pad, gynecomastia, or abdominal protuberance from visceral fat and loss of subcutaneous fat in the face, extremities, or buttocks).
- **Eyes**. Fundoscopic examination should be performed by an ophthalmologist to screen for cytomegalovirus retinitis in persons with advanced HIV (CD4 cell count <50 cells/mm^3).
- **Oropharynx**. Oral mucosa should be examined for evidence of thrush, hairy leukoplakia, mucosal Kaposi sarcoma, HSV infection, aphthous ulcers, and periodontal disease.
- **Lymph nodes**. Generalized lymphadenopathy from follicular hyperplasia is well described in HIV infection, but considering the higher risk of malignancies (e.g., lymphoma) or disseminated infections, asymmetric, bulky, or rapidly enlarging adenopathy requires further evaluation.
- **Hepatomegaly and splenomegaly**. Organomegaly can be seen in HIV infection, but could also occur as a result of other infections or malignancies.
- **Anogenital examination**. Rectal examination should be performed to evaluate for rectal masses, prostate size, external genital ulcers, or condylomatous lesions. Women should undergo pelvic examination to assess for abnormal vaginal discharge and cervical lesions.
- **Neurological examination**. General assessment of cognitive function, as well as motor and sensory testing should be performed. Patients may benefit from neuropsychological testing if there are signs of cognitive dysfunction.

Diagnostic Testing

Laboratories

- Table 12-4 lists recommended laboratory studies for patients presenting with HIV.

TABLE 12-4	RECOMMENDED LABORATORY STUDIES FOR PATIENTS PRESENTING WITH HIV INFECTION		
HIV-related tests		**Coinfection and comorbidity laboratory tests**	
CD4+ cell count	Every 3–6 mo	Chest radiography^d	If indicated
Plasma HIV RNA (viral load)	Every 3–6 mo	CMV (IgG) and other herpes virus screening^e	If indicated

HIV-related tests		Coinfection and comorbidity laboratory tests	
HIV genotype	At diagnosis, prior to cART initiation, then as needed	Cytology: Vaginal pap smear for women Rectal pap smear for men	Yearly
Coreceptor tropism[a]	Prior to use of CCR5 antagonist	*Toxoplasma gondii* (IgG)	On diagnosis, if negative, yearly
Safety monitoring laboratory tests		RPR	Every 6 mo
HLA-B*5701[b]	Once, prior to use of ABC	STD screening (chlamydia, gonorrhea)	Every 6–12 mo
Glucose-6-phosphate dehydrogenase[c]	Once, on diagnosis	Tuberculosis screening (PPD)[f]	Yearly
Complete blood count	Every 3–4 mo	Viral hepatitis screening: HBs-Ag, HBs-Ab, HCV-Ab, total HAV-Ab	On diagnosis, then yearly if indicated
Comprehensive metabolic panel	Every 3–4 mo	Serum testosterone[g]	If indicated
Fasting lipid profile	Yearly		
Urinalysis	Every 12 mo		

CMV, cytomegalovirus; cART, combination antiretroviral therapy; RPR, rapid plasma reagin; ABC, abacavir; STD, sexually transmitted disease; PPD, purified protein derivative.

[a]Coreceptor tropism assay should be performed when CCR5 antagonist is considered as part of cART.

[b]HLA-B*5701 should be tested when abacavir is considered as part of cART; patients who are positive for HLA-B*5701 haplotype are at higher risk for hypersensitivity reactions with abacavir.

[c]Glucose-6-phosphate dehydrogenase (G6PD) deficiency is found in 10–15% of black men and women and men from the Mediterranean, India, and Southeast Asia. In persons with low G6PD, dapsone or trimethoprim–sulfamethoxazole can cause hemolysis.

[d]Chest radiography recommended for patients with positive PPD. Consider to obtain baseline chest radiograph in patients with underlying lung disease for future comparison.

[e]CMV screening advocated for detection of latent CMV in low-risk patients. Varicella zoster virus screening for patients without history of chickenpox or shingles. Some experts recommend HSV-2 screening.

[f]Annual PPD is important since HIV-infected patients are prone to acquire tuberculosis regardless of the CD4 cell count.

[g]Consider checking testosterone level in males who complain of fatigue, weight loss, loss of libido or erectile dysfunction, depression, and reduced bone mineral density.

- **HIV genotype testing**
  - It is important to be aware of the most commonly encountered HIV drug resistance mutations and their effect on the choice of cART (Table 12-5). Baseline genotype resistance testing is recommended at the time of HIV diagnosis and prior to initiation of cART.
  - In persons failing cART, another genotype should be performed in order to optimize further treatment options.

TABLE 12-5	IMPORTANT HIV RESISTANCE MUTATIONS

NRTI resistance mutation

M184V	Commonly seen as the first drug resistance mutation in patients who are failing treatment on 3TC- or FTC-containing regimens. It confers resistance to 3TC and FTC, decreased susceptibility to ABC and ddI. Conversely, it confers hypersusceptibility to AZT, d4T, and TDF. This mutation decreases HIV replication capacity.
K65R	Confers resistance to TDF and cross-resistance to ABC, 3TC, and ddI. Conversely, K65R induces hypersusceptibility to AZT. It also decreases the replication capacity, which may be additive when M184V is present.
L74V	Confers resistance to ddI and ABC. Conversely, it confers hypersusceptibility to AZT and TDF. L74V causes less replication capacity than wild-type virus.
TAMs	Occurs with exposure to AZT or d4T. There are two pathways: first pathway involves M41L, L210W, and T215Y, which confers high-level resistance to AZT/d4Tand has more NRTI cross-resistance; second pathway involves D67N, K70R, and K219Q/E, which confers low-level resistance to AZT/d4T and has less NRTI cross-resistance.

NNRTI resistance mutation

K103N	Commonly seen and confers resistance to EFV and NVP. ETR is still effective and should be considered as an alternative.

Note: Other NNRTI mutations may confer resistance to ETR; use of weighted score system is recommended when the use of ETR is considered in patients with NNRTI drug resistance.

PI resistance mutations

D30N	This is a signature NFV mutation that causes high level of resistance to NFV
I50L	Signature ATV mutation that causes high-level resistance to ATV but increased susceptibility to other PIs.

NRTI, nucleoside reverse transcriptase inhibitor; 3TC, lamivudine; FTC, emtricitabine; ABC, abacavir; ddI, didanosine; AZT, zidovudine; d4T, stavudine; TDF, tenofovir; TAM, thymidine analog mutations; NNRTI, nonnucleoside reverse transcriptase inhibitor; EFV, efavirenz; NVP, nevirapine; ETR, etravirine; PI, protease inhibitor; NFV, nelfinavir; ATV, atazanavir.

○ However, in extensively treatment-experienced patients with multi-class drug resistance, additional phenotype resistance could be useful, especially when use of PIs is anticipated.

○ PIs have high genetic barriers for drug resistance (need multiple mutations to confer resistance), whereas some NRTIs (such as lamivudine [3TC]) and most NNRTIs (efavirenz [EFV] and nevirapine [NVP]) have low genetic barriers where a single mutation can result in resistance.

TREATMENT

• cART or highly active antiretroviral therapy (HAART) has evolved over the past decade with easily tolerated and once-daily regimens widely available for treatment-naïve patients in resource-rich countries.

• **When to start**. Due to many ongoing clinical trials and data from large cohort studies, **treatment recommendations change frequently**. Table 12-6 summarizes the most recent recommendations for initiating ART in treatment-naïve persons.[1] **The trend is to start treatment earlier,** based on the results of several large cohort studies that demonstrated reduced mortality.[2,3]

TABLE 12-6	RECOMMENDATION FOR TIMING OF INITIATING ANTIRETROVIRAL THERAPY IN TREATMENT-NAÏVE ADULTS WITH HIV-1 INFECTION WHO ARE READY TO BEGIN THERAPY

Recommended for patients with any CD4 cell count if

• Symptomatic HIV disease

• Pregnant women

• HIV-1 RNA >100,000 copies/mL

• Rapid decline in CD4 cell count, >100 cells/mm³ per year

• Active hepatitis B or C virus infection

• Active or high risk of cardiovascular disease

• HIV-associated nephropathy

• Symptomatic primary HIV infection

• Risk of secondary HIV transmission is high (e.g., serodiscordant couples)

Recommended

• Asymptomatic, CD4 cell count ≤500 cells/mm³

Considered

• Asymptomatic, CD4 cell count >500 cells/mm³

Elite controllers (HIV RNA <50 copies/mL off ART) or stable CD4 cell counts with low-level viremia could be monitored off cART.

cART, combination antiretroviral therapy.

Adapted from Thompson MA, Aberg JA, Cahn P, et al. Antiretroviral treatment of adult HIV infection: 2010 recommendations of the International AIDS Society-USA panel. *JAMA*. 2010;304:321-333.

Medications

What to start (see Tables 12-7 through 12-11).

TABLE 12-7	RECOMMENDED INITIAL REGIMENS FOR ANTIRETROVIRAL-NAÏVE PERSONS
Dual NRTI backbone	**Key third agent**
First line	
TDF/FTC (tenofovir/emtricitabine)	**NNRTI**
	EFV (efavirenz)
	PI
	ATV/r (atazanavir plus low-dose ritonavir)
	DRV/r (darunavir plus low-dose ritonavir)
	INSTI
	RAL (raltegravir)
Second line	
ABC/3TC (abacavir/lamivudine)	**PI**
AZT/3TC	LPV/r (lopinavir/ritonavir booster)
(zidovudine/lamivudine)	FPV/r (fosamprenavir/ritonavir booster)
	NNRTI
	NVP (nevirapine)

NRTI, nucleoside reverse transcriptase inhibitor; INSTI, integrase strand transfer inhibitor; PI, protease inhibitor; NNRTI, nonnucleoside reverse transcriptase inhibitor.

TABLE 12-8	NUCLEOSIDE/NUCLEOTIDE REVERSE TRANSCRIPTASE INHIBITORS			
	Dose	**Food restrictions**	**Side effects**	**Comments**
ABC	300 mg twice daily 600 mg once daily	None	Systemic hypersensitivity reaction	Baseline HLA-B5701 needed prior to initiation; if positive do not initiate Potential cardiovascular risk

ddI	Preferred as an enteric-coated formula (Videx EC) >60 kg: 400 mg once daily <60 kg: 250 mg once daily	On empty stomach	Pancreatitis, peripheral neuropathy, diarrhea	When co-administered with TDF adjust dose to 250 mg
FTC	200 mg once daily	None	Well tolerated	Closely related to 3TC; longer half-life compared with 3TC
3TC	150 mg twice daily 300 mg once daily	None	Well tolerated	
d4T	>60 kg: 40 mg twice daily <60 kg: 30 mg twice daily Extended release >60 kg: 100 mg once daily <60 kg: 75 mg once daily	None	Peripheral neuropathy, fat redistribution, lactic acidosis, pancreatitis; hyperlipidemia	Not recommended as first line
TDF	300 mg once daily	None	GI intolerance rare; renal toxicity, bone density loss	
AZT or ZDV	300 mg twice daily	None	Bone marrow suppression, GI intolerance	Recommended in pregnancy

ABC, abacavir; ddI, didanosine; TDF, tenofovir; FTC, emtricitabine; 3TC, lamivudine ; d4T, stavudine; GI, gastrointestinal; AZT or ZDV, zidovudine; NRTI, nucleoside reverse transcriptase inhibitors; EFV, efavirenz.

Commonly used co-formulated NRTIs in the US: TDF/FTC (300 mg/200 mg); ABC/3TC (600 mg/300 mg); AZT/3TC (150 mg/300 mg); ABC/3TC/AZT (300 mg/150 mg/300 mg); EFV/TDF/ FTC (600 mg/300 mg/200 mg).

TABLE 12-9	NONNUCLEOSIDE REVERSE TRANSCRIPTASE INHIBITORS			
	Dose	Food restrictions	Side effects	Comments
EFV	600 mg once daily	On empty stomach	CNS symptoms (dizziness, vivid dreams); false-positive cannabinoid test; hyperlipidemia	Teratogenic: avoid in women of childbearing potential
NVP	Start 200 mg once daily for 2 wk, then 200 mg twice daily	None	Rash, hepatotoxicity, hypersensitivity with liver failure	Avoid initiating in females with CD4 > 250 cells/mm^3 and males with CD4 > 400 cells/mm^3
ETR	200 mg twice daily	After meal	Rash, Stevens-Johnsons syndrome	Avoid concurrent use of all PIs except DRV
DLV	400 mg three times daily	None	Rash	Rarely used

EFV, efavirenz; CNS, central nervous system; NVP, nevirapine; ETR, etravirine; PI, protease inhibitor; DRV, darunavir; DLV, delavirdine.

TABLE 12-10	PROTEASE INHIBITORS			
	Dose	Food restrictions	Side effects	Comments
ATV	300 mg with 100 mg RTV once daily	Take with food	Benign elevation of indirect bilirubin	Must be boosted with RTV with concurrent use of TDF
	Unboosted: 400 mg once daily			
DRV	800 mg with 100 mg RTV once daily	Take with food	GI intolerance; headache	
	600 mg with 100 mg RTV twice daily			

LPV/r/ fixed-dose combination with RTV	400 mg with 100 mg RTV twice daily	None	GI intolerance (dose dependent), dyslipidemia, hyperglycemia	Twice-daily regimen recommended in pregnancy
	For treatment-naïve only: 800 mg with 200 mg RTV once daily			
FPV or fAPV	700 mg with 100 mg RTV twice daily	None	Rash, GI intolerance	
	1400 mg with 200 mg RTV once daily			
	Nonboosted: 1400 mg twice daily			
SQV	1,000 mg with 100 mg RTV twice daily	Take with food	GI intolerance, headache; PR/ QT interval prolongation	Requires RTV boosting Rarely used
NFV	Nonboosted: 1,250 mg twice daily	Take with food	Significant GI intolerance (diarrhea, nausea)	Only PI that does not require boosting
IDV	800 mg with 100 mg RTV twice daily	On empty stomach if taken without RTV	Nephrolithiasis, hyperbilirubinemia	Needs adequate hydration Rarely used
	800 mg three times daily			
TPV	500 mg with 200 mg RTV twice daily	Take with food	Hepatotoxicity, hyperlipidemia, GI intolerance, subarachnoid hemorrhage	Boosted with higher dose of RTV
RTV	Used as a boosting agent with other PIs (no longer used in full dose)		GI intolerance	Capsule form replaced by tablet not requiring refrigeration

ATV, atazanavir; RTV, ritonavir; TDF, tenofovir; DRV, darunavir; GI, gastrointestinal; LPV, lopinavir/r; FPV or fAPV, fosamprenavir; SQV, saquinavir; NFV, nelfinavir; PI, protease inhibitor; IDV, indinavir; TPV, tipranavir.

TABLE 12-11	OTHER ANTIRETROVIRAL CLASSES			
	Dose	Food restrictions	Side effects	Comments
Fusion inhibitor				
T-20	90 mg subcutaneous injection twice daily	No	Painful injection site reactions	Use of injection devices to reduce pain
CCR5 receptor antagonist				
MVC	300 mg twice daily	No	Generally well tolerated; hepatotoxicity	Baseline tropism testing is required prior to initiation
	150 mg twice daily with PIs (except TPV/r)			
	600 mg twice daily with EFV or ETR			Active against R5 virus only
	150 mg twice daily with EFV or ETR and PI			Recommended for treatment-naïve patients only
INSTI				
RAL	400 mg twice daily	No	Well tolerated	

T-20, enfuvirtide; MVC, maraviroc; PI, protease inhibitor; TPV, tipranavir; EFV, efavirenz; ETR, etravirine; INSTI, integrase strand transfer inhibitor; RAL, raltegravir.

- Selection of an antiretroviral regimen is individually based, with consideration of toxicity, tolerability, pill burden, drug interactions, comorbidities, and baseline genotype.
- **The combination of dual NRTI backbone and a potent third agent from another class** is recommended and once-daily regimen is preferred.
- Once effective cART is started, treatment interruption is strongly discouraged. Based on the SMART trial data, treatment interruption was associated with increased rates of opportunistic infections and death and increased rates of major cardiovascular, renal, and hepatic complications.[3]

First Line
- Dual NRTI backbone: A combination of **tenofovir/emtricitabine (TDF/FTC) is preferred**. Renal dysfunction and decreased bone mineral density have been observed with TDF use.
- NNRTI as a third agent. **EFV is the preferred NNRTI.** EFV is contraindicated in pregnant women due to teratogenicity (category D); therefore, use of a PI should be considered in women of childbearing age.

- PI as a third agent. Recommended agents are boosted atazanavir (ATV/r) or darunavir (DRV/r). Ritonavir is added as a boosting agent to most of the PIs. ATV requires acidic gastric pH for dissolution; thus, antacids such as proton pump inhibitors may impair the absorption of ATV.
- INSTI as a third agent. Raltegravir is the only FDA-approved drug in this class at present. It is given twice daily. RAL is well tolerated with a low side-effect profile.

Second Line
- Combination of abacavir (ABC)/3TC and zidovudine (AZT)/3TC as a dual NRTI backbone has become second line. ABC was associated with increased cardiovascular risk in long-term observational studies. When starting on ABC/3TC, baseline HLA-B*5701 testing should be done to avoid serious hypersensitivity reaction to ABC.
- There is extensive clinical experience with lopinavir (LPV)/r as a third agent, but risks of dyslipidemia and gastrointestinal side effects limit its use.
- MVC is frequently reserved for treatment-experienced patients. In order to use MVC, baseline viral tropism assay is needed and the viral population should be exclusively using CCR5 receptor.

Drug Interactions
- Many antiretrovirals utilize hepatic cytochrome P-450 pathway, particularly NNRTIs and PIs.
  - These can both inhibit and induce CYP isoenzymes. Therefore, drug interactions are common with other medication classes such as rifamycins, macrolides, statins, antifungals, anticonvulsants, and others.
  - Due to complexity of drug interactions and need for dose adjustment, it is best to refer to a drug interaction database or a specialized pharmacist. Some of the important drug interactions with antiretroviral medications are listed in Table 12-12.[4]

TABLE 12-12	IMPORTANT DRUG INTERACTIONS WITH ANTIRETROVIRAL MEDICATIONS

Statins: Do not co-administer PIs with **simvastatin, lovastatin**; the statin levels significantly increase causing myopathy and rhabdomyolysis. Rosuvastatin, atorvastatin, and pravastatin can be administered at the lowest possible dose with close monitoring.

Atorvastatin	Start with lowest possible dose
Pravastatin	Avoid using with DRV/r, or start with lowest possible statin dose; other PIs do not require dose adjustment
Rosuvastatin	Co-administration with FPV/r does not require dose adjustment. For other PIs, start with lowest possible statin dose

Acid Reducers: ATV needs acid environment (solubility depending on gastric pH), thus anything that may affect gastric pH should be avoided or used with caution.

PPIs	PPIs are not recommended in patients receiving ATV. PPIs should be administered at least 12 h prior to ATV/r
	Do not co-administer NFV and PPIs. DRV/r and TPV/r may reduce PPI level

(continued)

TABLE 12-12 (CONTINUED)

H$_2$ receptor antagonists	H$_2$ receptor antagonist single dose should not exceed a dose equivalent of famotidine 20 mg daily or total daily dose equivalent of famotidine 20 mg bid in PI-naïve patients. When using with ATV/r, administer simultaneously and/or >10 h after the H$_2$ receptor antagonist

Benzodiazepines: PIs increase concentration of benzodiazepines, use with caution. Do not use midazolam or triazolam with PIs.

Antidepressants: Antidepressant response should be monitored and titrated based on clinical assessment.

Anticonvulsants

Phenytoin	Phenytoin level reduced with most of the PIs. Consider alternative anticonvulsant (typically lamotrigine. Do not co-administer with ETR
Carbamazepine	Co-administration with boosted PIs will increase carbamazepine level and decrease PI levels. Do not co-administer with ETR
Phenobarbital	PI levels reduced substantially; consider alternative. Do not co-administer with ETR
Lamotrigine	Lamotrigine level is decreased with concurrent use of PIs. Titrate lamotrigine dose to effect
VPA	VPA level decreased by LPV/r and conversely LPV/r level increased by VPA. Monitor VAP level and response.

Antifungals (Azoles): Azoles have significant interactions with PIs and NNRTIs.

Itraconazole	Co-administration of itraconazole and PIs may result in increased itraconazole or PI levels. Itraconazole level should be monitored for dose adjustments
Posaconazole	Posaconazole increases ATV level, monitor for adverse events
Voriconazole	Voriconazole level is reduced with concomitant use of RTV. Voriconazole is contraindicated to co-administer with EFV as standard dose. If co-administration is necessary, adjust dose to voriconazole 400 mg twice daily and EFV 300 mg once daily

Inhaled Fluticasone

Concurrent use of RTV results in significant increased level of fluticasone (used in inhalers such as fluticasone/salmeterol or intranasal spray) causing systemic corticosteroid adverse effect. Avoid fluticasone, or give with caution.

Antimycobacterials

Do not co-administer rifampin and PIs. Rifabutin dose should be adjusted. Refer Chapter 13 for detailed dosing. Clarithromycin level may be increased with concurrent PIs; monitor for side effects. Clarithromycin level is reduced with concurrent use of NNRTIs; monitor for efficacy.

Hormonal Contraceptives

Boosted PIs significantly reduce the ethinyl estradiol level, thus alternatives or additional method of contraception should be used. ATV/r may be used if the oral contraceptives contain at least 35 µg of ethinyl estradiol. NVP decreases ethinyl estradiol level, thus alternative or additional method of contraception should be used. EFV may decrease ethinyl estradiol level. Depomedroxyprogesterone acetate is usually the common hormonal contraceptive choice.

Phosphodiesterase Type 5 Inhibitors: Concurrent use of PIs increases levels of medications in this class; start with lower dose and monitor for side effects.

Methadone: PIs decrease methadone levels; titrate the dose to avoid opiate withdrawal.

Herbals: St. John wort decreases the level of PIs and should not be co-administered.

DRV, darunavir; PI, protease inhibitor; FPV, fosamprenavir; ATV, atazanavir; PPI, proton pump inhibitors; NFV, nelfinavir; TPV, tipranavir; ETR, etravirine; VPA, valproic acid; LPV, lopinavir; NNRTI, nonnucleoside reverse transcriptase inhibitor; EFV, efavirenz; RTV, ritonavir; NVP, nevirapine.

Adapted from Panel on Antiretroviral Guidelines for Adults and Adolescents. Guidelines for the use of antiretroviral agents in HIV-1-infected adults and adolescents. Department of Health and Human Services. December 1, 2009; 1-161. http://www.aidsinfo.nih.gov/ContentFiles/AdultandAdolescentGL.pdf. Accessed May 7, 2012.

- NRTIs do not undergo hepatic transformation through the CYP metabolic pathway. INSTI is metabolized by glucuronidation that is mediated by the UDP-glucuronosyltransferase (UGT1A1) enzymes. Strong inducers of UGT1A1 enzymes (e.g., rifampin) can decrease the concentration of RAL. Other inducers of UGT1A1 such as EFV, tipranavir (TPV)/r, or rifabutin may reduce the RAL concentration.
- CCR5 antagonist MVC is a substrate of CYP3A enzymes and P-glycoprotein. MVC is neither an inducer nor an inhibitor of the CPY3A system, but its concentration can increase with CPY3A inhibitors, such as RTV and other PIs. In this case, MVC dose requires adjustment.

Management of HIV-Infected Patients in Critical Care Settings

- Among the common reasons for ICU admission among patients with HIV are respiratory failure due to bacterial pneumonias, *Pneumocystis* pneumonia, chronic obstructive pulmonary disease, and asthma exacerbation.[5] Immune reconstitution inflammatory syndrome should always be considered when cART was recently initiated.
- In patients already on cART, treatment should be continued unless the cART itself is believed to be causing harm. Common challenges in this setting are administration mode and absorption of cART, increased chance of drug interactions, and need for renal or hepatic adjustment (Table 12-13).
- If the patient is diagnosed with HIV infection during the hospitalization that required ICU care, consult an HIV specialist to discuss the indication and timing of cART.

TABLE 12-13	ANTIRETROVIRALS THAT CAN BE USED IN LIQUID FORMULATION

Liquid formulation

Abacavir	20 mg/mL
Emtricitabine	10 mg/mL
	200 mg of capsule = 240 mg of solution
Lamivudine	10 mg/mL
Stavudine	1 mg/mL
Zidovudine	50 mg/5 mL
Nevirapine	50 mg/5 mL
Lopinavir/ritonavir	400 mg lopinavir and 100 mg ritonavir per 5 mL
	Liquid contains 42.4% alcohol
Fosamprenavir	50 mg/mL
Ritonavir	600 mg/7.5 mL

Powder formulation

Didanosine	Either 10 or 20 mg/mL concentration
	10 mg/mL: Dilute the powder with water first and then equal parts with antacid (magnesium hydroxide)
	20 mg/mL: Dilute with only antacid (magnesium hydroxide). Unlabeled use
	Oral powder containing 50 mg per 1 g. Use water or milk to mix. Do not use antacids.
	More practically, 625 mg tablet could be dissolved to a small amount of water, but need to ingest immediately

Intravenous formulation

Zidovudine	10 mg/mL

Dissolves in water

Etravirine	Dissolve the dose (two 100 mg tablets) in a cup of water and ingest immediately
Nelfinavir	625 mg tablet could be dissolved in a small amount of water and ingested immediately

Instruction for opening capsules or crushing tablet available

Emtricitabine	Powder in the capsule is water soluble (no stability and pharmacokinetic information available)
Tenofovir	Dissolves in 100 mL of water (no stability and pharmacokinetic information available)

| Efavirenz | Liquid formulation is currently under investigation. Insoluble in water. Open the capsules and mix with 5 mL MCT oil (Captex) or 15 mL Orasweet and ingest immediately (no stability and pharmacokinetic information available) |
| Atazanavir | Open the capsules and mix with four ounces of applesauce and ingest immediately (bioavailability of atazanavir mixed with applesauce was 92% compared with ingestion of two 200 mg capsules) |

- ○ If the patient has AIDS-associated condition, initiation of cART should be considered, preferably within 2 weeks.
- ○ If the condition is not associated with AIDS but the CD4 cell count is ≤200 cells/mm^3, initiation of ART should be considered.[6]

SPECIAL CONSIDERATIONS

Antiretroviral Therapy in Specific Conditions

- • **Chronic kidney disease**. Renal dose adjustment is required for most of the NRTIs (except ABC). Possible backbone drugs are ABC, FTC, or 3TC, TDF is associated with proximal renal tubular injury and should be used with caution in patients with chronic kidney disease (CKD). Possible third agents would be PIs and NNRTIs and other classes (RAL and MVC) that do not require renal adjustment.
- • **Chronic HBV infection**. At least two HBV-active drugs should be used in cART. Typically regimens containing TDF/FTC are used in this setting. Potential third agents include EFV, RAL, or a boosted PI.
- • **Chronic HCV infection**. cART should be initiated in all HCV coinfected patients, regardless of CD4 cell count. If HCV infection is being treated with a ribavirin-containing regimen, concurrent AZT use should be avoided due to high rates of anemia; didanosine (ddI)/stavudine (d4T) should be avoided due to life-threatening mitochondrial toxicity, hepatomegaly, steatosis, pancreatitis, and lactic acidosis, and ABC could decrease response to HCV treatment.
- • **Management of pregnant women**
  - ○ **To prevent mother to child transmission, all HIV-infected pregnant women should receive cART during pregnancy regardless of HIV RNA and CD4 cell count**. Therapy is usually started in the second trimester. Close follow-up is imperative. The goal is to achieve an undetectable viral load before delivery.
  - ○ Avoid teratogenic drugs (e.g., EFV) or drugs with known adverse potential for the mother (e.g., combination of d4T/ddI).
  - ○ AZT is the only FDA-approved antiretroviral for HIV-infected pregnant women.
  - ○ **LPV/r + AZT/3TC is the preferred regimen during pregnancy**.
  - ○ NVP should be avoided if CD4 cell count is >250 cells/mm^3 due to increased risk of hepatotoxicity. Women already on NVP should continue regardless of the CD4 cell count.
  - ○ Intrapartum intravenous (IV) AZT is recommended for all HIV-infected pregnant women. AZT continuous IV infusion is administered with loading dose of 2 mg/kg over 1 hour, followed by 1 mg/kg/h until delivery.

TABLE 12-14 MANAGEMENT OF HIV-INFECTED PREGNANT WOMEN

1) *HIV-1-infected women on cART who became pregnant*

   a) Continue cART, but discontinue medications (with known adverse potential in pregnancy

   b) Perform HIV genotype resistance test if the women have detectable viremia on cART

   c) Continue cART during intrapartum period and postpartum

2) *HIV-1-infected women who are antiretroviral naïve and have indications for cART*

   a) Perform HIV genotype resistance test prior to initiating cART

   b) Initiate cART after the first trimester (14 wk gestation)

   c) If a woman requires immediate initiation of ART for her own health, initiate as soon as possible, including the first trimester

   d) Continue cART during intrapartum period and postpartum

3) *HIV-1-infected women who are antiretroviral naïve and do not require cART treatment for their own health*

   a) Initiate cART after the first trimester

   b) Decision to continue or discontinue cART after delivery should be individualized

4) *HIV-infected women who received no cART prior to labor*

   a) Use AZT only

   • IV AZT as continuous infusion during labor for a woman

   • Oral AZT for infant for 6 wk

   b) Use combination of AZT + single-dose NVP

   • IV AZT as a continuous infusion during labor, plus single-dose NVP at the onset of labor

   • Combination of oral AZT/3TC can be given for at least 7 d postpartum to reduce the chance of NVP resistance

   • Oral single-dose NVP plus oral AZT for 6 wk for infant

---

cART, combination antiretroviral therapy; AZT, zidovudine; NVP, nevirapine; 3TC, lamivudine.

Adapted from Panel on Treatment of HIV-Infected Pregnant Women and Prevention of Perinatal Transmission. Recommendations for use of antiretroviral drugs in pregnant HIV-1-infected women for maternal health and interventions to reduce perinatal HIV transmission in the United States. September 14, 2011;1-207. http://aidsinfo.nih.gov/contentfiles/PerinatalGL.pdf. Accessed May 7, 2012.

○ Elective cesarean delivery should be scheduled at 38 weeks gestation if plasma HIV-1 RNA remains >1,000 copies/mL near the time of delivery. For scheduled cesarean delivery, IV AZT should be started at least 3 hours prior.

○ Infants should be started on AZT as soon as possible after birth. AZT dosing for infants ≥35 weeks gestation at birth is 2 mg/kg orally within 6 to 12 hours of delivery, then every 6 hours for 6 weeks.

○ Breast-feeding should be avoided in developed countries with access to clean water and formula.

○ Table 12-14 provides further details on management of HIV-infected pregnant women.[7]

Immunization in HIV-Infected Patients

Table 12-15 summarizes the recommendations for immunization of HIV-infected patients. **Inactivated vaccines are generally acceptable, live vaccines are contraindicated in severely immunocompromised** (CD4 cell count <200 cells/mm^3).

TABLE 12-15 IMMUNIZATION IN HIV-INFECTED PATIENTS

Immunization	Special considerations
Inactivated vaccines	
Pneumococcal vaccine: 23 polyvalent polysaccharide pneumococcal vaccines. Some experts recommend deferring the vaccine until the CD4 cell counts are >200 cells/mm^3 for a better response.	Vaccinate every 5 y
Hepatitis A vaccine: Recommended for MSM, IVDU, persons with chronic liver disease, and those coinfected with HBV and/or HCV. Patients with CD4 cell count >200 cells/mm^3 or undetectable HIV RNA are more likely to achieve vaccine response.	Two doses given at 0 and 6–12 mo for HAVRIX, 0 and 6–18 mo for VAQTA
Hepatitis B vaccine: Recommended for those without evidence of past or present HBV infection. Standard dose of 20 µg may be used; however, we recommend routine use of higher dose (40 µg) as standard dose was inferior to higher dose to elicit vaccine response. Patients with CD4 cell counts of >200 cells/mm^3 and suppressed virus have higher chance of adequate vaccine response.	Three doses given at 0, 1, and 6 mo. Dose 40 µg. Vaccinated patients should be tested for HBs antibody response after the third dose. Consider repeating the series if no response and giving a booster if low response
Influenza vaccine: Inactivated influenza vaccine is recommended for all HIV-infected patients. Use of the intranasally administered, live, attenuated vaccine is not recommended.	Vaccinate annually
Tetanus toxoid: Principles are the same as HIV-negative persons. Substitute one-time dose of Tdap vaccine at time of next booster.	Every 10 y

(continued)

TABLE 12-15 (CONTINUED)

Human papillomavirus vaccine: Optional. Vaccine could be given to females aged 9–26 y, but may also be considered in other groups. Safety and immunogenicity in HIV-infected patients are unknown and studies are ongoing.	Three doses given at 0, 2, and 6 mo
Meningococcal vaccine: Optional. Conjugated meningococcal vaccine should be administered to persons with asplenia, with travel exposure, of college age, or living in dormitories	Single dose, repeat every 5 y if high risk
Polio vaccine: Optional. Live OPV is contraindicated. Immunize with IPV in selected patients at high risk.	IPV consists of three doses at 0, 4–8 wk, and 6–12 mo
Haemophilus influenzae type B vaccine: Optional. The incidence of Hib infection among HIV-infected adults is low. However, asplenic patients and those with history of recurrent *Haemophilus* infections should be considered for immunization.	Single dose
Live vaccines	
Varicella vaccine (Varivax): Varicella vaccine should be administered to HIV-infected patients with CD4 cell count >200 cells/mm^3 if no evidence of immunity to varicella.	Two doses at 0 and 4–8 wk
Zoster vaccine (Zostavax): Zostavax consists of attenuated varicella virus at a concentration at least 14 times that found in Varivax. Safety and immunogenicity studies among HIV-infected persons are ongoing.	Single dose for persons with history of varicella
MMR vaccine: MMR vaccine should be administered to HIV-infected patients with CD4 cell counts >200 cells/mm^3.	One or two doses (if two doses, minimum interval of 28 d)

MSM, Men who have sex with men; IVDU, intravenous drug user; HBV, hepatitis B virus; HCV, hepatitis C virus; OPV, oral polio vaccine; IPV, inactivated polio vaccine; Hib, *H. influenzae* type b.

COMPLICATIONS

Antiretroviral Toxicities

- **Lactic acidosis**. The clinical picture can range from asymptomatic hyperlactatemia to severe lactic acidosis with hepatomegaly and steatosis. Higher rates of lactic acidosis have been reported with the use of stavudine and didanosine. Suspected drugs should be discontinued and supportive care provided. Incidence of lactic acidosis has declined with the use of current NRTIs.

TABLE 12-16 CHOICE OF LIPID-LOWERING AGENTS

Serum LDL above threshold or triglyceride 200–500 mg/dL with elevated non-HDL cholesterol

- First choice: Pravastatin 20–40 mg PO once daily or atorvastatin 10 mg PO once daily

- Alternative choice: Fluvastatin 20–40 mg PO once daily, rosuvastatin 5 mg PO once daily

- Alternative classes: Fibrate or niacin

Serum triglycerides >500 mg/dL

- First-choice fibrate: Gemfibrozil 600 mg PO twice daily or fenofibrate 54–160 mg PO once daily

- Alternative to fibrate: Niacin or fish oil

LDL, low-density lipoprotein; HDl , high-density lipoprotein.

- **ABC hypersensitivity reaction**. Symptoms of hypersensitivity include fever, skin rash, fatigue, and gastrointestinal symptoms such as nausea, vomiting, diarrhea, or abdominal pain and respiratory symptoms such as pharyngitis, dyspnea, or cough. ABC may cause a fatal hypersensitivity reaction at re-challenge. To avoid these reactions, routine screening for the presence of HLA-B*5701 allele is recommended; the presence of the allele indicates high risk of ABC reactions.
- **Hepatotoxicity caused by NVP**. NVP can cause severe hepatotoxicity, which may be fatal. Females with CD4 cell count >250 cells/mm^3 or males with CD4 cell count >400 cells/mm^3 are at increased risk for developing hepatotoxicity. If used, NVP should be initiated at a lower dose with close monitoring of the liver function.
- **Nephrotoxicity caused by TDF**. TDF is associated with nephrotoxicity, particularly rare cases of proximal tubular toxicity (Fanconi syndrome) and requires frequent kidney function monitoring in persons with CKD.

Complications Associated with cART for HIV

- **Fat redistribution**. Lipodystrophy and lipohypertrophy are alterations in body fat distribution, such as accumulation of visceral fat in the abdomen, neck (buffalo hump), and pelvic areas and/or depletion of subcutaneous fat causing facial or peripheral wasting. PIs and NRTIs (stavudine, didanosine, and to a lesser extent AZT) are associated with these changes but other factors may also play a role.
- **Peripheral neuropathy**
  - HIV-associated neuropathy is a common neurological complication of HIV infection and its treatment. Diagnosis is made clinically and by excluding other possibilities for peripheral neuropathy.
  - HIV-associated neuropathy is common in advanced infection when CD4 cell count is low and HIV RNA is high. NRTIs such as d4T, ddI, and AZT are associated with this condition.
  - If onset of neuropathy is recent, optimizing cART can improve the symptoms to some extent.

- o Treatment is largely symptomatic and includes lamotrigine, gabapentin, and antidepressants (amitriptyline, duloxetine, and venlafaxine).
- **Cardiovascular disease** associated with HIV infection and cART
  - o A number of observational studies have demonstrated higher rates of cardiovascular disease in HIV-infected patients.
  - o Certain antiretrovirals are linked to increased cardiovascular risk in observational studies. Studies have shown increased atherogenic effects of some antiretrovirals.
  - o ABC is associated with increased risk of cardiovascular events. Some experts avoid ABC when patients have high underlying risk profile for cardiovascular disease. LPV, fosamprenavir, and indinavir may be associated with increased cardiovascular risk with cumulative use.
- **Dyslipidemia** associated with HIV infection and cART. Dyslipidemia is a common problem among HIV-infected patients (see table 12-16 for treatment recommendations).[8] Lipid abnormalities are frequently observed in persons with HIV independent of cART. Different antiretrovirals may induce various patterns of lipid abnormalities, for example, hypertriglyceridemia is associated with many PIs, and stavudine causes low-density lipoprotein elevation. Lastly, some NRTIs are considered "lipid neutral."

HIV-Associated Complications
- **HIV-associated nephropathy** (HIVAN)
  - o HIVAN is characterized by rapidly progressive renal dysfunction and massive proteinuria (1 to 3 g/d or more). Renal biopsy shows focal segmental glomerulosclerosis. Risk factors include African descent; diabetes; hypertension; hepatitis C infection; and CD4 cell count <200 cells/mm^3, HIV RNA level of >4,000 copies/mL.
  - o cART can halt the progression when started early; angiotensin converting enzyme inhibitors may be effective, although no prospective randomized controlled trials have been performed.
- **HIV-associated neurocognitive disorders** (HAND):
  - o With wide use of cART, the prevalence of HIV-associated dementia has diminished while less severe neurocognitive disorders have risen as individuals live longer.
  - o Patients with mild forms of HAND may complain of mild difficulties in concentration, attention, and memory while the neurologic examination is unremarkable. Whether HAND improves with better central nervous system penetrating cART is unclear.
- **HIV-associated thrombocytopenia**: Primary HIV-associated thrombocytopenia can present as the initial manifestation of HIV in 10% of cases. It is similar to idiopathic thrombocytopenic purpura. Timely initiation of cART will reverse HIV-associated thrombocytopenia.

MONITORING/FOLLOW-UP

- HIV RNA and CD4 cell count should be monitored closely, preferably 6 to 8 weeks after initiation of cART, and routinely monitored 3 to 4 times a year. Long-term treatment goal is to suppress HIV below the levels of detection and reconstitute CD4 cell count.
- Treatment failure. Treatment failure is defined as a suboptimal response to cART. Reasons for treatment failure include poor adherence, medication tolerability, and drug interactions.

- **Virologic failure**. Virologic failure is defined as inability to achieve or maintain HIV RNA levels below the limit of detection (<20 copies/mL).
  - Incomplete virologic response. Two consecutive plasma HIV RNA >200 copies/ mL after 24 weeks of cART.
  - Virologic rebound. Detection of HIV RNA after complete virologic suppression.
  - Antiretroviral regimens should be reviewed and genotype resistance testing should be obtained while the patient is still taking the failing regimen.
- **Immunologic failure**. Immunologic failure can be defined as a failure to achieve and maintain an adequate CD4 T-cell response despite virologic suppression but a specific cut-off is difficult to establish. Typically, CD4 cell counts increase by 100 to 150 cells/ mm^3 in antiretroviral-naïve persons. There is no consensus on how to manage immunologic failure and it is not clear if cART regimen adjustment makes a difference.

OUTCOME/PROGNOSIS

- Mortality continues to decline with wide use of potent cART that provides durable virologic suppression and reconstitution of the immune system. **Life expectancy in HIV infection is now comparable to any chronic disease**.
- An increasing proportion of deaths in HIV-infected patients are attributed to other causes, such as malignancies, HCV infection, and cardiovascular disease.
- HIV infection may be associated with accelerated aging. It is unclear if this is due to HIV infection–induced chronic inflammatory response or cART toxicities.

ADDITIONAL RESOURCES

- HIV management guideline available at http://aidsinfo.nih.gov/ (last accessed May 7, 2012)
- HIV knowledge base and drug interaction database: http://hivinsite.ucsf.edu/ (last accessed May 7, 2012)
- HIV resistance interpretation algorithms: http://hivdb.stanford.edu/ (last accessed May 7, 2012)
- Genotype interpretation algorithms and treatment guidelines at IAS-USA: http:// www.iasusa.org/ (last accessed May 7, 2012)
- Drug interaction charts: http://www.hiv-druginteractions.org/ (last accessed May 7, 2012)
- HIV primary care guidelines: http://www.hivma.org/ (last accessed May 7, 2012)
- Useful resource for patients: www.thebody.com (last accessed May 7, 2012), www. aidsmed.com (last accessed May 7, 2012), www.avert.org/ (last accessed May 7, 2012)

REFERENCES

1. Thompson MA, Aberg JA, Cahn P, et al. Antiretroviral treatment of adult HIV infection: 2010 recommendations of the International AIDS Society-USA panel. *JAMA.* 2010;304:321-333.
2. Kitahata MM, Gange SJ, Abraham AG, et al. Effect of early versus deferred antiretroviral therapy for HIV on survival. *N Engl J Med.* 2009;360:1815-1826.
3. El-Sadr WM, Lundgren JD, Neaton JD, et al. CD4+ count-guided interruption of antiretroviral treatment. *N Engl J Med.* 2006;355:2283-2296.

4. Panel on Antiretroviral Guidelines for Adults and Adolescents. Guidelines for the use of antiretroviral agents in HIV-1-infected adults and adolescents. Department of Health and Human Services. December 1, 2009; 1-161. http://www.aidsinfo.nih.gov/ContentFiles/AdultandAdolescentGL.pdf. Accessed May 7, 2012.

5. Huang L, Quartin A, Jones D, Havlir DV. Intensive care of patients with HIV infection. *N Engl J Med.* 2006;355:173-181.

6. Zolopa A, Andersen J, Powderly W, et al. Early antiretroviral therapy reduces AIDS progression/death in individuals with acute opportunistic infections: a multicenter randomized strategy trial. *PLoS One.* 2009;4(5):e5575.

7. Panel on Treatment of HIV-Infected Pregnant Women and Prevention of Perinatal Transmission. Recommendations for use of antiretroviral drugs in pregnant HIV-1-infected women for maternal health and interventions to reduce perinatal HIV transmission in the United States. September 14, 2011; 1-207. http://aidsinfo.nih.gov/contentfiles/PerinatalGL.pdf. Accessed May 7, 2012.

8. Dubé MP, Stein JH, Aberg JA, et al. Guidelines for the evaluation and management of dyslipidemia in human immunodeficiency virus (HIV)-infected adults receiving antiretroviral therapy: recommendations of the HIV Medical Association of the Infectious Disease Society of America and the Adult AIDS Clinical Trials Group. *Clin Infect Dis.* 2003;37(5):613-627.

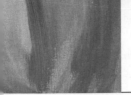

Opportunistic Infections Associated with HIV

13

Toshibumi Taniguchi and Jessica R. Grubb

- With progressive HIV disease, immunosuppression occurs, manifest by declining CD4 T-lymphocyte counts and a marked increase in the risk of opportunistic infections (OIs).
- With increased use of potent combined antiretroviral therapy (cART), the incidence of OIs has declined, resulting in a marked improvement in survival.
- OIs still occur in individuals presenting with advanced AIDS and in patients who are nonadherent or fail cART reconstitution.
- Prophylaxis for OIs can be divided into primary and secondary prophylaxis. Primary prophylaxis is instituted before an OI occurs. Institution mainly depends on the level of immunosuppression (Table 13-1). Secondary prophylaxis is instituted after treatment of an episode of infection.
- **Immune reconstitution inflammatory syndrome** (IRIS) describes clinical findings associated with immune reconstitution that occur in patients with advanced HIV disease who experience paradoxical worsening of an underlying OI after initiation of cART. Progression of known OIs, development of new OIs, and drug toxicity may make the diagnosis of IRIS more difficult. If IRIS occurs, ART should be continued unless there is a reason to stop (e.g., life-threatening illness or danger of permanent sequelae). Addition of low-dose steroids might decrease the degree of inflammation.
- Timing of starting cART with active OIs.
  AIDS Clinical Trials Group (ACTG) A5164 showed survival benefit in patients who were started on cART within 2 weeks of treatment of OIs excluding tuberculosis (TB).[1] Other studies also suggest survival benefits when patients are treated earlier versus later for TB.[2,3] Some experts recommend initiating cART immediately after starting the treatment of OIs, while others may wait a few days for the patient to stabilize.

FUNGAL INFECTIONS

PNEUMOCYSTIS PNEUMONIA

GENERAL PRINCIPLES

- Pneumocystis pneumonia (PCP) is a fungal infection caused by *Pneumocystis jirovecii.*
- Before the use of cART and primary PCP prophylaxis, PCP occurred in 70% to 80% of patients with AIDS. The incidence of PCP has declined dramatically, although it is still one of the most common OI in advanced HIV disease.
- Risk factors are CD4 cell count <200 cells/mm^3, history of oropharyngeal candidiasis, or prior PCP.

TABLE 13-1	COMMON OPPORTUNISTIC INFECTION PRIMARY PROPHYLAXIS		
Opportunistic infection	Indication for prophylaxis	Medications	Discontinue prophylaxis
Pneumocystis pneumonia	CD4 <200 cells/mm^3 or oropharyngeal candidiasis or CD4 <14%	TMP/SMX DS PO once daily or three times weekly Alternatives: Dapsone 100 mg PO once daily Atovaquone 1,500 mg PO once daily	CD4 >200 cells/mm^3 for >3 mo
Toxoplasmosis	CD4 <100 cells/mm^3 and anti-*Toxoplasma* IgG positive	TMP/SMX DS PO once daily Alternatives: Dapsone 200 mg PO once weekly + pyrimethamine 50 mg PO once weekly + leucovorin 25 mg PO once weekly. Atovaquone 1,500 mg PO once daily +/– (pyrimethamine 25 mg PO once daily + leucovorin 10 mg PO once daily)	CD4 >200 cells/mm^3 for >3 mo
MAC	CD4 <50 cells/mm^3 after ruling out active MAC infection	Azithromycin 1,200 mg PO once weekly Alternatives: clarithromycin, rifabutin (rule out active TB)	CD4 >100 cells/mm^3 for >3 mo

TMP/SMX, trimethoprim–sulfamethoxazole; MAC, *Mycobacterium avium* complex.

DIAGNOSIS

Clinical Presentation
- Symptoms are often present for weeks and may include progressive fatigue, exertional dyspnea, nonproductive cough, fever, pleuritic chest pain, and hypoxemia.
- Lung examination is usually normal, although fine bibasilar rales may be heard. There may be a decline in oxygen saturation with exertion.

Diagnostic Testing
- **Lactate dehydrogenase** (LDH) may be elevated, but is nonspecific and sensitivity depends on severity of the pulmonary disease. The arterial blood gas helps determine whether to hospitalize the patient, to administer adjunctive corticosteroids, or to assess response to treatment. Use of polymerase chain reaction (PCR) technology is under investigation.
- **Chest radiographs** are initially normal in up to 25% of the patients. The most common findings are diffuse, bilateral, interstitial, or alveolar infiltrates progressing from perihilar to peripheral regions. Pneumatoceles are associated with prolonged, indolent disease and predispose to pneumothoraces. In patients at high-risk

suspicion for PCP but with normal chest radiographs, **high-resolution chest CT scan** may reveal ground glass opacities.
- Diagnosis of PCP relies on **microscopic visualization** of the cysts and/or trophozoite forms on stained respiratory specimens.
  - Sputum induction is usually attempted, followed by bronchoscopy with bronchoalveolar lavage (BAL) with or without transbronchial biopsies.
  - Sensitivity of sputum induction varies depending on the quality of the sample and experience of the laboratory, making **BAL the diagnostic procedure of choice** for obtaining adequate specimens.
  - Specimens can be stained by methenamine silver or toluidine blue or Giemsa, but **direct fluorescent antibody staining** is the most common technique used.

TREATMENT

- Treatment duration is 21 days, but response is gradual. Trimethoprim–sulfamethoxazole (TMP-SMX) is recommended as first-line treatment for PCP (Table 13-2).

TABLE 13-2	TREATMENT OF PNEUMOCYSTIS PNEUMONIA

Not acutely ill (able to take oral medication, Pao$_2$ >70 mm Hg)
- TMP-SMX two DS tabs PO every 8 h.

Acutely ill (not able to take oral medication, Pao$_2$ <70 mm Hg)
- TMP-SMX (5 mg/kg of TMP component per day) intravenously every 6–8 h.
- Prednisone taper is administered when Pao$_2$ <70 mm Hg or alveolar-arterial oxygen gradient >35 mm Hg. Prednisone is given 40 mg PO twice daily for 5 d, then 40 mg PO once daily for 5 d and 20 mg PO once daily for 11 d. (If oral medication is not feasible, IV methylprednisolone can be administered as 75% of prednisone dose.)

Alternative regimens
- Clindamycin 600 mg IV every 8 h (or 300–450 mg PO four times daily) plus primaquine 30 mg PO once daily.
- Atovaquone 750 mg PO twice daily. Only for PCP of mild-to-moderate severity.
- Pentamidine 4 mg/kg/d IV once daily. Adverse reaction can be life threatening and may include pancreatitis, hypotension, hypoglycemia, renal insufficiency, cardiac arrhythmias (including torsade de pointes).

Secondary prophylaxis
- TMP-SMX should be given at the completion of PCP treatment. Regimen is the same as the primary prophylaxis.
- Secondary prophylaxis may be discontinued with CD4 cell count >200 cells/mm^3 for more than 3 mo.

TMP/SMX, trimethoprim–sulfamethoxazole; PCP, pneumocystis pneumonia.

- Glucose-6-phosphate dehydrogenase deficiency should be assessed prior to the use of dapsone or primaquine to avoid severe hemolytic anemia.
- TMP-SMX is still the drug of choice for the pregnant patient.
- Some evidence has been found for person-to-person transmission of *P. jirovecii*, but there is no clear evidence of benefit from isolating patients with PCP.[4]

CANDIDIASIS

GENERAL PRINCIPLES

- **Oropharyngeal candidiasis is the most common OI in HIV-infected patients.** It is most often observed in patients with CD4 cell count <200 cells/mm^3.
- *Candida albicans* is the most common pathogen; however, *Candida tropicalis*, *Candida krusei*, and *Candida dubliniensis* have been reported.
- Infections by *Candida glabrata* and *Candida parapsilosis* tend to occur in patients with prior antifungal exposure.

DIAGNOSIS

- **Oropharyngeal candidiasis.** Patients experience burning pain in the mouth and altered taste sensation. "Thrush" is a removable white creamy plaque on any oral mucosal surfaces. These plaques have an erythematous base when scraped.
- **Esophageal candidiasis.** Patients may present with dysphagia or odynophagia, with or without oropharyngeal lesions. Diagnosis is made by direct visualization of the esophagus by endoscopy. **This is an AIDS-defining condition**.
- **Vulvovaginal candidiasis.** Patients present with itching, vaginal erythema with white discharge, dyspareunia, dysuria, and erythema of the labia and vulva.

TREATMENT

- **Oropharyngeal candidiasis.** Patients respond well to **topical antifungal therapy**. Clotrimazole oral troches (10 mg five times daily) or nystatin oral suspension (500,000 units/5 mL four times daily) may be used. Patients with moderate to severe disease, recurrent infections, and advanced immunosuppression (CD4 <100 cells/mm^3) should be treated with **oral azoles** (fluconazole 200 mg loading dose, followed by 100 to 200 mg once daily for 7 to 14 days after clinical improvement).
- **Esophageal candidiasis.** Fluconazole (400 mg loading dose, followed by 200 to 400 mg PO or IV once daily) is recommended for esophageal candidiasis. Those refractory to fluconazole after 1 week may be switched to voriconazole or posaconazole (oral therapy) or echinocandins (e.g., caspofungin) if IV is required. Amphotericin B is an alternative option, but toxicity limits its use. Pregnant patients should be treated with amphotericin B since azoles are teratogenic; safety data are not available for echinocandins.
- **Vulvovaginal candidiasis. Topical antifungal therapy** such as clotrimazole, miconazole, butoconazole, or tioconazole cream is used. **Oral fluconazole** 150 mg as a single dose is also effective. Complicated cases may require prolonged therapy, either with topical treatment >7 days or two doses of fluconazole 150 mg given 72 hours apart.

CRYPTOCOCCOSIS

GENERAL PRINCIPLES

- Cryptococcal infection is the most common systemic fungal infection in HIV-infected patients.
- While cryptococcal disease may occur at any CD4 cell count, over 75% of meningitis occurs in patients with CD4 cell count <50 cells/mm^3.

DIAGNOSIS

Clinical Presentation

- **Cryptococcal meningitis** has an indolent course and is generally a manifestation of disseminated disease. Symptoms include headache, malaise, and prolonged fever. Meningeal irritation is uncommon. The headache often worsens with sneezing or coughing.
- Pulmonary symptoms, with abnormal chest radiograph, and prostatitis may occur; the prostate may serve as a nidus for recurrence.
- Other sites of extraneural involvement include joints, oral cavity, pericardium, myocardium, skin, mediastinum, and genitourinary tract.

Diagnostic Testing

- A positive cerebrospinal fluid (CSF) culture for *Cryptococcus neoformans* is the gold standard. Lumbar puncture is necessary.
- Brain imaging is often obtained prior to lumbar puncture, which may show cerebral atrophy and ventricular enlargement.
- Latex agglutination test for **cryptococcal polysaccharide antigen** is highly sensitive and specific in both serum and CSF.
- If serum cryptococcal antigen is positive in a suspected case, lumbar puncture should still be performed. Opening pressure should always be documented and is of prognostic significance. Elevation of intracranial pressure may require repeated CSF drainage.

TREATMENT

- Standard treatment is **amphotericin B** 0.7 to 1.0 mg/kg/d IV (lipid formulation of amphotericin 4 to 6 mg/kg/d IV) plus **flucytosine** (5-FC) 100 mg/kg/d PO divided over 4 doses for 2 weeks (induction therapy) followed by **fluconazole** 400 mg PO once daily for 8 weeks (consolidation therapy).
- Flucytosine blood level should be monitored to avoid toxicity; peak level 2 hours after dose should not exceed 75 µg/mL.
- Close monitoring is required for any clinical signs of increased pressure or with intracranial pressure of >25 cm H$_2$O. One approach is to remove the volume of CSF that halves opening pressure (typically 20 to 30 mL).
- For patients intolerant of amphotericin B, fluconazole 400 to 800 mg once daily (PO or IV) plus flucytosine 100 mg/kg/d PO divided over four doses for 4 to 6 weeks can be used.
- **Secondary prophylaxis** with fluconazole 200 mg PO once daily should be given upon completion of treatment. It can be discontinued when the CD4 cell count is >200 cells/mm^3 for >6 months.

SPECIAL CONSIDERATIONS

- The optimal timing of cART in HIV-infected patients presenting with cryptococcal meningitis remains controversial. ACTG A5164 showed survival benefit of early initiation of cART (within 2 weeks). However, a study from Zimbabwe showed increased mortality when cART was started within 72 hours of diagnosis of cryptococcal meningitis.[5] Further studies are needed.
- In asymptomatic patients with positive serum cryptococcal antigen, blood cultures should be obtained and lumbar puncture be performed. If the CSF is positive, the patient should be treated for meningitis. If CSF is negative, the patient should receive fluconazole 400 mg PO once daily until CD4 cell count >100 cells/mm^3 for 3 months.

HISTOPLASMOSIS

GENERAL PRINCIPLES

- In the pre-cART era, histoplasmosis occurred in about 5% of HIV-infected patients in endemic regions (Ohio and Mississippi River valleys). Nearly all cases were disseminated at the time of diagnosis.
- The incidence has declined dramatically with the use of cART, but patients in endemic regions with CD4 cell counts <100 cells/mm^3 are at increased risk for histoplasmosis.
- Dissemination can result from primary infection or reactivation of *Histoplasma capsulatum*.

DIAGNOSIS

Clinical Presentation
- Fever, weight loss, and respiratory symptoms occur.
- Hepatosplenomegaly, lymphadenopathy, and skin lesions may be found.
- Neurological disease is seen in 10% of disseminated histoplasmosis, presenting as subacute meningitis or focal brain lesions.
- Disseminated disease can cause sepsis-like syndrome and acute respiratory distress syndrome. It may also cause adrenal insufficiency.

Diagnostic Testing
- Chest radiograph on presentation may show streaky infiltrates but may be normal 50% of the time.
- An elevated LDH (>600 units/L) may suggest histoplasmosis in patients with persistent fevers.
- Diagnosis is made by isolation of *H. capsulatum* from blood, bone marrow, lung tissue, or lymph nodes.
- Sensitivity of serologic tests may decrease with profound immunosuppression. Rapid diagnosis of disseminated histoplasmosis can be made by detection of polysaccharide antigen in the urine (sensitivity 90%) and blood (sensitivity 75%); however,

there is cross-reactivity with *Penicillium marneffei*, *Paracoccidioides brasiliensis*, and *Blastomyces dermatitidis* antigens. Monitoring antigen levels may detect early relapse.

TREATMENT

- Standard therapy is **itraconazole**. For additional details, see "*Histoplasma capsulatum*" in Chapter 15.
- Itraconazole levels should be monitored for optimal treatment. Serum concentrations of itraconazole + hydroxyitraconazole should be >1 μg/mL.
- Secondary prophylaxis can be discontinued with >12 months of itraconazole therapy, negative blood cultures, *Histoplasma* serum antigen <2 units, CD4 cell count >150 cells/mm³, and ART use for >6 months. Secondary prophylaxis should be resumed if CD4 count drops to <150 cells/mm³.

COCCIDIOIDOMYCOSIS

GENERAL PRINCIPLES

- *Coccidioides immitis* and *Coccidioides posadasii* are soil-dwelling dimorphic fungi.
- Most cases in HIV-infected patients occur in endemic areas (Southwestern United States, Northern Mexico, and portions of Central and South America).

DIAGNOSIS

- The main clinical syndromes are pneumonia, skin manifestations, meningitis, and liver or lymph node involvement.
- Patients can be asymptomatic and have positive coccidioidal serology tests.
- Focal pneumonia can occur in patients with CD4 cell count >250 cells/mm³, whereas other manifestations occur with lower CD4 counts.
- Diagnosis is confirmed by culture of the organism or by demonstration of the typical spherule on histopathologic examination of involved tissue.
- Serologic tests are specific and tend to reflect active disease, although they are less frequently positive in patients with low CD4 cell counts.
- Complement fixation IgG antibody is frequently detected in CSF in coccidioidal meningitis.

TREATMENT

- Standard therapy is amphotericin B or an azole antifungal agent. See "*Coccidioides immitis*" in Chapter 15.
- Secondary prophylaxis in mild infection may be discontinued if treated for >12 months and CD4 cell counts are >250 cells/mm³ and receiving cART.
- Unlike histoplasmosis or cryptococcosis, secondary prophylaxis of severe infection and meningitis should be continued indefinitely regardless of the CD4 cell count.

BACTERIAL INFECTIONS

MYCOBACTERIUM AVIUM COMPLEX

GENERAL PRINCIPLES

- Disseminated *Mycobacterium avium* complex (MAC) infection is an important OI in patients with advanced HIV infection (CD4 cell counts <50 cells/mm^3).
- Localized MAC infection may occur with higher CD4 cell counts, especially among patients who have immune reconstitution with use of cART.

DIAGNOSIS

Clinical Presentation

- Symptoms of disseminated MAC are nonspecific. Fever and malaise are most frequent. Night sweats, abdominal pain, organomegaly, lymphadenopathy, diarrhea, and weight loss are also seen.
- Focal inflammatory lymphadenitis may develop shortly after initiation of cART.

Diagnostic Testing

- Common laboratory abnormalities include anemia, neutropenia, and elevated alkaline phosphatase.
- Diagnosis is established by culturing the organism from blood or bone marrow although it often takes weeks for the organism to grow. Blood cultures using special media (BACTEC or DuPont Isolator systems) yield the highest sensitivity.
- Specific DNA probes for MAC are available, differentiating MAC from other mycobacteria within hours when there is sufficient mycobacterial growth in broth or agar.
- With high suspicion of disseminated MAC infection but negative blood cultures, bone marrow, liver, or lymph node biopsy may yield acid-fast bacteria or granulomas.

TREATMENT

- Combination therapy is necessary to decrease the risk of drug resistance (Table 13-3).
- **Clarithromycin** 500 mg PO twice daily (or clarithromycin extended release formulation 1,000 mg PO once daily) and **ethambutol** 15 mg/kg PO once daily are recommended agents.[6]
- Adding **rifabutin** 300 mg PO once daily may be beneficial, but clinicians should evaluate potential interactions with other agents. Increased levels of rifabutin and decreased levels of clarithromycin may occur when given together. Uveitis may occur with this combination.
- Azithromycin 500 to 600 mg PO once daily may be substituted if the patient is intolerant to clarithromycin. However, some studies suggest inferiority of azithromycin to clarithromycin.[7] Adding a third or fourth agent may be considered in severe cases.
- Without immune reconstitution, treatment is lifelong. After immune reconstitution, at least 12 months of MAC treatment and 6 months of immune reconstitution (CD4 >100 cells/mm^3) is suggested.

TABLE 13-3   TREATMENT OF TUBERCULOSIS

Treatment for drug-susceptible active TB

Initial phase (2 mo)

INH + (RIF or RFB) + PZA + EMB (If drug susceptibility shows sensitivity to INH and RIF and PZA, then EMB may be discontinued before 2 mo of treatment is completed.)	Pulmonary TB	6 mo
	Pulmonary TB with cavitary lung lesions and positive culture after 2 mo of TB treatment	9 mo

Continuation phase

INH + (RIF or RFB) once daily or three times weekly or twice weekly (if CD4 count >100 cells/mm^3)	Extrapulmonary TB with CNS, bone, or joint infections	9 to 12 mo
	Extrapulmonary TB in other sites	6 to 9 mo

Treatment of drug-resistant active TB

Resistant to INH	(RIF or RFB) + EMB + PZA	6 mo
	(RIF or RFB) + EMB	12 mo
	FQ may strengthen the regimen for patients with extensive disease	
Resistant to rifamycins	INH + PZA + EMB + FQ for 2 mo, followed by 10–16 mo with INH + EMB + FQ	12–18 mo
	Amikacin or capreomycin may be included in the first 2–3 mo for patients with rifamycin resistance and severe disease	

MDR or XDR TB

Therapy should be individualized based on resistance pattern

TB, tuberculosis; INH, isoniazid; RIF, rifampin; RFB, rifabutin; PZA, pyrazinamide; EMB, ethambutol; CNS, central nervous system; FQ, fluoroquinolones; MDR, multidrug resistant; XDR, extensively drug resistant.

MYCOBACTERIUM TUBERCULOSIS

GENERAL PRINCIPLES

- HIV-infected patients are at substantially increased risk for developing TB regardless of CD4 cell count.
- After HIV seroconversion, rapid depletion of TB-specific T helper cells is seen.

- **TB is the leading cause of AIDS-related death worldwide**, especially in sub-Saharan Africa. The emergence of drug-resistant TB has further increased the high mortality.

DIAGNOSIS

Clinical Presentation

- The clinical presentation depends on the level of immunosuppression. Patients with higher CD4 cell counts (>200 to 300 cells/mm^3) will have classic TB with apical cavitary lung disease, respiratory symptoms, fever, night sweats, and weight loss.
- As immunity wanes, atypical chest radiographic features and extrapulmonary TB are more common.
- The most common sites of extrapulmonary involvement are blood and extrathoracic lymph nodes, followed by bone marrow, genitourinary tract, and the central nervous system (CNS).

Diagnostic Testing

- Cultures of *Mycobacterium tuberculosis* from appropriate specimens are required for diagnosis.
- The sputum acid-fast bacillus (AFB) smear for AFB is approximately 50% sensitive in HIV-infected patients.
- Rapid growth detection is enabled by newer liquid culture methods like BACTEC and MIGIT systems. Nucleic acid–based amplification test (NAAT) assays are used for rapid detection of TB in patients with positive AFB smears. In patients with negative AFB smears, the sensitivity of NAAT assays is low and positive tests should be interpreted with caution.
- Drug-susceptibility testing helps guide treatment and decreases the transmission of drug-resistant TB.
- Chest radiographs should be obtained; upper lung field involvement and pulmonary cavitation are both suggestive of TB.

TREATMENT

Primary Tuberculosis

- For details regarding TB treatment, see the Tuberculosis section in Chapter 5.
- Optimal timing of ART in patient with active TB infection remains controversial, although data suggest survival benefit in early initiation of ART after starting TB therapy.
- There are important drug interactions to consider in HIV-infected persons with TB. Where available, rifabutin is substituted due to rifampin's potent induction of cytochrome P450 CYP3A, lowering the concentration of protease inhibitors and nonnucleoside reverse transcriptase inhibitors.
- Directly observed therapy is recommended for all HIV patients undergoing treatment for active TB.

Latent Tuberculosis

- All HIV-infected patients should be tested for latent TB infection (LTBI) at the time of HIV diagnosis and once every year.
- Diagnosis of LTBI can be made by tuberculin skin test (TST); **induration >5 mm is considered positive**.

TABLE 13-4	DOSE ADJUSTMENT WITH RIFABUTIN/RIFAMPIN AND CONCURRENT ART
ART	**Rifabutin-related dose adjustment**
Boosted protease inhibitors	Decrease rifabutin to 150 mg PO three times weekly or 150 mg PO every other day
EFV	Increase rifabutin to 450–600 mg PO once daily
NVP and ETR	No need for rifabutin dose adjustment
ETR coadministered with boosted protease inhibitors	Do not use rifabutin
RAL and MVC	Under investigation
ART	**Rifampin-related dose adjustment**
Boosted protease inhibitors	Do not use rifampin
EFV	Increase EFV to 800 mg PO once daily

ART, antiretroviral therapy; EFV, efavirenz; NPV, nevirapine; ETR, etravirine; RAL, raltegravir; MVC, maraviroc.

- Interferon-gamma release assay is another test with better specificity than TST.[8]
- In any HIV-infected patient, LTBI should be treated once active TB has been ruled out.
- Isoniazid (INH) 300 mg PO once daily or 900 mg PO twice weekly (both with pyridoxine 50 mg PO once daily) for 9 months should be used as treatment.
- If INH is not tolerated, rifampin 600 mg PO once daily or rifabutin (dose adjusted based on the concomitant ART, Table 13-4) for 4 months may be used.
- For known exposure to drug-resistant TB, consultation with public health authorities is recommended.

SYPHILIS

- See Syphilis section in Chapter 11 for diagnosis and treatment recommendations.
- The presentation of syphilis in HIV-infected patients may be atypical, with more organ involvement, atypical rashes, and rapid progression to neurosyphilis.
- Primary syphilis in HIV-infected patients may manifest with the classic chancre, a painless nodule that rapidly ulcerates, or with multiple or atypical chancres. The primary lesion may be absent or missed. More rapid progression to secondary syphilis is observed in HIV-infected patients, especially among those with advanced immunosuppression.
- Neurosyphilis can occur at any stage of syphilis and may be asymptomatic. CSF examination should be considered in patients with neurologic symptoms or in patients with syphilis regardless of the stage, if serum rapid plasma reagin is >1:32, or with a CD4 cell count <350 cells/mm^3. CSF VDRL is specific but not sensitive; therefore, a negative test does not exclude the diagnosis of neurosyphilis.

BARTONELLOSIS

GENERAL PRINCIPLES

- *Bartonella* spp. can cause a wide variety of infections including cat scratch disease, endocarditis, bacillary angiomatosis (BA), and bacillary peliosis hepatis (BP). The latter two occur only in immunosuppressed persons.
- BA is a unique vascular proliferative lesion caused by *Bartonella quintana* or *Bartonella henselae* and usually occurs in advanced HIV infection with CD4 cell counts <50 cells/mm^3. These lesions can form in different organs, including skin, bone, brain, lymph nodes, bone marrow, and gastrointestinal and respiratory tract.
- BP is a histopathologically different vascular proliferative response that can be seen in the liver and spleen.

DIAGNOSIS

- Diagnosis can be confirmed by histopathological examination of biopsied tissue.
- **Upon visual inspection, BA is indistinguishable from Kaposi sarcoma** (KS); therefore, any new vascular lesion should be biopsied.
- BA lesions show characteristic vascular proliferation, and a modified silver stain (e.g., Warthin-Starry stain) usually reveals numerous bacilli. Gram stain and acid-fast stains are negative.
- Antibodies to *B. henselae* can be measured using indirect immunofluoresence. A new enzyme immunoassay is more sensitive.
- Blood collection tubes containing ethylenediaminetetraacetic acid can be used to isolate *Bartonella* spp. from blood.
- PCR for Bartonella DNA is sensitive but is not widely available.

TREATMENT

- **Erythromycin** 500 mg PO four times daily or **doxycycline** 100 mg PO twice daily is recommended. Considering the poor tolerability of erythromycin, some experts recommend doxycycline over erythromycin. Clarithromycin and azithromycin are alternatives.
- CNS involvement of severe bartonellosis should be treated with doxycycline 100 mg IV every 12 hours with 300 mg IV every 12 hours.
- Duration of therapy should be at least 3 months. BP should probably be treated with IV for the first several weeks and then switched to PO for at least 4 months and possibly indefinitely.
- Relapse can occur after the primary treatment; long-term suppression with doxycycline or a macrolide should be given if relapse occurs.
- Long-term suppression can be discontinued after the patient has received 3 to 4 months of treatment and when the CD4 cell count is >200 cells/mm^3 for more than 6 months.

PROTOZOAL INFECTIONS

TOXOPLASMA GONDII

GENERAL PRINCIPLES

- Toxoplasmosis occurs due to reactivation of the intracellular protozoan parasite *Toxoplasma gondii*, generally when the CD4 cell count is <100 cells/mm^3.
- All patients with HIV infection should be screened for *T. gondii* antibodies at baseline and yearly if negative.
- Counseling on prevention is needed for seronegative patients. Ingestion of undercooked or raw meat, vegetables or other products containing tissue cysts, and direct contact with cat feces are the major routes of transmission.

DIAGNOSIS

Clinical Presentation

- Toxoplasmic encephalitis (TE) is the most common presentation. Patients present with headache, weakness, confusion, seizures, and coma depending on the location of the lesion.
- Disseminated toxoplasmosis, which involves the heart, lung, colon, skeletal muscles, and other organs, is rare.

Differential Diagnosis

- Both CNS lymphoma and TE can present with ring-enhancing brain lesions. It is difficult to distinguish between the two based on imaging alone.
- After obtaining appropriate diagnostic testing, empiric therapy for TE may be started and response assessed.
- TB, fungal infections, nocardiosis, syphilis, KS, chagoma, and other brain tumors are other possibilities.

Diagnostic Testing

- The presence of **IgG *T. gondii*–specific antibodies** is a marker for potential development of toxoplasmosis as most infections are due to reactivation. Therefore, a patient with negative *T. gondii* IgG is unlikely to have TE. The level of antibody does not predict reactivation or severity of disease.
- **Multiple ring-enhancing brain lesions** often associated with edema are characteristic. MRI is more sensitive than CT scan for detection of brain lesions. Primary CNS lymphoma cannot be distinguished from TE solely on the basis of imaging. Thallium single-photon emission computed tomography and fluorodeoxyglucose positron emission tomography may be useful in distinguishing between TE and CNS lymphoma, but their value has not been established in HIV-infected patients.
- Definitive diagnosis is made by demonstrating numerous *T. gondii* tachyzoites or cysts in a **brain biopsy**. Brain tissue should also be checked by PCR for *T. gondii* DNA. Response to empiric therapy can be helpful when biopsy is not possible.

- CSF may show mild mononuclear pleocytosis and elevated protein. Wright-Giemsa stain of centrifuged preparation of CSF may reveal tachyzoites. *T. gondii* DNA should also be assessed by PCR. The sensitivity of CSF PCR for *T. gondii* is between 50% and 98% and the specificity is almost 100%.[9]

TREATMENT

- Treatment of toxoplasmosis is summarized in Table 13-5.
- **Alternative regimens are clearly inferior** and should be reserved for patients who cannot tolerate the standard regimens.

TABLE 13-5	TREATMENT OF TOXOPLASMOSIS

Standard regimens

- Pyrimethamine 200 mg PO loading dose followed by 50 mg (<60 kg) or 75 mg (>60 kg) once daily *plus* leucovorin (folinic acid) 10–25 mg PO once daily *plus* sulfadiazine 1,000 mg (<60 kg) or 1,500 mg (>60 kg) PO every 6 h.
  - If the patient cannot tolerate sulfadiazine, use clindamycin 600 mg IV or PO every 6 h

Alternative regimens

- Pyrimethamine *plus* leucovorin *plus* one of the following:
  - Atovaquone 750 mg PO every 6 h or 1,500 mg PO twice daily
  - Azithromycin 1,200–1,500 mg once daily
- TMP-SMX (5 mg/kg TMP and 25 mg/kg SMX) IV or PO twice daily

Other consideration

Corticosteroids are used for significant edema and/or mass effect

Duration of therapy

At least 6 wk of treatment regimen followed by chronic maintenance therapy (secondary prophylaxis)

Secondary prophylaxis

- Pyrimethamine 25–50 mg PO once daily *plus* sulfadiazine 2,000–4,000 mg PO daily (in two to four divided dose) *plus* leucovorin 10–25 mg PO once daily
- Alternatives:
  - Clindamycin 600 mg PO every 8 h *plus* pyrimethamine 25–50 mg PO once daily *plus* leucovorin 10–25 mg PO once daily
  - Atovaquone 750 mg PO every 6–12 h and/or ([pyrimethamine 25 mg PO once daily *plus* leucovorin 10 mg PO once daily] *or* sulfadiazine 2,000–4,000 mg PO daily)

—

TMP-SMX, trimethoprim–sulfamethoxazole.

DIARRHEA CAUSED BY PROTOZOAL INFECTIONS

- Diarrhea is one of the most common symptoms of HIV-infected patients.
- Acute diarrhea may be caused by bacteria (*Campylobacter jejuni, Clostridium difficile, Salmonella, Shigella*, etc.) or enteric viruses.
- Patients with CD4 cell count <200 cells/mm^3 may have chronic diarrhea with *Cryptosporidium, Cyclospora, Isospora, Microspora*, cytomegalovirus (CMV), or MAC. *Giardia* and *Entamoeba histolytica* can cause persistent diarrhea regardless of CD4 cell counts.
- TMP-SMX prophylaxis has greatly reduced the incidence of diarrheal illness in HIV-infected patients.

CRYPTOSPORIDIOSIS

GENERAL PRINCIPLES

- This is a highly infectious parasite (size 4 to 6 μm) that may be fatal in HIV-infected individuals.
- Transmission is primarily via fecal–oral route.
- Numerous US waterborne outbreaks have affected non–HIV-infected persons.

DIAGNOSIS

- Symptoms include diarrhea, nausea and vomiting, abdominal pain, and weight loss.
- Fulminant and extraintestinal disease can be seen in patients with CD4 cell counts <50 cells/mm^3. Infection of the biliary tree causes sclerosing cholangitis and acalculous cholecystitis.
- Laboratory studies reveal an elevated alkaline phosphatase.
- Ultrasonography may demonstrate gallbladder wall thickening and dilated bile ducts.
- Modified acid-fast stain and enzyme immunoassays of the stool or other tissue specimens are used.

TREATMENT

- Reconstitution of immune system with cART is key to treatment of cryptosporidium.
- **There is no reliable therapy for cryptosporidiosis.**
- Nitazoxanide has been approved for children of age <11 but its effectiveness in immunosuppressed adults is questionable. Paromomycin has transient or no benefit.

MICROSPORIDIOSIS

GENERAL PRINCIPLES

- Microsporidia is the smallest (1 to 5 μm) protozoal pathogen in this section.
- Two species are important to be aware of in HIV-infected patients.
  - ○ *Enterocytozoon*: Causes 90% of intestinal microsporidiosis. *Enterocytozoon bieneusi* is also associated with cholangitis and cholecystitis.
  - ○ *Encephalitozoon*: *Encephalitozoon hellem* and *Encephalitozoon cuniculi* can disseminate to lungs and kidneys and often spare the intestine. *E. hellem* causes punctuate keratoconjunctivitis. *Encephalitozoon intestinalis* causes diarrhea, accounting for 10% of microsporidial diarrhea.

DIAGNOSIS

- Microscopic examination of stool, tissue, or corneal scraping using modified tri-chrome stains can establish the diagnosis.
- Transmission electron microscopy is considered the gold standard but is time consuming.

TREATMENT

- **Albendazole** 400 mg PO twice daily for 2 to 4 weeks is the recommended treatment.
- For *E. bieneusi*, albendazole is only partially active. The treatment of choice is fuma-gillin (or TNP-470, a synthetic analog of fumagillin), which is not available in the United States.

ISOSPORIASIS

- *Isospora belli* is an acid-fast coccidian protozoan (20 to 30 μm) that causes a **diar-rheal illness indistinguishable from cryptosporidiosis**.
- Disseminated disease can also occur.
- There is a higher prevalence in developing countries.
- Treatment consists of **TMP-SMX** DS 1 tablet PO four times daily for 10 days fol-lowed by every 12 hours for 3 weeks. Relapse rates are high; therefore, long-term maintenance therapy (TMP-SMX 1 DS tablet three times weekly) is recommended until immune reconstitution (CD4 cell count >200 cells/mm^3 for >6 months).
- Alternatively, pyrimethamine 75 mg PO once daily plus leucovorin 10 mg PO once daily may be used if patients cannot tolerate TMP-SMX. Chronic maintenance ther-apy is with pyrimethamine 25 mg PO once daily plus leucovorin 5 mg PO once daily.

CYCLOSPORIASIS

- *Cyclospora cayetanensis* is an acid-fast coccidian (8 to 10 μm) transmitted by the fecal–oral route and by contaminated water or food. It causes a diarrheal illness in advanced HIV-infected patients.
- The only treatment is **TMP-SMX** DS 1 tablet four times daily for 10 days followed by 1 DS tablet three times weekly indefinitely.
- Ciprofloxacin can be tried in patients intolerant to TMP-SMX, but is inferior.

VIRAL INFECTIONS

CYTOMEGALOVIRUS

GENERAL PRINCIPLES

- With widespread use of cART, there has been a marked decline in CMV disease, although patients with CD4 cell counts <50 cells/mm^3 are still at risk.
- The risk of developing disease and death in advanced HIV-infected patients is cor-related with the quantity of CMV DNA measured by PCR.

DIAGNOSIS

Chorioretinitis

- Ocular disease occurs in patients with advanced HIV infection.
- CMV chorioretinitis is due to reactivation and may not be associated with viremia.
- Routine biannual ophthalmologic examinations are recommended for all patients with CD4 cell count <50 cells/mm^3.
- Symptoms include decreased visual acuity, presence of "floaters," or unilateral visual field loss.
- Diagnosis is made by ophthalmologic examination, revealing large creamy to yellowish white granular areas with perivascular exudates and hemorrhages. Lesions occur in the periphery but can progress to involve the macula and optic disk in 2 to 3 weeks.

CMV Neurological Disease

- Polyradiculopathy, encephalitis, mononeuritis multiplex, and painful neuropathy can all be caused by CMV infection.
- **Polyradiculopathy** presents with low back pain radiating to the perianal area and progressive lower extremity weakness, hypo- or aflexia and variable sensory deficit with preserved proprioception and vibratory sensation, or bladder/anal sphincter dysfunction causing urinary retention/fecal incontinence.
  - ○ Diagnosis is based on clinical presentation.
  - ○ MRI may reveal enhancement of leptomeninges and clumping of lumbosacral roots.
  - ○ CSF is usually positive for CMV antigen or DNA.
- **Encephalitis** presents with rapidly progressive cognitive impairment and mental status changes. MRI may reveal meningeal or periventricular enhancement.
- **Mononeuritis multiplex** causes multifocal, patchy, asymmetrical sensory and motor deficits. Biopsy of the involved peripheral nerve can confirm the diagnosis.
- **CMV colitis and esophagitis**
  - ○ CMV colitis occurred in 5% to 10% of AIDS patients in the pre-cART era, but is now uncommon.
  - ○ Diarrhea, weight loss, anorexia, abdominal pain, and fever are present.
  - ○ Diagnosis is made by endoscopic biopsy. Endoscopy reveals mucosal ulceration and submucosal hemorrhage, although 10% of those with histologic evidence of CMV colitis may have normal-appearing mucosa. Biopsy shows characteristic CMV inclusions (owl eye), CMV antigen, or nucleic acid.
  - ○ Esophagitis is also diagnosed by endoscopic biopsy.
- **CMV pneumonitis** is less common than in transplant recipients. Isolation of CMV from pulmonary secretions is common, but the true pathogenic role of CMV in pneumonia is not well established. Diagnosis is established by finding pathognomonic intranuclear inclusion bodies in biopsy.

TREATMENT

- Treatment of CMV neurological disease should be initiated promptly.
  - ○ Combination of **ganciclovir** IV plus **foscarnet** IV to stabilize disease and maximize response. Continue until symptomatic improvement.

- ○ Maintenance therapy with valganciclovir PO plus foscarnet IV should be continued until evidence of immune reconstitution.
- Treatment of CMV chorioretinitis is presented in Table 13-6.
- Treatment of CMV colitis and esophagitis consists of ganciclovir IV or foscarnet IV for 21 to 28 days or until resolution of signs and symptoms. Oral valganciclovir may be used when symptoms (and oral absorption) improve. Maintenance therapy is usually unnecessary, unless there is relapse.
- Treatment for CMV pneumonitis should be considered in patients with histologic evidence or when CMV is the only pathogen identified in a progressive, deteriorating pneumonia not responding to other treatments. Ganciclovir IV can be used.

TABLE 13-6   **TREATMENT OF CYTOMEGALOVIRUS CHORIORETINITIS**

For small peripheral lesions

- Valganciclovir 900 mg PO twice daily for 14–21 d, then 900 mg PO once daily

For immediate sight-threatening lesions

- Ganciclovir intraocular implant + valganciclovir 900 mg PO (twice daily for 14–21 d, then once daily)

- One dose of intravitreal ganciclovir (2 mg in 0.05–0.1 mL) may be given until the implant can be placed.

- Alternatives
  - ○ Ganciclovir 5 mg/kg IV every 12 h for 14–21 d, then 5 mg/kg IV once daily
  - ○ Ganciclovir 5 mg/kg IV every 12 h for 14–21 d, then valganciclovir 900 mg PO once daily
  - ○ Foscarnet 60 mg/kg IV every 8 h or 90 mg/kg IV every 12 h for 14–21 d, then 90–120 mg/kg IV once daily
  - ○ Cidofovir 5 mg/kg/wk IV for 2 wk, then 5 mg/kg every other week with saline hydration before and after therapy and probenecid 2 g PO 3 h before the dose followed by 1 g PO 2 h after the dose and 1 g PO 8 h after the dose (total of 4 g)

Secondary prophylaxis (until immune reconstitution)

- Valganciclovir 900 mg PO once daily

- Ganciclovir implant (may be replaced every 6–8 mo if CD4 cell count remains <100 cells/mm^3) plus valganciclovir 900 mg PO once daily

- Alternatives for secondary prophylaxis
  - ○ Ganciclovir 5 mg/kg IV five to seven times weekly
  - ○ Foscarnet 90–120 mg/kg IV once daily
  - ○ Cidofovir 5 mg/kg IV every other week with saline hydration and probenecid

VARICELLA-ZOSTER VIRUS

GENERAL PRINCIPLES

- Reactivation of varicella-zoster virus (VZV) infection is more frequent among HIV-infected persons than among age-matched non–HIV-infected controls.
- Most herpes zoster–related complications, including disseminated disease, occur in patients with CD4 cell count <200 cells/mm^3.

DIAGNOSIS

- Patients may present with typical, single-dermatome shingles. Disseminated skin involvement and organ involvement are more common in immunocompromised hosts.
- VZV-related neurologic disease includes CNS vasculitis, multifocal leukoencephalitis, ventriculitis, myelitis and myeloradiculitis, optic neuritis, cranial nerve palsies and focal brain stem lesions, and aseptic meningitis.
  - **HIV-associated zoster ophthalmicus** occurs with reactivated infection involving the ophthalmic division of the trigeminal nerve, which may cause keratitis and retinitis.
  - **Acute retinal necrosis** (ARN) is a necrotizing herpetic retinopathy characterized by marked anterior and intermediate uveitis, retinal arteritis, papillitis of the optic disk, and retinal and choroidal occlusive vasculitis. Retinal detachment is common. ARN can occur regardless of CD4 cell count. It is also seen with CMV or HSV infections.
  - **Progressive outer retinal necrosis (PORN)** is caused almost exclusively by VZV and occurs in severely immunosuppressed patients with CD4 cell count <50 to 100 cells/mm^3. PORN presents with pain in the eye with movement as a result of optic nerve involvement. Retinal findings are multifocal necrotic lesions that rapidly coalesce. There is no or minimal vitreous inflammation. Most patients with PORN will become blind within 1 month due to retinal detachment, optic neuropathy, or widespread retinal necrosis.

TREATMENT

- For uncomplicated varicella (primary infection), oral **acyclovir** 20 mg/kg/d (commonly 800 mg PO five times daily), **valacyclovir** 1 g PO three times daily, or **famciclovir** 500 mg PO three times daily for 5 to 7 days are used.
- For recurrent infection, oral valacyclovir, famciclovir, or acyclovir for 5 to 7 days is recommended.
- If cutaneous lesions are extensive or with concerns for visceral involvement, IV acyclovir should be initiated.
- ARN requires aggressive treatment with high-dose IV acyclovir (10 mg/kg every 8 hours) or foscarnet for 10 to 14 days followed by prolonged oral valacyclovir (1 g PO three times daily for 6 weeks), and early laser retinopexy to prevent extension of peripheral detachments may result in good vision.
- Treatment for PORN consists of combination IV ganciclovir and foscarnet, plus intravitreal ganciclovir and/or foscarnet. Optimal cART is recommended. Prognosis is poor.

SPECIAL CONSIDERATIONS

- **Postexposure prophylaxis.** HIV-infected patients who are susceptible to VZV should receive varicella-zoster immune globulin within 96 hours of close contact with a person who has active varicella or herpes zoster.
- **Vaccination.** The live attenuated varicella vaccine can be safely given to HIV-infected patients with CD4 cell count >200 cells/mm^3.

PROGRESSIVE MULTIFOCAL LEUKOENCEPHALOPATHY

GENERAL PRINCIPLES

- Progressive multifocal leukoencephalopathy (PML) is characterized by deep white matter changes due to focal demyelination caused by infection of oligodendrocytes by the JC polyoma virus.
- In the pre-cART era, PML occurred in approximately 4% of AIDS patients and progressed to death within months from diagnosis.
- Despite the fact that the incidence of PML has declined with cART, morbidity and mortality associated with PML remains high.
- PML may occur in patients with high CD4 count and even on cART.

DIAGNOSIS

Clinical Presentation
- Clinical presentation varies from diffuse encephalopathy to focal deficits.
- Initial symptoms may begin as partial neurologic deficits and may evolve to hemiparesis. Symptoms tend to progress over several weeks to months.
- Seizures may develop in up to 20% of affected patients.

Diagnostic Testing
- Definitive diagnosis is made by a **brain biopsy**. However, PML is usually diagnosed with a combination of clinical and neuroimaging findings.
- **MRI** lesions are hyperintense on T2-weighted and fluid-attenuated inversion recovery sequences and hypointense on T1-weighted sequence.
- PCR detection of JC virus from CSF has sensitivity of 72% to 92% and specificity of 92% to 100% in patients not on cART.[10] Immune recovery decreases the sensitivity of the test.

TREATMENT

- **No established treatment exists for PML.**
- Patients should be started on cART immediately. Immune reconstitution (IRIS) can cause a paradoxical response.
- Corticosteroids have been used in this setting to control the local inflammation and reduce cerebral edema although data are limited.

HEPATITIS B

GENERAL PRINCIPLES

- Liver disease has emerged as a leading cause of death in HIV-infected patients.
- Coinfection of hepatitis B virus (HBV) and HIV accelerates progression of liver disease to end-stage liver disease.
- HIV can cause HBV reactivation with higher HBV DNA levels and higher incidence of chronicity.

DIAGNOSIS

- All HIV-infected patients should be tested for HBV infection. Hepatitis B surface antigen (HBsAg), hepatitis B core antibody (anti-HBc total), and hepatitis B surface antibody (anti-HBs total) should be measured.
- Patients with chronic HBV infection should be tested for HBeAg, antibody to HBeAg (anti-HBe), and HBV DNA level. HBeAg-positive patients tend to have higher HBV DNA than those with negative HBeAg.
- Some patients have isolated anti-HBc positivity; check HBV DNA levels in these cases for occult HBV infection.

TREATMENT

- Anti-HBV therapy is indicated for HBeAg-positive patients with abnormal alanine aminotransferase (ALT) levels and HBV DNA levels >20,000 IU/mL and for HBeAg-negative patients with abnormal ALT levels and HBV DNA levels >2,000 IU/mL.
- Anti-HBV therapy should also be considered in patients with low but detectable HBV DNA levels who have substantial histologic inflammation or fibrosis on liver biopsy.
- Some other treatment considerations:
  - Consider treatment for both HIV and HBV if there is low-level HBV viremia, inflammation or fibrosis on liver biopsy, or falling CD4 counts.
  - If treatment of HIV is needed but not HBV, use either tenofovir/emtricitabine (TDF/FTC) or TDF/lamivudine (3TC) as ART NRTI backbone. **Avoid using only one active agent for HBV to prevent HBV-resistant mutants**.
  - If treatment for HBV is needed, treat for HIV as well. NRTI backbone of TDF plus FTC or 3TC should be used. If TDF cannot be used, another agent with anti-HBV activity should be added. Avoid using only one active agent for HBV.
  - Treating only HBV is not recommended. In special circumstances where HIV treatment is not desirable, pegylated interferon α-2a could be used for the treatment of HBV infection, as it does not lead to emergence of HIV resistance.
  - Need to discontinue FTC, 3TC, or TDF: Exacerbation of liver dysfunction may be seen with discontinuation of anti-HBV agents. Monitor the clinical course and liver function tests closely and consider treating with different anti-HBV agents such as interferon, adefovir, or telbivudine.

GENERAL PRINCIPLES

- Hepatitis C virus (HCV) is transmitted by contaminated blood or blood products. **HIV is an important cofactor for HCV progression**.
- HCV-coinfected patients have a higher rate of fibrosis progression, decompensated liver disease, and higher morbidity and mortality.
- HCV coinfection also increases the risk of hepatotoxicity from cART, although the benefit of cART outweighs the risk of liver injury. Some experts advise starting cART in the presence of HCV.
- Coinfected patients should be immunized against hepatitis A virus (HAV) as they are at increased risk for developing fulminant HAV hepatitis.

DIAGNOSIS

Clinical Presentation

- Patients are usually asymptomatic until cirrhosis develops.
- Jaundice, encephalopathy, ascites, splenomegaly, or gastrointestinal bleeds secondary to portal hypertension may occur with disease progression.
- Extrahepatic manifestations of HCV infection include mixed cryoglobulinemia, membranous proliferative glomerulonephritis, and porphyria cutanea tarda.

Diagnostic Testing

- Diagnosis is made by detection of antibody to HCV in blood. If serologic test results are negative but the suspicion of HCV infection is high, plasma HCV RNA should be tested.
- Plasma HCV RNA should be tested in all seropositive patients and in seronegative patients where suspicion for HCV is high.
- Quantitative HCV RNA level does not correlate with the degree of liver damage, but provides information about the response to HCV treatment.
- HCV genotype should be performed because it predicts the response to interferon-based treatment.
- Liver biopsy is the definitive method to assess liver fibrosis, but is expensive and loses sensitivity due to sampling error. The overall risks and benefits from this procedure should be considered. Other methods to assess liver fibrosis include the use of serum fibrosis markers and transient elastography.[11,12]
- The Model for End-Stage Liver Disease (MELD) score should be calculated every 3 to 6 months in patients with cirrhosis. Coinfected patients with MELD score >12 should be considered for liver transplantation.

TREATMENT

- Peginterferon and ribavirin are the mainstay of HCV treatment. Table 13-7 summarizes the current recommendations. Addition of a newer third agent, such as boceprevir or telaprevir, is currently being studied in HIV/HCV-coinfected patients.

TABLE 13-7	TREATMENT OF HCV INFECTION	
Genotype 1, 4, 5, or 6	Peginterferon alfa-2a 180 µg SQ once weekly or Peginterferon alfa-2b 1.5 mg/kg SQ once weekly plus Ribavirin PO (weight-based dosing) <75 kg: 600 mg every morning and 400 mg every evening ≥75 kg: 600 mg BID	Duration: 48 wk Some experts recommend extending treatment for 72 wk when patient does not achieve undetectable HCV RNA level at 4 wk
Genotype 2 or 3	Peginterferon alfa-2a 180 µg SQ once weekly or Peginterferon alfa-2b 1.5 mg/kg SQ once weekly plus Ribavirin PO 400 mg BID	Duration: 48 wk Some experts recommend shortening treatment to 24 wk when patient achieves undetectable HCV RNA level at 4 wk, unless the patient has advanced cirrhosis or some other unfavorable prognostic factors

HCV, hepatitis C virus.

- Treatment of HCV infection should be offered when the benefits outweigh the risks of treatment, usually including these situations:
  - HCV genotype 2 or 3 infection
  - HCV genotype 1 infection with HCV RNA level <800,000 IU/mL
  - Significant hepatic fibrosis (bridging fibrosis or cirrhosis)
  - Stable HIV infection not requiring ART
  - Acute HCV infection (<6 months duration)
  - Cryoglobulinemic vasculitis
  - Cryoglobulinemic membranoproliferative glomerulonephritis
  - Strong motivation to treat their HCV infection
- Factors associated with the likelihood of achieving a sustained virologic response (SVR) should be evaluated. SVR is the absence of HCV RNA at the end of treatment and 6 months later.
  - CD4 cell count. Response to HCV treatment depends on immune status. Some experts recommend starting cART for HIV infection and waiting until the CD4 cell count is >200 to 350 cells/mm^3.
  - Types of ART. Zidovudine is associated with increased incidence of anemia and didanosine with mitochondrial toxicity and abacavir interacts with ribavirin; therefore, these agents should be avoided.
  - Genotype. Genotypes 2 and 3 have better rates of SVR compared with genotype 1.
  - HCV RNA level.

- In HCV infection with genotype 1, baseline HCV RNA levels of <400,000 IU/mL had higher chance of achieving SVR than those with >400,000 IU/mL in the APRICOT trial.[13]
  - Undetectable HCV RNA level 4 weeks after starting treatment (rapid virologic response, or RVR) is a powerful positive predictor for achieving SVR.
  - Undetectable HCV RNA level at 12 weeks is early virologic response (EVR). Partial EVR is achieving HCV RNA level decrease by at least 2 logs 12 weeks after starting treatment. Absence of EVR is a powerful negative predictor for achieving SVR.
  - Genetic polymorphism near IL28B: Single nucleotide polymorphism (SNP) near IL28B is strongly associated with SVR when peginterferon and ribavirin are used for treatment in monoinfected HCV patients. Homozygous C/C genotype at this SNP is associated with increased SVR.[14] The C/C allele is found most commonly in Asia, followed by Europe and is relatively uncommon in Africa.
- Treatment of HCV is not recommended for coinfected patients with high-risk conditions such as the following:
  - Pregnancy or lack of reliable birth control
  - Advanced HIV infection, not controlled with ART
  - Hepatic decompensation
  - Severe, uncontrolled comorbid medical conditions (cancer or cardiopulmonary disease)
  - Severe, active depression with suicidal ideation, until successfully treated
  - Significant hematologic abnormalities (hemoglobin <10.5 g/dL, absolute neutrophil count <1,000/µL, platelet count <50,000/µL)
  - Renal insufficiency (creatinine >1.5 mg/dL or creatinine clearance <50 cc/min); can use pegylated interferon only
  - Active, uncontrolled autoimmune conditions (e.g., sarcoidosis, systemic lupus erythematosus, or rheumatoid arthritis) due to increased risk of exacerbation from interferon

MONITORING/FOLLOW-UP

Patients with HCV-related cirrhosis are at risk for developing hepatocellular carcinoma (HCC). Screening for HCC with liver ultrasound every 6 to 12 months is recommended.

HUMAN PAPILLOMAVIRUS INFECTION

- Human papillomavirus (HPV) is a common sexually transmitted virus and the cause of cervical cancer. Other types of lesions caused by HPV infection include genital, anal, and oral warts. Anal and some oropharyngeal cancers are caused by HPV.
- **Women with HIV infection have a sevenfold higher rate of cervical cancer**.
- Most infections resolve or become latent and undetectable; persistent infection with oncogenic types is required to develop cancerous lesions.
- There are more than 100 HPV serotypes.
  - The most important serotypes are type 16 and 18, which account for approximately 50% and 10% to 15% of cervical cancer, respectively.
  - HPV types 6 and 11 cause 90% of genital warts.
- Two **vaccines** are now available:

○ A quadrivalent HPV vaccine targets types 6, 11, 16, and 18.
○ A bivalent vaccine targets types 16 and 18.
○ A 9-valent HPV vaccine designed to target HPV types 6, 11, 16, 18, 31, 33, 45, 52, and 58 is currently under phase III trial.
○ HPV vaccine is indicated for young women under age 26, including those with HIV. It can also be given to young men.

HUMAN HERPESVIRUS 8 DISEASE

GENERAL PRINCIPLES

- Human herpesvirus (HHV) 8 is associated with KS as well as **primary effusion lymphoma** (PEL) and **multicentric Castleman disease** (MCD).
- HHV-8 seroprevalence in the general population of the United States is 1% to 5%; men who have sex with men have a seroprevalence of 20% to 70%.
- The incidence of KS in the pre-cART era was about 20%, which has since dramatically declined.
- PEL is an uncommon AIDS-related lymphoma, associated with HHV-8 and presenting as a body cavity effusion. It can occur in patients with any CD4 cell count.
- MCD is a lymphoproliferative disorder associated with HHV-8. The incidence of MCD has been increasing with the use of cART. It can occur at any CD4 cell count. MCD has been linked with overexpression of interleukin (IL)-6.

DIAGNOSIS

- KS is a multicentric tumor that initially presents as purplish nodules on the skin or mucous membranes.
  ○ Patients with CD4 cell count >300 cells/mm^3 may develop limited cutaneous lesions.
  ○ Oral lesions are common on the hard palate and gingival margins and are often asymptomatic.
  ○ Lymphatic and visceral sites of disease are common, with 40% having gastrointestinal involvement at diagnosis. Lymph node involvement may result in edema of the legs and scrotum.
  ○ Biopsy should be performed to distinguish from BA.
- PEL originates on serosal surfaces such as pleura, pericardium, peritoneum, joint spaces, and meninges and produces a symptomatic serous effusion with high-grade malignant lymphocytes, but without detectable mass.
  ○ Diagnosis is made by fluid cytology; the presence of HHV-8 in the nuclei of the malignant cell is diagnostic. This could be detected with immunohistochemical staining for latent viral gene product (latency-associated nuclear antigen LANA-1).
- MCD is characterized by polyclonal hypergammaglobulinemia, generalized lymphadenopathy, hepatosplenomegaly, constitutional symptoms (e.g., fever, weakness, and weight loss), and autoimmune hemolytic anemia. KS is also commonly found in patients with MCD.

TREATMENT

- All HIV-infected patients presenting with KS should be started on cART as the lesions may regress in response to HIV treatment. Management of KS is largely palliative. In advanced KS or with lesions associated with pain, extremity edema, soft tissue infection, and GI and respiratory symptoms, therapy is recommended.
  - Local therapies include radiotherapy, intralesional chemotherapy with vinblastine, cryotherapy, and alitretinoin gel.
  - Systematic therapies include chemotherapy and interferon α. First-line chemotherapy is liposomal doxorubicin. For poor response or relapse, paclitaxel has been shown to have a high response rate.[15] Other agents are etoposide and vinorelbine.
- The overall prognosis of PEL is poor. All patients should receive cART. There are only limited data regarding chemotherapy in patients who fail cART alone. Patients may be treated with liposomal doxorubicin with or without bortezomib and prednisone.
- Treatment for MCD has not been well established, although there are anecdotal reports of use of steroids, chemotherapy (e.g., vinblastine, etoposide, cyclophosphamide/hydroxydaunorubicin/vincristine/prednisone [CHOP]), antiviral therapy (such as ganciclovir, foscarnet, and cidofovir), inhibitor of IL-6 (tocilizumab), and monoclonal anti-CD20 antibody (rituximab). Rituximab seems to be the most promising.[16]

MALIGNANCIES IN HIV-INFECTED PATIENTS

- Malignancies that occur in HIV-infected patients can be categorized as AIDS-associated malignancies and non–AIDS-associated malignancies.
- **AIDS-associated malignancies include cervical cancer, KS, non-Hodgkin's lymphoma, and primary brain lymphoma, which define AIDS**. The incidence of AIDS-associated malignancies has dramatically declined with the widespread use of potent cART.
- Non–AIDS-associated malignancies are an increasingly important cause of morbidity and have emerged as one of the leading causes of mortality for HIV-infected patients.
  - **The most common non–AIDS-associated malignancies are anal cancer, Hodgkin's lymphoma, and oropharyngeal cancer**. Risks of these malignancies significantly increase with declining CD4 cell count, but do not seem to be associated with high HIV viral loads.
  - In a retrospective cohort study, the incidence of melanoma was higher in HIV-infected patients, regardless of CD4 cell counts, and the incidence of lung cancer and colorectal cancer was higher in immunocompromised patients with CD4 cell count <200 cells/mm^3.[17] Another prospective cohort study showed increased incidence of liver and renal cancers and leukemia. Conversely, this study showed that the incidence of prostate cancer was lower in HIV-infected population.[18]

REFERENCES

1. Zolopa A, Andersen J, Powderly W, et al. Early antiretroviral therapy reduces AIDS progression/death in individuals with acute opportunistic infections: a multicenter randomized strategy trial. *PLoS One*. 2009;4:e5575.
2. Abdool Karim SS, Naidoo K, Grobler A, et al. Timing of initiation of antiretroviral drugs during tuberculosis therapy. *N Engl J Med*. 2010;362:697-706.

3. Blanc FX, Sok T, Laureillard D, et al. Significant enhancement in survival with early (2 weeks) vs. late (8 weeks) initiation of highly active antiretroviral treatment (HAART) in severely immunosuppressed HIV-infected adults with newly diagnosed tuberculosis. Program and abstracts of the XVIII International AIDS Conference; July 18–23, 2010; Vienna, Austria. Abstract THLBB106.

4. Kovacs JA, Masur H. Prophylaxis against opportunistic infections in patients with human immunodeficiency virus infection. *N Engl J Med.* 2000;342:1416-1429.

5. Makadzange AT, Ndhlovu CE, Takarinda K, et al. Early versus delayed initiation of antiretroviral therapy for concurrent HIV infection and cryptococcal meningitis in sub-Saharan Africa. *Clin Infect Dis.* 2010;50:1532-1538.

6. Benson CA, Williams PL, Currier JS, et al. A prospective, randomized trial examining the efficacy and safety of clarithromycin in combination with ethambutol, rifabutin, or both for the treatment of disseminated *Mycobacterium avium* complex disease in persons with acquired immunodeficiency syndrome. *Clin Infect Dis.* 2003;37:1234-1243.

7. Ward TT, Rimland D, Kauffman C, et al. Randomized, open-label trial of azithromycin plus ethambutol vs. clarithromycin plus ethambutol as therapy for *Mycobacterium avium* complex bacteremia in patients with human immunodeficiency virus infection. Veterans Affairs HIV Research Consortium. *Clin Infect Dis.* 1998;27:1278-1285.

8. Menzies D, Pai M, Comstock G. Meta-analysis: new tests for the diagnosis of latent tuberculosis infection: areas of uncertainty and recommendations for research. *Ann Intern Med.* 2007;146:340-354.

9. Mesquita RT, Ziegler AP, Hiramoto RM, et al. Real-time quantitative PCR in cerebral toxoplasmosis diagnosis of Brazilian human immunodeficiency virus-infected patients. *J Med Microbiol.* 2010;59:641-647.

10. Cinque P, Scarpellini P, Vago L, et al. Diagnosis of central nervous system complications in HIV-infected patients: cerebrospinal fluid analysis by the polymerase chain reaction. *AIDS.* 1997;11:1-17.

11. Parkes J, Roderick P, Harris S, et al. Enhanced liver fibrosis test can predict clinical outcomes in patients with chronic liver disease. *Gut.* 2010;59:1245-1251.

12. Castera L, Forns X, Alberti A. Non-invasive evaluation of liver fibrosis using transient elastography. *J Hepatol.* 2008;48:835-847.

13. Dore GJ, Torriani FJ, Rodriguez-Torres M, et al. Baseline factors prognostic of sustained virological response in patients with HIV-hepatitis C virus co-infection. *AIDS.* 2007;21:1555-1559.

14. Dayyeh BK, Gupta N, Sherman KE, et al.; AIDS Clinical Trials Group A5178 Study Team. IL28B alleles exert an additive dose effect when applied to HCV-HIV coinfected persons undergoing peginterferon and ribavirin therapy. *PLoS One.* 2011;6:e25753.

15. Cianfrocca M, Lee S, Von Roenn J, et al. Randomized trial of paclitaxel versus pegylated liposomal doxorubicin for advanced human immunodeficiency virus-associated Kaposi sarcoma: evidence of symptom palliation from chemotherapy. *Cancer.* 2010;116:3969-3977.

16. Hoffmann C, Schmid H, Müller M, et al. Improved outcome with rituximab in patients with HIV-associated multicentric Castleman disease. *Blood.* 2011;118:3499-3503.

17. Silverberg M, Chao C, Leyden WA, et al. HIV infection, immunodeficiency, viral replication, and the risk of cancer. *Cancer Epidemiol Biomarkers Prev.* 2011;20:2551-2559.

18. Patel P, Hanson DL, Sullivan PS, et al. Incidence of types of cancer among HIV-infected persons compared with the general population in the United States, 1992–2003. *Ann Intern Med.* 2008;148(10):728-736.

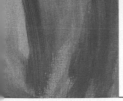

Infection in Non-HIV Immunocompromised Hosts

14

Cynthia Johnson and Carlos Santos

HEMATOPOIETIC STEM CELL TRANSPLANTATION

THE PROCEDURE

- There are three **major types** of hematopoietic stem cell transplant (HSCT).
  - **Autologous** refers to the patient serving as his or her own source of stem cells. This is commonly used for the treatment of malignant diseases to facilitate cytotoxic chemotherapy.
  - **Allogeneic** indicates that the source of stem cells is a human leukocyte antigen (HLA)–matched donor (e.g., family member or unrelated volunteer donor) or banked cord blood cells. This is commonly used for the treatment of malignant diseases involving the hematopoietic system (e.g., acute and chronic leukemia).
  - **Syngeneic** involves using stem cells harvested from an identical twin. It is ideal for the treatment of nonmalignant marrow disorders. It is less optimal for the treatment of malignant diseases given the absence of allogeneic graft versus malignancy effect.
- The three **major steps** of HSCT are as follows:
  - **Stem cell harvest and manipulation**. Stem cells are obtained either directly from the bone marrow or by apheresis of peripheral blood after stem cell mobilization with chemotherapy, or administration of granulocyte colony-stimulating factor (G-CSF) or plerixafor. Hematopoietic potency is measured by the proportion of cells expressing the CD34 antigen, an antigen expressed on the cell surface of primitive hematopoietic progenitors. A high CD34 count portends faster neutrophil recovery. Immune potency is indicated by the proportion of lymphocytes (CD3+ cells). A high proportion of lymphocytes, natural killer (NK) cells, and dendritic cells predicts rapid immune reconstitution. The stem cell graft is sometimes manipulated prior to transplantation. Most commonly, T-cell depletion is performed to reduce the risk of graft-versus-host disease (GVHD). However, T-cell depletion may also result in a greater risk of graft rejection, a higher risk of cancer relapse, and slower posttransplant T-cell reconstitution.
  - **Conditioning**. Prior to the infusion of the stem cell graft, a conditioning regimen is chosen based on the type of stem cell graft and reason for HSCT. Patients with cancer receive cytotoxic chemotherapy with or without total body irradiation. Most commonly, prospective allogeneic HSCT recipients are given an intensive myeloablative regimen consisting of cyclophosphamide, total body irradiation, and antithymocyte globulin (ATG). Nonmyeloablative regimens are increasingly being used, however, and are especially indicated for elderly patients and individuals with numerous comorbidities who may not tolerate intensive conditioning regimens.

○ **Stem cell graft infusion and posttransplant care**. The duration of neutropenia after stem cell graft infusion varies according to the type of HSCT performed (10 to 14 days for autologous, 15 to 30 days for allogeneic with an ablative regimen, 5 to 7 days for allogeneic with a nonablative regimen). An immunosuppressive regimen commonly consisting of a calcineurin inhibitor (cyclosporine or tacrolimus) plus a short course of methotrexate is given to allogeneic HSCT recipients to prevent both stem cell graft rejection and GVHD. The immunosuppressive regimen is typically tapered over 4 to 6 months and discontinued unless GVHD occurs. **Immune reconstitution after allogeneic HSCT may take a year or more.** Autologous HSCT does not require posttransplant immunosuppression and therefore takes only 3 to 9 months for immune recovery. While there is currently no definitive laboratory marker for immune reconstitution, several studies have shown that **CD4+ cell counts are the most accessible and predictive marker for restoration of immune competence after HSCT**.

INFECTION RISK

- The risk and type of infection with HSCT differs depending on the type of transplant, type of stem cell graft, conditioning regimen, immunosuppressive regimen, and development of posttransplant complications such as GVHD.
- **Allogeneic HSCT**, especially transplants from **unrelated** or **mismatched donors**, results in slower immune reconstitution and elevated infection risk.
- **Myeloablative conditioning regimens** result in rapid-onset neutropenia, prolonged neutropenia, and more mucosal injury compared with nonmyeloablative regimens and therefore have a higher risk of neutropenic infections, especially typhlitis.
- **Antithymocyte globulin** results in profound T-cell immunodeficiency; **methotrexate** results in delayed neutrophil recovery and more mucosal injury; these drugs elevate the risk of invasive fungal infections (IFIs) and herpesvirus infections.
- **Central venous catheters** breach the skin barrier and predispose patients to bacterial and yeast infections. Catheter-associated infections are the leading cause of bloodstream infections in HSCT recipients, particularly during the pre-engraftment period and in patients with GVHD.
- **GVHD** results in markedly elevated infection risk, because of prolonged and intensive administration of immunosuppressive medications.
- The types of infections at various times after HSCT are outlined in Table 14-1.

COMMON INFECTIOUS COMPLICATIONS AFTER HSCT

NEUTROPENIC FEVER

GENERAL PRINCIPLES

- Fever frequently occurs in patients with neutropenia and may be a sign of infection. Likely **sites of infection include the lungs, central venous catheters, genitourinary tract, bloodstream, skin, and intestine**. Overt inflammation is usually not present, and a high index of suspicion must be maintained while searching for foci of infection.

TABLE 14-1	TYPES OF INFECTIONS IN HSCT RECIPIENTS[a]		
Type of pathogen	**Early pre-engraftment (<2–4 wk):** Neutropenia, barrier breakdown from mucositis and central venous catheters.	**Early post-engraftment (<3 mo):** Impaired cellular and humoral immunity, NK cell recovery first, then CD8+ T-cell recovery with restricted T-cell repertoire.	**Late post-engraftment (>2–3 mo)[b]:** Impaired cellular and humoral immunity (B-cell and CD4– T-cell recovery, diversified repertoire).
Bacteria	**Gram positive:** Including CONS, *Staphylococcus aureus*, viridans *Streptococcus*. Risk factors: mucositis and central venous catheter use. **Gram negative:** Including *Legionella*, *Pseudomonas aeruginosa*, *Enterobacter*, and *Stenotrophomonas maltophilia*. Risk factors: mucositis/cutaneous injury and neutropenia. ***Clostridium difficile*:** Risk factors, antibiotic use, neutropenia.	**Gram positive:** Including *Listeria*. Risk factor: central venous catheter use. **Gram negative:** including *Legionella*. Risk factors: enteric involvement of GVHD and use of central venous catheters. ***Mycobacterium*:** Rare. Due to reactivation in TB or MAC; new exposure with atypical mycobacterium.	**Encapsulated bacteria:** Including *Streptococcus pneumoniae*, *Haemophilus influenzae*, *Neisseria meningitidis*. Risk factors, immunoglobulin deficiency, hyposplenism, severe chronic GVHD (poor opsonization). **Gram positive:** Including *Staphylococcus*, *Nocardia*. **Gram negative:** Including *Pseudomonas*. Risk factor, chronic GVHD.
Viruses	**HSV:** Due to viral reactivation. Decreased incidence with acyclovir prophylaxis. **Respiratory viruses:** Including RSV, parainfluenza, rhinovirus, influenza, human metapneumovirus. Follow community outbreak patterns.	**CMV:** Risk factors, acute GVHD, older age, total body irradiation conditioning, matched unrelated donor, and impaired CMI. Decreased incidence with prophylaxis. **EBV:** Risk factors, mismatched donors and T-cell–depleted grafts	**CMV:** Risk factors, GVHD, impaired CMI, and viral latency pretransplant. **EBV:** Including PTLD. Risk factors, mismatched donors, and T-cell–depleted grafts. **VZV:** Decreased incidence with acyclovir prophylaxis. Risk factors: viral latency or infection pretransplant, total body irradiation, *(continued)*

TABLE 14-1 (CONTINUED)

	BK virus: Risk factors, GVHD, cyclophosphamide conditioning regimens.	antithymocyte globulin therapy, GVHD, and lymphopenia.
	Respiratory viruses: Including RSV, influenza, parainfluenza, rhinovirus, human metapneumovirus. Follow community outbreak patterns.	**Respiratory viruses, Adenovirus**: Due to reactivation. Risk factor: GVHD. **HBV, HCV**: Due to reactivation.
	Adenovirus: Due to reactivation. Risk factor, acute GVHD.	**Other viruses**: Measles, mumps, rubella, parvovirus B19, BK/JC virus, HHV-8. Due to loss of specific B-cell immunity.
	HHV-6: Related to anti-CD3 mAb use, GVHD.	
	Enteric viruses: Including coxsackie, echovirus, rotavirus, norovirus. Usually summer/fall months.	
Fungi	**Aspergillus**: Risk factors, GVHD, diminished CMI, older age, corticosteroid therapy, graft failure, cytopenia, iron overload.	**Aspergillus, other molds**: Risk factors, GVHD, older age, corticosteroid therapy, graft failure, cytopenia, iron overload.
	Other molds: Including *Fusarium*, *Mucorales*. Risk factors with allogeneic HSCT: GVHD, CMV infection pretransplantation.	*Pneumocystis jirovecii*: Related to GVHD. Decreased incidence with prophylaxis.
	Candida: Decreased incidence with antifungal prophylaxis.	
	Candida: Due to mucositis, antibiotic use, and neutropenia. Decreased incidence with antifungal prophylaxis, except triazole-resistant species (*Candida krusei*, *Candida glabrata*).	
	Molds: Including *Aspergillus*, *Fusarium*, *Zygomycetes*, others. Risk factors with allogeneic HSCT: prolonged neutropenia, older age, HLA match, delayed engraftment.	

| Parasites | *Pneumocystis jiroveci*: Related to GVHD. Decreased incidence with prophylaxis use. |
| | *Toxoplasma*: Due to reactivation. Risk factors: T-cell depletion, severe immunosuppressed allogeneic HSCT |

---

[a]Based primarily on studies with myeloablative regimens. Paradigm for the early pre-engraftment period differs significantly for nonmyeloablative regimens, but is similar in the post-engraftment period.

[b]Late post-engraftment infections are usually only seen in allogeneic HSCT and not autologous HSCT due to posttransplant immunosuppressive regimens and chronic GVHD.

HSCT, hematopoietic stem cell transplantation; NK, natural killer; CONS, coagulase-negative staphylococci; GVHD, graft-versus-host disease; CMI, cell-mediated immunity; HSV, herpes simplex virus; CMV, cytomegalovirus; EBV, Epstein-Barr virus; VZV, varicella zoster virus; RSV, respiratory syncytial virus; HHV, human herpes virus; mAb, monoclonal antibody; TB, *Mycobacterium tuberculosis*; MAC, *Mycobacterium avium* complex; PTLD, posttransplant lymphoproliferative disorder; HBV, hepatitis B virus; HCV, hepatitis C virus.

- Frequently identified causative organisms include coagulase-negative staphylococci, enterococci, streptococci, several gram-negative bacilli, and anaerobes. Infections caused by *Candida*, *Aspergillus*, and other molds are less common but may occur.

DIAGNOSIS

A thorough workup must be initiated and should include two separately drawn blood cultures, urinalysis and urine culture, chest radiograph, and liver function tests and abdominal imaging as indicated.[1]

TREATMENT

- Timely and appropriate administration of broad-spectrum antibiotics should be provided, with the choice of therapy determined by the most likely site of infection, causative organisms, and institutional bacterial and fungal susceptibility patterns. This typically involves the use of a third- or fourth-generation cephalosporin or a carbapenem, with vancomycin added if indicated.[2]
- In 21% of cancer patients with neutropenic fever, serious medical complications occur, with mortality correlating with the duration and severity of neutropenia and the time elapsed until the first dose of antibiotics is administered.[3] The overall mortality rate is 4% to 30%.
- **In adult patients expected to be neutropenic 7 days or more, it is recommended that antibacterial prophylaxis with a fluoroquinolone be initiated.**[2,4] Antibacterial prophylaxis is usually started at the time of stem cell transplantation and continued until recovery from neutropenia or initiation of empiric antibacterial therapy for neutropenic fever. Growth factors such as granulocyte macrophage colony-stimulating factor (GM-CSF) and G-CSF have been shown to reduce the duration of neutropenia after HSCT, but have not been shown to reduce mortality.

NON-NEUTROPENIC FEVER
- Fever without localizing signs occurring after engraftment is typically from an infectious cause.
  - A thorough search for the causative agent should be performed and should include routine, anaerobic, mycobacterial, and fungal cultures of blood; urinalysis and urine cultures; blood samples for cytomegalovirus (CMV) detection; and CT scans of the sinuses, chest, abdomen, and pelvis.
  - Usual causative agents are enumerated in Table 14-2.
- **Fever occurring at the time of engraftment is usually secondary to engraftment syndrome**.
  - Engraftment syndrome consists of fever occasionally accompanied by rash, pneumonitis, hyperbilirubinemia, or diarrhea.
  - Infections must be excluded with a full septic workup.
  - If no infections are identified, then a trial of short-course high-dose corticosteroids should be considered.

TABLE 14-2	DIFFERENTIAL DIAGNOSIS OF CLINICAL MANIFESTATIONS OF DISEASE AFTER HSCT BY TIME PERIOD		
Illness	Early pre-engraftment (<2–4 wk)	Early post-engraftment (<3 mo)	Late post-engraftment (>2–3 mo)
Bloodstream infections	Bacteria, *Candida* (especially associated with central venous catheters and those receiving TPN)	Bacteria (especially CONS) *Candida*	Encapsulated organisms including *Streptococcus pneumoniae*, *Neisseria meningitidis*
Bone marrow suppression	Drug toxicity, CMV, HHV-6, acute GVHD, graft failure	CMV, HHV-6, acute GVHD, graft failure, drug toxicity	Parvovirus, CMV, graft failure, HHV-6, drug toxicity, chronic GVHD
CNS disease	**Focal:** Bacteria, molds, *Candida*, stroke, drug toxicity	**Focal:** bacteria, toxoplasmosis, molds, tumor relapse	**Focal:** bacteria, molds, PML, tumor relapse, drug toxicity
	Diffuse: Bacteria, HSV, *Candida*, drug toxicity	**Diffuse:** HHV-6, CMV, *Cryptococcus*, drug toxicity	**Diffuse:** VZV, drug toxicity
Diarrhea/colitis	*Clostridium difficile*, *Candida*, enteric viruses, neutropenic enterocolitis (typhlitis), noninfectious (mucosal injury from conditioning regimen, GI bleed, infarct)	*C. difficile*, CMV, enteric viruses, adenovirus, acute GVHD, GI bleed, infarct, drug toxicity	CMV, EBV, adenovirus, *C. difficile*, enteric viruses, drug toxicity, chronic GVHD, GI bleed, infarct
Esophagitis	Drug toxicity, *Candida*, HSV	Drug toxicity, CMV	Drug toxicity
Neutropenic fever: severity risk related to duration and degree of neutropenia, degree of mucosal damage	Usually bacteria including *Staphylococcus epidermidis*, viridans streptococci, *Staphylococcus aureus*, *Enterobacter*, *Escherichia coli*, *Klebsiella*, *Pseudomonas*; *Candida*, *Aspergillus*; HSV; respiratory viruses; tumor fever; drug fever; acute GVHD; PE	Bacteria, CMV, adenovirus, PCP, *Aspergillus* and other molds, chronic disseminated candidiasis, respiratory viruses, acute GVHD, drug fever	CMV, VZV, EBV, PCP, molds, encapsulated bacteria, chronic GVHD, drug fever

(continued)

TABLE 14-2 (CONTINUED)

Non-neutropenic fever	Engraftment syndrome, acute GVHD, drug fever, bacteria, respiratory viruses	CMV, sinusitis, central line infection, fungal infection, drug fever	CMV, sinusitis, central line infection, fungal infection, drug fever
Hemorrhagic cystitis	Cyclophosphamide toxicity, adenovirus	CMV, cyclophosphamide toxicity, adenovirus	BK virus
Hepatitis	Bacteria, HSV, chronic disseminated candidiasis, veno-occlusive disease (sinusoidal obstructive syndrome) from conditioning regimen, drug toxicity, iron overload	Acute GVHD, HSV, CMV, HHV-6, PCP, chronic disseminated candidiasis, drug toxicity, iron overload	HBV, HCV, EBV, VZV (fulminant hepatitis, even in absence of rash), veno-occlusive disease, drug toxicity, chronic GVHD, iron overload
Mucositis	HSV, *Candida*, drug toxicity (conditioning regimen), acute GVHD, viridans *Streptococci*	HSV, *Candida*, acute GVHD	*Candida*, HSV, chronic GVHD
Nephritis	Bacteria	CMV, adenovirus	BK/JC viruses
Ocular disease	Candida, molds	CMV, PCP, toxoplasmosis	VZV
Pneumonia: Focal infiltrate	Bacteria, *Aspergillus*, or other molds (halo sign or cavitary lesions), chemotherapy, PE, aspiration pneumonitis	Bacteria, *Aspergillus* or other molds, *Legionella*, PCP, TB, *Nocardia*, MAC, tumor relapse	Bacteria, *Aspergillus*, or other molds, PCP, *Legionella*, *Nocardia*, VZV, EBV-associated lymphoma
Diffuse	ARDS from conditioning regimen, pulmonary edema from CHF (cardiotoxic drugs) or volume overload, acute GVHD, radiation pneumonitis, hemorrhagic alveolitis, hypersensitivity drug reaction, respiratory viruses, HSV	Respiratory viruses, CMV, PCP, adenovirus, *Legionella*, Mycoplasma, TB, MAC, Cryptococcus, acute GVHD, idiopathic interstitial pneumonitis, radiation pneumonia, hemorrhagic alveolitis, pulmonary veno-occlusive disease	CMV, respiratory viruses, PCP, adenovirus, chronic GVHD, bronchiolitis obliterans with organizing pneumonia, alveolar proteinosis

| Rash | HSV, *Candida*, bacteria, molds, drug toxicity, acute GVHD | Acute GVHD, bacteria, *Candida*, molds, CMV, HHV-6, atypical mycobacteria, drug toxicity | VZV, molds, drug toxicity, chronic GVHD |

HSCT, hematopoietic stem cell transplant; TPN, total parenteral nutrition; CONS, coagulase-negative staphylococci; PML, progressive multifocal leukoencephalopathy; GVHD, graft-versus-host disease; CNS, central nervous system. HSV, herpes simplex virus; HHV, human herpes virus; CMV, cytomegalovirus; VZV, varicella zoster virus; GI, gastrointestinal; EBV, Epstein-Barr virus; PE, pulmonary embolism; PCP, *Pneumocystis jiroveci* pneumonia; HBV, hepatitis B virus; HCV, hepatitis C virus; TB, *Mycobacterium tuberculosis*; MAC, *Mycobacterium avium* complex; ARDS, acute respiratory distress syndrome; CV, cardiovascular.

GENERAL PRINCIPLES

- Pneumonia commonly occurs in HSCT recipients. A myriad of infectious causes of pneumonia exist, and these vary by time period after transplantation and type of infiltrate (Table 14-2). Multiple pathogens are frequently present.
  - **Focal infiltrates** are typically due to bacteria (e.g., *Streptococcus pneumoniae*, *Pseudomonas aeruginosa*), *Nocardia*, *Aspergillus*, and other molds. Noninfectious causes include aspiration, wedge infarction from pulmonary embolism, and chemotherapy-induced micronodules.
  - **Diffuse infiltrates** are typically due to respiratory viruses (e.g., influenza, parainfluenza, adenovirus, and respiratory syncytial virus [RSV]), CMV, *Pneumocystis jirovecii* pneumonia (PCP), and *Legionella*. Noninfectious causes include adult respiratory distress syndrome, pulmonary edema, and hemorrhagic alveolitis.

DIAGNOSIS

- A chest radiograph or CT scan of the chest should be performed for patients with suspected pneumonia.
- Blood and sputum cultures, nasopharyngeal swab for viral immunofluorescence assay and culture, blood CMV quantitation, urine *Legionella* antigen, and serum galactomannan determination should be performed as indicated.
- Bronchoscopy with bronchoalveolar lavage (BAL) is often useful and should be considered especially for patients who fail standard therapy.
- Nodules may be biopsied with CT guidance in the absence of severe thrombocytopenia.

TREATMENT

- Empiric treatment should be targeted toward the most likely pathogens.
- Antibiotic choice is guided by the institutional bacterial susceptibility patterns and the patient's own microbiome.
- If bacterial pneumonia is suspected, **third- or fourth-generation cephalosporins with or without vancomycin is typically started**. If *Legionella* is suspected, azithromycin or a quinolone may be added.
- If fungal pneumonia is suspected, amphotericin B or a broad-spectrum azole is typically started.
- Treatment for viruses, PCP, mycobacteria, or *Nocardia* is typically withheld until such infections are proven to be present due to potential harm from polypharmacy.

GENERAL PRINCIPLES

- Diarrhea commonly ensues after HSCT and has myriad causes (Table 14-2).
- In the **pre-engraftment period**, typical causes are mucosal injury from conditioning chemotherapy, *Clostridium difficile* enterocolitis, viral enteritis, and neutropenic enterocolitis (typhlitis).

- In the **post-engraftment period**, usual causes are GVHD, CMV, adenovirus, and *C. difficile* enterocolitis. Rarely, pathogenic bacteria (e.g., *Salmonella*, *Shigella*, *Yersinia*, and *Campylobacter*) and parasites (e.g., *Cryptosporidium* and *Giardia*) are encountered.

DIAGNOSIS

- A CT scan of the abdomen and pelvis should be performed for patients with moderate to severe diarrhea.
- Stool cultures, stool *C. difficile* toxin testing, and stool examination for ova and parasites should be performed as indicated.
- Transaminases and blood CMV quantitation should be done. It is important to note, however, that **CMV** enteritis is a predominantly local disease, and virus may not be detectable in the systemic circulation.
- Persistent diarrhea in the post-engraftment period should prompt consideration of a colonoscopy given that GVHD and infectious agents such as CMV exist with equal probability and may at times coexist.

TREATMENT

- Empiric treatment against *C. difficile* should be considered.
- If proven, neutropenic enterocolitis warrants broad-spectrum antibiotic therapy.
- Treatment for other conditions such as CMV enterocolitis and GVHD are typically withheld until a definite diagnosis is made.

HERPES SIMPLEX VIRUS

GENERAL PRINCIPLES

- The incidence of herpes simplex virus (HSV) disease has decreased with antiviral prophylaxis. Prior to routine administration of antiviral prophylaxis, up to 80% of HSCT recipients developed HSV reactivation.
- HSV disease usually occurs in HSCT recipients with chronic GVHD.
- **All HSV-seropositive HSCT recipients should receive acyclovir or valacyclovir during the pre-engraftment and early post-engraftment period.**
- Use of HSV prophylaxis is not indicated for HSV-seronegative recipients, even if the donor is HSV seropositive.
- Use of ganciclovir for CMV prophylaxis protects against HSV reactivation as well.

DIAGNOSIS

- Patients generally present with oral ulcers; however, this can progress to severe mucositis and esophagitis.
- Disseminated disease occurs rarely, with viral replication in the lungs, liver, gastrointestinal tract, and central nervous system (CNS).
- Genital HSV accounts for only a small percentage of HSV reactivation cases.
- An HSV polymerase chain reaction (PCR) swab should be done for all suspected mucocutaneous lesions. Blood and cerebrospinal fluid (CSF) HSV PCR should be

performed for suspected disseminated disease. Viral inclusions are typically noted on histopathologic samples of infected organs.

TREATMENT

Acyclovir remains the treatment of choice. In cases of acyclovir resistance, foscarnet or cidofovir can be used.

VARICELLA ZOSTER VIRUS

GENERAL PRINCIPLES

- The incidence of varicella zoster virus (VZV) disease has decreased with **antiviral prophylaxis**. However, it remains common and occurs in up to 40% of HSCT recipients, usually starting after prophylactic antivirals have been discontinued.
- VZV disease usually occurs within the first 12 months post-engraftment or in HSCT recipients with chronic GVHD.
- **All VZV-seropositive HSCT recipients should receive acyclovir or valacyclovir for at least 12 months after engraftment.** Prophylactic antivirals should be continued in the presence of chronic GVHD.
- Use of ganciclovir for CMV prophylaxis protects against VZV reactivation as well.
- **VZV-seronegative HSCT recipients who are exposed to persons with active VZV disease should ideally receive intravenous varicella zoster immunoglobulin (VZIG) within the first 96 hours postexposure.** However, VZIG is no longer available in the United States. VariZIG, an intramuscularly dosed formulation of concentrated VZV IgG, is available through an expanded access protocol sponsored by Cangene Corporation/FFF Enterprises (1-800-843-7477); delivery within 24 hours can be arranged.

DIAGNOSIS

- Most commonly, VZV reactivation presents as a cutaneous infection, with involvement of single dermatome. Occasionally, multiple dermatomes are affected.
- Rarely, disseminated VZV infection, with involvement of the lungs, liver, gastrointestinal tract, and skin, and meningoencephalitis or myelitis can occur.
- Cutaneous lesions consistent with herpes zoster usually do not need confirmatory testing for a definitive diagnosis.
- Suspected cases of VZV dissemination or CNS disease should have blood and CSF sent for VZV detection using nucleic acid detection.
- Viral inclusions are typically noted on histopathologic samples of infected organs.

TREATMENT

Acyclovir is the treatment of choice; in cases of acyclovir resistance, foscarnet or cidofovir can be used.

CYTOMEGALOVIRUS

GENERAL PRINCIPLES

- The incidence of CMV disease among HSCT recipients has decreased with the advent of **preemptive treatment** for asymptomatic CMV infection. Without prophylaxis, up to 35% of patients develop CMV disease.
- All allogeneic and autologous HSCT recipients who are CMV seropositive and at high risk should undergo blood screening for CMV viremia using a nucleic acid test or pp65 antigen on a weekly basis. **Two consecutive positive tests should prompt preemptive therapy**.
  - ○ Ganciclovir is the preferred antiviral choice; alternatives are valganciclovir, foscarnet and cidofovir.
  - ○ A minimum of 2 weeks of treatment and a negative indicator test are required before the antiviral drug can be discontinued.
- **Risk factors** for CMV disease include the following:
  - ○ Among **allogeneic** HSCT recipients, CMV seropositivity in either the donor or the recipient, high-dose corticosteroid use, T-cell depletion, acute and chronic GVHD, and the use of mismatched or unrelated donors.
  - ○ Among **autologous** HSCT recipients, CD34+ selection, high-dose corticosteroid use, and the use of total body irradiation or fludarabine as part of the conditioning regimen.
- **CMV disease** usually occurs within the first 100 days post-engraftment. However, widespread use of preemptive therapy has led to an increasing incidence of late-onset (>100 days post-engraftment) CMV disease.
- CMV disease may coexist with other conditions, such as GVHD. Coinfections with bacteria, *P. jirovecii*, and *Aspergillus* are not uncommon.

DIAGNOSIS

- HSCT recipients commonly develop pneumonia.
- Patients may also develop esophagitis, gastritis, enterocolitis, and hepatitis.
- Rarely, meningoencephalitis and retinitis may ensue.
- Diagnosis depends on demonstrating viral replication in the presence of a clinical syndrome consistent with invasive CMV disease.
- Suspected cases of CMV pneumonia should have BAL specimens sent for **shell vial viral culture**. However, caution must be taken in interpreting the results, since CMV shedding into the respiratory tract is common and does not necessarily correlate with disease. A negative shell vial viral culture, however, makes a diagnosis of CMV pneumonia highly unlikely.
- An assay to detect CMV in blood, using **nucleic acid testing or pp65 antigen determination**, should be done. Pneumonia, hepatitis, and disseminated disease generally have detectable viremia; gastrointestinal disease, however, is usually local and can have no detectable viremia.
- Histopathologic evidence for CMV disease, such as nuclear inclusions, is usually evident in affected organs. Gastrointestinal disease usually requires a biopsy for proof of CMV disease.

TREATMENT

- Treatment entails the administration of **ganciclovir** as first-line therapy. Valganciclovir, foscarnet, and cidofovir are alternatives.
- Intravenous immunoglobulin (IVIG) or pooled CMV immunoglobulin is usually indicated for the treatment of CMV pneumonia.
- Drug-resistant viruses are increasingly recognized. Failure to decrease viral replication after 1 to 2 weeks of drug administration should prompt UL97 and UL54 mutational analysis to determine antiviral drug resistance.

HUMAN HERPES VIRUS 6

- Human herpes virus (HHV) 6 is the cause of **roseola**, a febrile childhood rash. Like all herpesviruses, **it is capable of establishing latency**. Nearly all children are infected with HHV-6 by age 3.
- HHV-6 reactivation is common among allogeneic HSCT recipients in the early posttransplant period. The clinical significance of HHV-6 viremia is unknown, but has been associated with fever, rash, hepatitis, idiopathic pneumonia syndrome, bone marrow suppression, and delayed platelet and monocyte engraftment.
- Uncommonly, **acute limbic encephalitis** is associated with HHV-6 reactivation in the CNS. This usually occurs in the early post-engraftment period; is more common with umbilical cord blood, use of anti-CD3 monoclonal antibodies, or HLA-mismatched grafts; and can lead to profound memory loss, seizures, mild CSF pleocytosis, and significant mesial temporal lobe abnormalities on MRI.
- Treatment with **ganciclovir and foscarnet** has been used with mixed success in case reports.

RESPIRATORY VIRUS INFECTIONS

- Respiratory virus infections occur in up to 20% of HSCT recipients; 30% to 40% of patients who initially present with upper respiratory tract infection develop lower respiratory tract disease. Risk factors for progression to lower respiratory tract disease include age greater than 65, use of myeloablative conditioning, severe neutropenia or lymphopenia, and an underlying diagnosis of leukemia.
- The etiology of respiratory virus infections should be determined by nasopharyngeal viral swab or BAL.
- **The most common viral etiologies of respiratory disease in HSCT recipients are influenza, parainfluenza, RSV, and adenovirus.**[5] Emerging viruses such as human metapneumovirus, coronavirus, enteroviruses, and rhinovirus are increasingly being recognized.
- Symptoms for viral respiratory infections are similar; dyspnea may indicate progression to lower tract disease or bacterial superinfection.
- HSCT recipients typically have prolonged shedding of virus and require extended isolation precautions.

INFLUENZA

GENERAL PRINCIPLES

- **All HSCT candidates, recipients, household contacts, and health care workers should receive the annual inactivated trivalent influenza vaccine.** Among HSCT recipients, the vaccine should be administered 6 months posttransplantation, given an absent immune response in the early period.

- **Chemoprophylaxis** should be considered for unvaccinated HSCT candidates, recipients, household contacts, and health care workers who are exposed to influenza.
- Complications of influenza virus infection are common in HSCT recipients and include a high rate of progression to pneumonia, bacterial or fungal superinfection, and death. Risk factors for complications include those with absolute lymphopenia, those using steroids, and those who were infected with influenza sooner after transplantation.

DIAGNOSIS

Diagnosis can be made by nucleic acid testing, direct fluorescent antibody (DFA), or virus culture of nasopharyngeal swab or BAL fluid.

TREATMENT

- Treatment options include neuraminidase inhibitors **oseltamivir and zanamivir**
- There is increasing resistance to M2 inhibitors amantadine and rimantadine.
- Antiviral choice depends on annual viral strain susceptibility and guidelines from the Centers for Disease Control and Prevention.
- Immunosuppressed hosts still benefit from treatment even if begun after 48 hours of the onset of symptoms.
- Some experts recommend prolonging therapy to 10 days, if patients are still symptomatic after 5 days of treatment.

PARAINFLUENZA

- Parainfluenza virus occurs year-round and can range from asymptomatic infections to severe pneumonia and respiratory failure among HSCT recipients. Other manifestations include Guillain-Barré syndrome, acute disseminated encephalomyelitis, and parotitis.
- Coinfections with bacterial and fungal organisms are common; lower respiratory tract disease portends a very poor prognosis.
- Diagnosis is typically made by DFA or viral culture of nasopharyngeal swab or BAL fluid.
- Treatment options are limited; intravenous and oral **ribavirin** has been used with mixed results.

RESPIRATORY SYNCYTIAL VIRUS

GENERAL PRINCIPLES

- RSV infections in HSCT recipients usually manifest as upper respiratory tract symptoms but can lead to severe lower respiratory tract infections.[5]
- Lower tract infections are associated with high morbidity and mortality and are frequently associated with significant copathogens.
- **Risk factors** for severe disease include pre-engraftment, lymphopenia, and preexistent obstructive airway disease.

DIAGNOSIS

Diagnosis should be sought by DFA or viral culture of nasopharyngeal swab or BAL fluid.

TREATMENT

- Treatment options include aerosolized ribavirin, IVIG, and RSV monoclonal antibody palivizumab. No randomized controlled trials have been done to define the best treatment option.
- **Aerosolized ribavirin** has been most frequently described; however, it needs to be administered in a negative pressure room, because of its potential for teratogenicity. It is likely most useful in preventing progression of upper airway infection to lower tract disease.
- Intravenous or oral ribavirin has been proposed as an alternative; systemic ribavirin use must be weighed against unqualified efficacy and potential risk.
- Palivizumab is typically reserved for RSV treatment or prophylaxis in pediatric patients.

ADENOVIRUS

GENERAL PRINCIPLES

- Adenovirus most commonly causes upper or lower respiratory tract infection, but can also cause conjunctivitis, hepatitis, enteritis, and hemorrhagic cystitis.
- Adenovirus infection in HSCT recipients is relatively common, with high mortality rates with fulminant hepatitis and disseminated disease.
- Risk factors for severe disease include T-cell-depleted grafts, HLA-mismatched transplants, GVHD, and use of anti-T-cell agents including ATG and alemtuzumab.

DIAGNOSIS

- Diagnosis is typically made by DFA, nucleic acid testing, or viral culture. Nucleic acid testing is most sensitive.
- Detection of adenovirus at two or more sites is predictive of invasive disease in HSCT recipients.

TREATMENT

- Treatment options include cidofovir, ribavirin, vidarabine, and IVIG.
- **Cidofovir** is most often used and has seen mixed results in case reports; care must be taken to avoid irreversible nephrotoxicity.
- Vidarabine has in vitro activity against adenovirus and has been used to treat hemorrhagic cystitis.
- Decreasing immunosuppression, if possible, should be attempted.

INVASIVE FUNGAL INFECTIONS

- IFIs may be caused by endemic or opportunistic fungi with a wide variety of clinical presentations from nonspecific respiratory illness to fulminant pneumonia.

- HSCT patients are more susceptible to ubiquitous opportunistic fungi due to immunosuppressive regimens.
- **The most common IFIs encountered in HSCT recipients are *Aspergillus* (43%), *Candida* (28%), other molds such as *Fusarium* and *Scedosporium* (16%), and zygomycetes (8%).**[6]
- Risk factors in general include antibiotic use, central line placement, neutropenia, GVHD, and prolonged corticosteroid use.
- Topical agents may reduce colonization of mouth and skin, but do not prevent locally invasive or disseminated fungal infections.
- Patients at high risk for IFIs (i.e., patients with prolonged neutropenia and patients with GVHD necessitating corticosteroid use) should receive triazole prophylaxis; most commonly, **fluconazole** is used.

ASPERGILLOSIS

GENERAL PRINCIPLES

- Invasive aspergillosis is the most common fungal infection in HSCT patients.
- Pathogenic mold infections among HSCT result from respiratory exposure as well as contaminated water.
- Risk factors for invasive aspergillosis include HSCT recipients (highest risk), prolonged neutropenia, corticosteroid use, GVHD, CMV disease, and older age. Patients with chronic lung diseases such as chronic obstructive pulmonary disease and those using corticosteroids are at considerably higher risk for chronic necrotizing aspergillosis and invasive pulmonary aspergillosis.
- First-line **prophylactic antifungal therapy** in allogeneic HSCT recipients remains **fluconazole** with a demonstrable survival benefit.[7-9]
  ○ In patients with prior invasive aspergillosis despite fluconazole prophylaxis, voriconazole may be used as secondary prophylaxis.
  ○ The use of laminar airflow or high-efficiency particulate air filtration for patients who receive bone marrow transplants and other high-risk patients prevents invasive aspergillosis.

DIAGNOSIS

- *Aspergillus* infection mainly manifests as pulmonary diseases, from hypersensitivity to angioinvasion, causing four main syndromes: allergic bronchopulmonary aspergillosis, chronic necrotizing *Aspergillus* pneumonia, aspergilloma, and invasive pulmonary aspergillosis.
- In severely immunocompromised patients, *Aspergillus* can hematogenously disseminate and can lead to endophthalmitis, endocarditis, and abscesses in the heart, kidney, liver, spleen, soft tissue, and bone.
- Diagnosis of infection can be accomplished by culture and galactomannan assay in serum or BAL fluid and is suggested by certain radiographic features.
- The **galactomannan assay** is specific and shows higher sensitivity in the detection of *Aspergillus* in HSCT patients than in solid organ transplant (SOT) recipients.
  ○ Serum galactomannan sensitivity and specificity are between 70% and 80%, but can be confounded by neutropenic status and concurrent use of antifungals where sensitivity can fall to less than 30%.[10]

- ○ Galactomannan assay on BAL fluid likely has better sensitivity and greater specificity.[11] Confounding factors include timing of bronchoscopy with regard to infection course and processing of BAL samples.
- Typical appearance of invasive aspergillosis on CT scan involves nodular lesions with a halo sign or cavity. However, neutrophil count, GVHD, and immunosuppression can affect the appearance on CT with tree-in-bud opacities and other lesions reported.

TREATMENT

- The drug of choice for the treatment of invasive aspergillosis is **voriconazole** due to higher tolerance and improved survival with its use when compared with amphotericin B.[12]
  - ○ Serum levels must be monitored.
  - ○ Side effects include visual disturbances, rash, and liver function test abnormalities.
- **Liposomal amphotericin B** is an alternative in patients unable to tolerate voriconazole, with improved outcomes with earlier initiation of treatment.
- **Posaconazole** can also be used for patients who cannot tolerate voriconazole as primary or salvage therapy. Absorption requires adequate caloric intake, and serum levels must also be monitored.
- **Caspofungin** has also been reported to be an effective primary therapy and salvage therapy in HSCT recipients.
- Dual therapy with voriconazole plus caspofungin or liposomal amphotericin B plus caspofungin can be considered in patients with refractory or progressive disease. However, there is no evidence at this time that combination therapy is more effective for primary treatment.

CANDIDA

- Invasive candidiasis is usually caused by dissemination of endogenous *Candida* colonizing the gastrointestinal tract.
- Risk factors include neutropenia, severe mucositis, central venous catheters, broad-spectrum antibiotics, severe gastrointestinal GVHD, and prior colonization with *Candida*.
- An erythematous, maculopapular rash can sometimes be the first sign of disseminated infection.
- **Antifungal prophylaxis with triazole antifungals** has significantly decreased the morbidity and mortality from invasive *Candida*.
  - ○ However, an increased incidence of infection with **fluconazole-resistant *Candida***, including *Candida krusei* and some *Candida glabrata* strains, has been noted.
  - ○ Autologous HSCT recipients are at lower risk for invasive candidiasis and generally do not require routine prophylaxis for *Candida*.
  - ○ **Fluconazole** is the drug of choice for *Candida* prophylaxis and is usually initiated when starting conditioning regimens.[2,4,7-9] High-dose fluconazole treatment does not seem to show any increased benefit over regular doses of 200 mg/d, but dosages less than 200 mg/d have variable efficacy and are not recommended.
- The **echinocandins** (i.e., caspofungin, micafungin, and anidulafungin) are first-line treatments for candidemia in HSCT recipients. Refractory cases, or cases with valvular or CNS disease, require treatment with amphotericin B.

MUCORALES

GENERAL PRINCIPLES

- **Mucormycosis** refers to infections with fungi in the order of Mucorales, of which *Rhizopus* species are most common. These organisms are ubiquitous in nature, and most people are exposed daily. The usual route of exposure is inhalation of spores.
- Mucormycosis is a fungal emergency, with 0.1% to 2% of HSCT recipients developing infection and fatality rates high (36% to 91%).[13] Even if successfully treated, infection can result in serious disfigurement among survivors.
- Infection rates have been increasing over the last two decades, especially among patients with hematological malignancies and HSCT recipients and patients where early diagnosis is difficult and infection can progress rapidly.
- **Types of infection** include pulmonary, rhinocerebral disease, cutaneous, gastrointestinal, and CNS.
  - ○ Disseminated infections can occur, usually following pulmonary or rhinocerebral disease.
  - ○ **Pulmonary infection** usually occurs in diabetic patients or immunocompromised hosts, especially those with neutropenia. **This is the most common form of infection in HSCT recipients**, followed by disseminated disease. In HSCT recipients, pulmonary mucormycosis often occurs after resolution of neutropenia and after engraftment and is associated with corticosteroid therapy for GHVD.
  - ○ Rhinocerebral disease usually occurs in diabetic patients; this is rare among HSCT patients.
  - ○ Cutaneous involvement has been reported in HSCT recipients and those with hematologic malignancies. It can also be found at the site of central catheter placement.
  - ○ CNS mucormycosis usually results from dissemination from pulmonary or rhinocerebral courses.

DIAGNOSIS

Clinical Presentation
- Clinical features vary depending on the type of infection.
- Symptoms of pulmonary infection include fever that does not resolve with antibiotics, dyspnea, cough, and pleuritic chest pain. Angioinvasion and the resultant tissue necrosis can lead to hemoptysis and may be fatal with major blood vessel involvement.
- Rhinocerebral mucormycosis may present with facial pain, black necrotic lesions, discharge from the nasal and palatal mucosa, fever, periorbital cellulitis, proptosis, and visual deficits.

Diagnostic Testing
- Establishing **diagnosis** can be difficult as clinical presentation may mimic other IFIs and *Mucorales* are environmental isolates and frequent contaminants/colonizers.
- **The gold standard for diagnosis requires a positive culture or histopathology from a sterile site** such as needle aspirate, tissue biopsy, or pleural fluid. Culture is unreliable: tissue processing that includes grinding kills the organism, and the mold often fails to grow. Therefore, biopsy with histopathology is the most sensitive and specific test.

- Probable infection is indicated with positive culture from nonsterile site (for example, BAL fluid) in a patient with appropriate risk factors and clinical/CT evidence consistent with *Mucorales* disease.
- Chest CT is the best test for determining the extent of pulmonary disease. Radiographic findings can include cavitations, lobar consolidation, isolated masses, nodular disease, or wedge-shaped infarcts. More than 10 pulmonary nodules, pleural effusion, or concurrent invasive sinusitis can help distinguish *Mucorales* from *Aspergillus*.[14]

TREATMENT

- Successful treatment requires a four-pronged approach: rapid diagnosis, correction of the underlying risk factors, aggressive surgical debridement, and appropriate antifungal therapy.
- **Rapid diagnosis is crucial as delay in initiation of appropriate antifungal therapy is associated with increased mortality**.
- Tight diabetic control and rapid correction of underlying ketoacidosis, dose reduction or discontinuation of corticosteroids or other immunosuppressants, and consideration of G-CSF in neutropenic patients are important measures also.
- **Surgical debridement** of infected and necrotic tissue has been shown to be an independent variable for favorable outcome and should be performed for rhinocerebral disease and considered in other types of infection including pulmonary infection, if possible. Due to the superficial nature of cutaneous disease, early diagnosis and surgical debridement with skin grafting yield very favorable outcomes.
- The optimal dose of any antifungal for treating these infections has not been established, though treatment length is usually 3 to 6 weeks.
- High doses of **lipid formulations of amphotericin B** (liposomal amphotericin B or amphotericin B lipid complex at 5 to 7.5 mg/kg/d) are the drug of choice for treatment of *Mucorales* infections. They also have excellent lung penetration versus amphotericin B deoxycholate and lower side-effect profiles, with improved survival demonstrated.[14]
- Voriconazole is not active in vitro. Posaconazole has in vitro activity, but serum concentrations achievable in patients are typically below MIC_{90}, so neither is recommended for first-line monotherapy.
- Posaconazole, however, has been used as an alternative for those who cannot tolerate amphotericin B or as salvage therapy.

FUSARIUM

GENERAL PRINCIPLES

- *Fusarium* species are found commonly in the soil and on plants and pathogenesis relies on three factors: colonization, tissue damage, and immunosuppression.
- In immunocompromised populations, it is primarily a nosocomial disease. Reservoirs for nosocomial infection include hospital water systems and patient-to-patient contact.
- Fusariosis is rare among SOT recipients, tends to remain localized, and has better mortality rates in this group.
- Pathogenesis of fusariosis may also be related to several virulence characteristics of the individual *Fusarium* strains, including mycotoxins that are thought to cause

leukopenia and production of cyclosporine in some species to suppress the host immune system. However, there are no studies examining whether these molecules are expressed in the setting of invasive disease.

- Risk factors include HSCT patients, severity and duration of immunosuppression, indwelling catheters, neutropenia (especially in the early pre-engraftment period), corticosteroid therapy (especially in the post-engraftment period in the setting of chronic GVHD), colonization, tissue damage, or receipt of a graft from an HLA-mismatched or unrelated donor.
- Prevention relies on treating cutaneous damage prior to initiation of immunosuppression and decreasing environmental exposure to *Fusarium*. No antifungal has been used successfully for *Fusarium* prophylaxis.

DIAGNOSIS

Clinical Presentation

- The clinical presentation includes refractory fever, skin lesions, and sinopulmonary infections.
- Type of skin lesions includes purpura, macules, target lesions, and multiple tender subcutaneous nodules.
- *Fusarium* skin lesions in immunocompetent hosts are fewer in number and localized and typically follow skin breakdown.
- The characteristic skin lesion in disseminated fusariosis is the "ecthyma gangrenosum–like" lesions, red or gray macules with central ulceration, or black eschar.
- The high incidence of skin lesions in the setting of disseminated disease contrasts with the low incidence and fewer number of skin lesions in disseminated aspergillosis.

Diagnostic Testing

- Diagnosis can be made by biopsy of skin lesions during disseminated fusariosis.
- The clinical and radiographic features of invasive mucormycosis and fusariosis are similar and nonspecific. Hence, it is almost impossible to establish a diagnosis on clinical grounds, and recovery of *Fusarium* from cultures of appropriate specimens is essential for a definite diagnosis.
- A thorough workup includes blood culture analysis, radiographic evaluation of the sinuses and lungs (using computed tomography), and skin biopsy for cultures, histopathologic examination, and fungal staining.
- In contrast to other types of invasive molds, *Fusarium* can frequently be recovered from blood specimens in the setting of disseminated disease, and fungemia may be the only manifestation of the infection.[15] Cultures often become positive relatively early in the course of the disseminated disease.

TREATMENT

- There is no optimal treatment for Fusarium. It is **highly resistant to most antifungal agents**.
- The mainstay in the treatment of fusariosis has traditionally been **lipid formulations of amphotericin B**. However, the in vitro susceptibility of *Fusarium* to amphotericin B is mediocre.
- Ketoconazole, miconazole, fluconazole, and itraconazole have no in vitro activity against *Fusarium*.

- Similarly, *Fusarium* is inherently resistant to the echinocandins caspofungin, micafungin, and anidulafungin.
- **Voriconazole appears to be more effective than liposomal amphotericin B both in vitro and in vivo for both primary therapy and salvage therapy in most species** and has a decreased side-effect profile.[16] Voriconazole is currently approved for the treatment of refractory fusariosis.
- Posaconazole is also active against *Fusarium* species both in vitro and in animal models. **Posaconazole may be useful with salvage therapy in refractory cases.**
- Surgical resection of infected necrotic tissue is a significant component of therapy for fusariosis, along with prompt removal of central venous catheters and reversal of underlying immunosuppression.
- Corticosteroid therapy should be decreased or discontinued, if feasible. Increasing neutrophil count by administration of recombinant G-CSF and GM-CSF or white cell transfusion should be considered.

INFECTIOUS COMPLICATIONS ASSOCIATED WITH SOLID ORGAN TRANSPLANTATION

- Improved immunosuppressive regimens have reduced the incidence of graft rejection but have increased the risk of infection and virally mediated malignancies. Early and specific diagnosis of invasive infection along with rapid, aggressive treatment is essential to good clinical outcomes.
- Etiology of infection includes both common, community-acquired diseases and diseases affecting immunocompromised hosts.
  - Increased use of antimicrobial prophylaxis has changed the epidemiology of infections in SOT recipients and will likely continue to evolve.
  - The incidence of CMV and PCP has been significantly decreased in this population.
  - Unfortunately, this has also caused increased antimicrobial resistance in these hosts.
- Clinical diagnosis can be complicated by the **diminution or complete absence of the usual signs and symptoms of inflammation or infection, resulting in advanced or disseminated infection at the time of clinical presentation.**
  - Additionally, alterations in anatomy due to organ transplantation can impair diagnosis; noninfectious causes of fever including graft rejection, drug toxicities, and autoimmune reactions can mimic infectious processes.
  - Serologic testing is usually not useful in diagnosis due to delayed seroconversion in these immunosuppressed individuals. Fortunately, the recent availability of quantitative antigen or nucleic acid–based assays facilitates early diagnosis; however, invasive diagnostic procedures including tissue biopsies and advanced imaging procedures are often necessary for diagnosis.
- Once diagnosis is established, choice of antimicrobials is complicated by the frequency of drug interactions with immunosuppressive medications.
- Antimicrobial therapy alone is inadequate in patients with undrained fluid collections, hematomas, or devitalized tissues, which require early, aggressive surgical debridement.

- The risk of infection is mainly determined by two factors: the epidemiologic exposures and the net state of immunosuppression.
  - To assess **epidemiologic exposures**, one must have a detailed history of potential pathogen encounters and risk factors for both the recipient and the donor, including contact with common community-acquired pathogens for their specific region.
  - The **net state of immunosuppression** takes into account the type, dose, duration, and sequence of immunosuppressive therapies; underlying diseases or comorbid conditions; the presence of devitalized tissues or fluid collections in the transplanted organ; invasive devices (central venous catheters, urinary catheters, drains, etc); the state of the host's immune system, including neutropenia and hypogammaglobulinemia; metabolic problems (uremia and malnutrition); and infection with immunomodulating viruses such as CMV, Epstein-Barr virus (EBV), HHV-6, hepatitis B virus (HBV), and hepatitis C virus (HCV).
- The differential diagnosis can be altered by the use of antimicrobial prophylaxis.
- Reactivation of infections can be derived from either the donor or the recipient, so it is important to screen for multiple diseases prior to transplantation to ensure a preventative strategy is developed.
- Additionally, some asymptomatic infections can be unveiled or their course accelerated with the use of immunosuppressive medications, including West Nile virus, HSV, HCV, and lymphocytic choriomeningitis virus.
- The risk and etiologies of infection posttransplantation can be divided into three time periods: **early posttransplantation** (first month), **intermediate period** (1 to 6 months), and **late period** (greater than 6 months) (see Table 14-3). This time line may vary between transplant centers using different immunosuppressive regimens, between different types of transplantation, and with different patient populations but can serve as a general guide.

HERPES SIMPLEX VIRUS

GENERAL PRINCIPLES

- Disease in SOT recipients differs in that they **shed virus more frequently, have more frequent and severe manifestations of disease, and may present atypically**, delaying diagnosis.
- Disease usually results from **reactivation of the virus**, although disease has been documented from allograft or primary infection. It typically occurs within the first month posttransplant.
- Risk factors include HSV-seropositive recipients with an incidence around 35% to 68% without prophylaxis; therefore, the serostatus of all SOT recipients should be checked prior to transplant.[17]
- Prevention by use of **prophylactic ganciclovir, acyclovir, valacyclovir, and valganciclovir** should be considered for all seropositive organ recipients not receiving CMV prophylaxis. CMV reactivation prophylaxis generally covers HSV also.
  - Prophylaxis should be continued at least 1 month. If they continue to experience frequent symptomatic reactivation, suppressive therapy should be continued.
  - **Suppressive therapy** can be given safely for several years and is associated with less acyclovir resistance than intermittent therapy.

TABLE 14-3   INFECTIONS IN SOLID ORGAN TRANSPLANT PATIENTS GROUPED BY TIME AFTER INFECTION

Early posttransplant period (<1 mo)	Intermediate period (1–6 mo)	Late posttransplant period (>6 mo)
Caused by donor- or recipient-derived infections; infectious complications of transplant surgery and hospitalization	Caused by activation of latent infections. Highest risk of opportunistic infections	Usually caused by community-acquired infections as decreased immunosuppression; rare infections from transplanted organ
Antimicrobial-resistant infections acquired during hospitalization, including MRSA, VRE, non-*albicans Candida*, resistant *Aspergillus*	**With prophylaxis (i.e., PCP, CMV, HSV, HCV):**	**Reduced immunosuppression:**
	Polyomavirus infections (BK), nephropathy	CMV (colitis, retinitis)
	Infectious diarrhea: *C. difficile* colitis; *Cryptosporidium, Microsporidia*, CMV, rotavirus	Hepatitis (HBV, HCV)
Aspiration		HSV encephalitis
Catheter infection	HCV infection	Community-acquired (West Nile)
Wound infection		BK virus (PML)
Anastomotic leaks and ischemia	Respiratory viruses including adenovirus, influenza, RSV, parainfluenza	Skin cancer
Clostridium difficile colitis		EBV-associated lymphoma, PTLD
	Cryptococcus neoformans	Community-acquired pneumonia: respiratory viruses, pneumococcus, Legionella, etc.
	Latent infection with protozoal diseases, i.e., toxoplasmosis, *Leishmania*, Chagas disease	Urinary tract infection
	Mycobacterium tuberculosis and nontuberculosis mycobacterium	Aspergillus, atypical molds, *Mucor, Nocardia, Rhodococcus*
Donor-derived infections: bacterial and fungal disease	**Without prophylaxis:**	**Higher immunosuppression due to inadequate graft function:**
	PCP	
Endemic infections (e.g., histoplasmosis, tuberculosis)	Herpesviruses (EBV, HSV, VZV, CMV)	Opportunistic infections: PCP, *Cryptococcus*, nocardiosis, etc.
	HBV infection	

(uncommon) Graft-associated infections including HSV, LCMV, rhabdovirus, West Nile virus, HIV, Trypanosoma cruzi, toxoplasmosis

Recipient-derived infections (colonization): Aspergillus, Pseudomonas

Endemic fungal infections including histoplasmosis, coccidioidomycosis, blastomycosis

Listeria, Nocardia, Toxoplasma, Strongyloides, Leishmania, T. cruzi

Severe community-acquired infections, especially influenza, Listeria

PML, progressive multifocal leukoencephalopathy; MRSA, methicillin-resistant *Staphylococcus aureus*; VRE, vancomycin-resistant *Enterococcus*; HSV, herpes simplex virus; LCMV, lymphocytic choriomeningitis virus; HIV, human immunodeficiency virus; PCP, *Pneumocystis jirovecii* pneumonia; HCV, hepatitis C virus; CMV, cytomegalovirus; RSV, respiratory syncytial virus; HBV, hepatitis B virus; VZV, varicella zoster virus; EBV, Epstein-Barr virus; PTLD, posttransplantation lymphoproliferative disorder.

DIAGNOSIS

- The clinical presentation is usually **vesicles or ulcerative disease in the orolabial, genital, or perianal region**.
- Visceral and disseminated disease (esophagitis, hepatitis, and pneumonitis) can also occur. Usual presentation with dissemination is fever, leukopenia, and hepatitis. Pneumonitis is more common in lung–heart transplants.
- **Diagnosis can be made by PCR** (more sensitive than tissue culture), which is the test of choice, DFA testing of lesions and other samples, and culture.

TREATMENT

- Treatment regimen depends on the severity and location of disease and should be continued until complete resolution of all lesions.
  - ○ Limited mucocutaneous disease can be treated with oral **acyclovir, valacyclovir, or ganciclovir**.
  - ○ **IV acyclovir** should be rapidly initiated with disseminated or visceral disease or extensive cutaneous disease.[17]
  - ○ Consideration should be given to decreasing immunosuppressive regimen.
- **With patients not responding to appropriate therapy with acyclovir, resistance should be considered**. Workup in these cases should include laboratory confirmation of HSV with acyclovir sensitivities performed. If resistance is found, foscarnet or cidofovir can be used.

CYTOMEGALOVIRUS

GENERAL PRINCIPLES

- CMV seroprevalence ranges from 30% to 97% in the general population and is one of the main causes of morbidity in SOT patients.[18] In the absence of prophylaxis, CMV occurs in the first 3 months after transplant.
- **CMV tends to invade the allograft and has been implicated in acute and chronic graft injury and increased risk of graft rejection**.
- The greatest risk factor for CMV disease is organ transplantation from seropositive donors to seronegative recipients. Other risk factors include the net state of immunosuppression; antilymphocyte antibodies, especially during antirejection therapy; and lung, small intestines, and pancreas transplant recipients.
- Preventative strategies include either prophylaxis or preemptive therapy. There currently is no consensus on the best method.
  - ○ **Prophylaxis** involves giving antiviral regimen for all at-risk patients beginning shortly posttransplant and continuing usually for 3 to 6 months. Benefits include preventing reactivation of other herpesviruses and have been **demonstrated to decrease graft loss and improve survival**.[18] Unfortunately, late-onset CMV disease may occur once off prophylaxis and is associated with higher mortality.
  - ○ **Preemptive therapy** involves weekly monitoring of CMV replication by pp65 antigen assay or PCR, with valganciclovir or IV ganciclovir initiated in those with signs of early CMV replication. Benefits for preemptive therapy include decreased drug costs and toxicity; however, this requires close monitoring.

- **Prophylaxis** for naive kidney and liver transplant, heart transplant, pancreas or pancreas/kidney transplant recipients and all intestinal transplant recipients includes **valganciclovir, oral ganciclovir, or IV ganciclovir,** with prophylaxis started within postoperative day 10 for 3 to 6 months.[18] In seropositive recipients, regimen can be given for 3 months.
  - In naive lung and heart–lung transplant recipients, IV ganciclovir or oral valganciclovir can be used for at least 6 months. Seropositive recipients follow the same regimen as heart transplant recipients above.
  - For heart or lung transplant recipients, CMV immunoglobulin can also be added.
  - Prophylaxis should also be given to patients receiving antilymphocyte therapies.
  - CMV prophylaxis is unnecessary in seronegative donors with seronegative grafts, but they should receive CMV-negative blood or leukodepleted blood products to prevent primary CMV infection.

DIAGNOSIS

- Symptoms can include a viral syndrome of fever, malaise, leukopenia, and thrombocytopenia or invasive diseases such as hepatitis, pneumonitis with nonproductive cough, retinitis, colitis, adrenalitis with adrenal insufficiency, or meningoencephalitis due to CMV vasculitis.
- **Diagnosis is usually made with the pp65 antigen assay or PCR**, both of which have higher sensitivity and specificity than culture methods.
- Higher viral loads by PCR are associated with tissue invasive disease, with the lower loads usually indicating asymptomatic infection.
- Levels can be followed with the antigen assay or with PCR to guide management and monitor treatment response, although standardization varies among institutions.
- Histopathology can also be used but requires an invasive procedure.

TREATMENT

- Treatment is **IV ganciclovir** until symptoms resolve and viremia is undetectable, usually 2 to 4 weeks.[18]
- **Oral valganciclovir** can also be used in mild-to-moderate CMV disease with similar efficacy.
- Addition of CMV immunoglobulin can be considered.
- For ganciclovir-resistant CMV, a few studies in SOT patients have shown positive results with foscarnet, although nephrotoxicity is a significant side effect.

EPSTEIN-BARR VIRUS AND POSTTRANSPLANT LYMPHOPROLIFERATIVE DISORDER

GENERAL PRINCIPLES

- In SOT recipients, **EBV is usually transmitted from a seropositive donor graft or when nonleukoreduced blood products are used**. Therefore, EBV serostatus should be determined prior to transplantation in order to determine EBV risk stratification.

- Median time of onset of primary EBV infection is 6 weeks after SOT, with reactivation events usually occurring at 2 to 3 months posttransplantation.
- **EBV is connected with most posttransplant lymphoproliferative disorder (PTLD) cases**, and the incidence of PTLD is increasing among organ transplant recipients.
  - The highest rate of PTLD in SOT occurs in the first year posttransplantation.
  - EBV genome is found in the majority of B-cell PTLD diagnosed within the first year after SOT, but a quarter to one-third of late PTLD cases are EBV B-cell negative. EBV-negative PTLD is more likely to occur more than 1 year after SOT.
- **Risk factors** for early PTLD disease include primary EBV infection, young age, CMV mismatch or CMV disease, seronegative recipients (immune naive) with seropositive donor organs, and polyclonal antilymphocyte antibodies.
  - Risk factors for late disease include the duration of immunosuppression, older recipient age, and type of transplant.
  - Type of organ transplanted changes the risk stratification, with small intestinal transplant recipients at greatest risk (up to 32%) and renal transplant patients at low risk (1% to 2%).[19]
- PTLD can also occur in HSCT recipients, primarily those with profound T-cell cytopenia (after T-cell depletion, use of anti-T-cell antibodies, and umbilical cord blood transplants) or chronic GVHD. In HSCT patients, EBV viral load increases are highest in patients at risk for PTLD; therefore, quantitative viral load surveillance may identify high-risk patients.
- Other than limiting immunosuppression where possible, **there is no accepted prophylaxis for PTLD**.

DIAGNOSIS

Clinical Presentation

- Disease syndromes linked with EBV after SOT including a **mononucleosis-like syndrome** with early disease, manifesting as fever, malaise, exudative pharyngitis, lymphadenopathy, hepatosplenomegaly, and atypical lymphocytosis.
- EBV is also associated with **organ-specific diseases** including hepatitis, pneumonitis, gastrointestinal symptoms that can lead to bleeding or perforation, and hematologic abnormalities including leukopenia, thrombocytopenia, and hemolytic anemia. All these syndromes can present similarly to PTLD.
- PTLD ranges from indolent to fulminant and extent of the disease can range from localized nodular lesions that can affect the allograft to widely disseminated disease and is characterized by lymphoproliferation after transplantation.
- No staging system currently exists for PTLD.
- Recurrence of PTLD occurs in around 5% of cases.[19]

Diagnostic Testing

- Diagnosis of PTLD requires tissue examination, which should be checked for EBV-specific nucleic acids by **RNA hybridization as well as immunostaining for EBV-specific latent antigens**.
- CMV infection status should also be determined.
- **Serology is unreliable** in immunocompromised individuals due to alterations in humoral response and should not be used to diagnose EBV or PTLD in this population.

- The role of EBV viral load remains uncertain as there lacks standardization between laboratories.
- In lung and heart–lung transplant recipients, determination of EBV load in BAL fluid may be a good predictor of PTLD.[19]
- Total body CT scan can be considered for initial assessment of PTLD.
- Head CT/MRI is included as presence of CNS lesions will influence treatment and outcome.
- Pulmonary lesions on chest radiograph will likely require high-resolution CT for better delineation prior to biopsy.
- Ultrasound or CT of the abdomen or GI endoscopy can be performed with suspected intraabdominal lesions.
- Positron emission tomography (PET) scanning is also starting to be used.

TREATMENT

- **Treatment usually starts with reductions in immunosuppression, which can result in regression of PTLD in 50% of patients.**[19,20]
- Surgical resection and local radiation therapy have been used as adjunct treatments.
- Although there is no evidence to support the use of antiviral agents, ganciclovir and acyclovir have been used. Ganciclovir in vitro has 10 times greater efficacy against EBV and is therefore preferred.
- Increasing evidence supports the use of **rituximab**, the humanized chimeric monoclonal antibody against CD20, to treat refractory PTLD.[19,21,22] To benefit from this therapy, there must be demonstrated CD20 markers in PTLD tissue samples. Side effects include tumor lysis syndrome, CMV reactivation, protracted hypogammaglobulinemia, and intestinal perforation with bowel PTLD.
- In patients with high viral load on diagnosis, response to therapy can be determined by following decline and clearance of EBV. With the exception of those on rituximab, this usually corresponds to clinical and histological regression.
- Factors associated with poor outcomes in PTLD patients include poor performance status, multiple sites of disease, CNS disease, EBV-negative PTLD, non-B-cell PTLD, and coinfection with HBV or HCV.

VARICELLA ZOSTER VIRUS

GENERAL PRINCIPLES

- Zoster is frequent in SOT patients with an incidence of around 10% in the first 4 years posttransplant.[23]
- Prevention can be accomplished with oral acyclovir or other regimen for CMV or HSV prophylaxis. Insufficient data exist to recommend long-term suppression.
- **Prior to transplantation, VZV-naive patients should be vaccinated with the varicella virus vaccine** if no other contraindications exist at least 2 to 4 weeks prior to transplant and 4 to 6 weeks in end-stage organ disease due to decreased seroconversion rates. Zoster vaccine should not be used as it contains 15 times more live virus.
- **Postexposure prophylaxis** should be given to naive SOT recipients with significant exposure to an infected individual (i.e., household contact, significant face-to-face contact, or roommate in the hospital).[23]

○ Options include passive immunoprophylaxis with VZIG and/or antiviral therapy. Unfortunately, VZIG is no longer available in most hospitals, must be given within 96 hours of exposure, and does not prevent disease but decreases severity when able to be given.
○ Antiviral therapy as postexposure prophylaxis has not been evaluated in clinical trials of SOT patients, but is an alternative when VZIG is not available, and comprises a 7- to 10-day course of valacyclovir or acyclovir.

DIAGNOSIS

- Zoster presents with painful vesicular lesions involving ≤2 adjacent dermatomes.
- Dissemination is uncommon but can occur. Neuralgia can precede the development of vesicles.
- **Diagnosis can be made clinically in typical cases or by PCR** (the most sensitive test) or direct fluorescent assay in those with atypical cases or suspected disseminated or visceral disease. Viral culture is slower and less sensitive.

TREATMENT

- **Treatment with IV acyclovir should be initiated early in SOT patients with primary varicella, as they are at risk for severe disease.**[23]
- Reduction of immunosuppression should be considered, with steroid dose left in place or increased for stress response.
- IVIG or VZIG has not shown any significant benefit.
- Localized dermatomal zoster can be treated with oral valacyclovir or famciclovir on an outpatient basis with close monitoring. However, VZV reactivation in the trigeminal ganglion (herpes zoster ophthalmicus) or in the geniculate ganglion (Ramsay-Hunt syndrome) should receive IV acyclovir as it can lead to blindness or facial palsy and hearing loss, respectively.
- Disseminated disease should be treated with IV acyclovir.

POLYOMAVIRUS INFECTIONS

GENERAL PRINCIPLES

- Polyomavirus infections can be detected in almost 60% of renal transplant recipients and are **a significant cause for graft failure**. Infectious nephropathy can occur in 1% to 10% of cases.[24]
- While JC virus and SV40 can cause nephropathy in this population, **the usual cause is BK virus**.
- BK virus infection has been associated with two **major complications in transplant recipients**: (1) nephropathy, usually in renal transplant patients, with a rate of 1% to 10%; and (2) hemorrhagic cystitis, usually affecting allogeneic HSCT patients at rates of 5% to 15%.[24]
  ○ It is also less commonly associated with pneumonitis, hemophagocytic syndrome, retinitis, and encephalitis.
  ○ In renal allograft recipients, it can also cause hemorrhagic cystitis, asymptomatic viruria, interstitial nephritis, ureteric obstruction, and increased creatinine.

- Primary BK virus infection is usually asymptomatic and occurs in the first decade of life. Latent infection is then usually established in the renourinary tract.
- Asymptomatic BK viruria occurs in immunocompetent hosts intermittently at a low rate, but in immunocompromised individuals, particularly after SOT or HSCT, higher levels of BK virus replication occurs.
- 30% to 50% of renal transplant patients with high-level BK viruria progress to viremia and nephropathy.[24]
- The virus directly causes loss of renal tubular epithelial cells, and inflammation elicited by necrosis and denudation of tubular basement membrane leads to infiltration by lymphocytes, tubular atrophy, and fibrosis.
- Graft loss after nephropathy is currently <10%.
- Independent **risk factors** for BK virus–associated nephropathy include ATG induction therapy, tacrolimus, mycophenolate mofetil, ischemia–perfusion injury during transplant, HLA mismatch, and corticosteroid.[24]
- To prevent nephropathy, kidney transplant recipients should be regularly screened for BK virus replication to identify at-risk individuals prior to significant allograft damage.

DIAGNOSIS

- The first clinical sign of BK-associated nephropathy is frequently a gradual increase in serum creatinine, but indicates extensive tubular damage and inflammation.
- Definitive diagnosis is made by histological examination of tissue and identification of BK virus–associated cytopathic changes. A minimum of two biopsies must be taken due to the focal nature of the destruction.

TREATMENT

- Treatment of BK nephropathy in renal transplant patients without signs of acute graft rejection is to **reduce immunosuppression**.[24,25] The primary goal is to control BK virus replication and preserve renal allograft function, which can be monitored by serum creatinine, BK viral load, and allograft histology.
- BK virus–specific immune recovery generally takes 1 to 2 months.
- In patients with sustained high-level plasma BK virus load despite reduced immunosuppression, **antiviral therapy can be considered**, but there are no randomized controlled trials with these medications and BK virus infection.
  - **Cidofovir** has been used for BK-associated nephropathy, but studies show conflicting results with regard to clinical efficacy. One study did show that while the rate of BK virus clearance was not improved with cidofovir versus placebo, graft survival improved significantly (graft loss 15% vs. 73% in untreated).[24,26]
  - Leflunomide has both antiviral and immunosuppressive properties, making it an attractive therapeutic candidate for patients with BK-associated nephropathy and acute rejection. Unfortunately, there is not much evidence regarding its efficacy, and there are significant toxic side effects.
  - IVIG has also been used, but no studies have compared this therapy with others.
- There are no evidence-based recommendations for treatment of BK-associated nephropathy in patients with concurrent acute rejection.

INVASIVE FUNGAL INFECTIONS

- Liver transplant patients have higher rates of fungal infection than other SOT recipients, with incidences up to 40% and mortality rates that can approach 100%.[27]
- Risk factors for invasive infections in liver transplant patients include elevated serum creatinine, long operative times, retransplantation, iron overload, and *Candida* colonization at the time of transplantation.
- Commercial renal transplant recipients are also a population with higher rates of IFIs, the most common being *Aspergillus*, followed by mucormycosis.
- Regarding cryptococcal infections, see Chapter 13.[28]

CANDIDIASIS

GENERAL PRINCIPLES

- **Candida infections are the most common IFI in SOT patients**, accounting for over half of cases, and overall rates of invasive candidiasis have increased slightly over time.
- Invasive candidiasis usually occurs within the first 3 months posttransplant, earlier than other invasive mycoses.
- With the exception of the liver transplant population, there have been limited studies on **prophylaxis** in SOT patients, making prophylaxis controversial. **In liver transplant patients, prospective randomized controlled trials have shown that antifungal prophylaxis in high-risk patients reduces the rate of invasive candidiasis**.
  - In this population, prophylaxis should be given to those with at least two of the following risk factors: retransplantation, prolonged or repeat surgery, renal failure, high transfusion requirement (>40 units of blood products), choledocojejunostomy, and *Candida* colonization preoperatively.[29]
  - There is no consensus on duration, but 4 weeks is the current recommendation.
  - **Fluconazole** is the treatment of choice, unless at risk for *Aspergillus*, in which case an antifungal with activity against both agents should be used.
  - Of note, fluconazole prophylaxis has also been shown to increase the rate of non-*albicans Candida* infections.
- With small bowel transplant patients, although there are a lack of clinical data to support the use of prophylaxis, due to the high rates of *Candida* infection, as high as 28% in some studies, antifungal prophylaxis is routinely used with either fluconazole or, if non-*albicans Candida* is suspected, lipid formulations of amphotericin B.[29] Prophylaxis is recommended for at least 4 weeks or until the anastomosis has completely healed.

DIAGNOSIS

- Diagnosis is made by recovery of *Candida* from a sterile body site/fluid.
- Cultures are sensitive for isolation of *Candida* only about 70% of the time.[29]
- There are FDA-approved assays available for adjunctive diagnosis, but they have not been extensively used clinically.
- The $(1{\Rightarrow}3)$-β-D-glycan assay has a sensitivity of 70% and a specificity of 87%.[29,30]

- Identification of the specific *Candida* species responsible for infection is important for choice of therapy. Susceptibility testing is usually not necessary as susceptibility can generally be predicted based on species and local susceptibility profiles, but may be beneficial with *C. glabrata* with suspected azole resistance or in cases of treatment failure.

TREATMENT

- There are no randomized studies in SOT patients examining treatment modalities, so recommendations are similar to those in other patients.[29]
- In general, an **echinocandin** is the treatment of choice (e.g., caspofungin loading dose of 70 mg, then 50 mg daily).[29,31]
  - Possible alternatives are lipid formulation amphotericin B, fluconazole, and voriconazole, depending on individual patient factors.
  - *C. glabrata* may be resistant to fluconazole and voriconazole, in which case an echinocandin is preferred. *C. krusei* may also be relatively resistant to fluconazole but is susceptible to voriconazole. Susceptibility testing can be done to guide therapy.
  - *Candida parapsilosis* may be less responsive to the echinocandins.
- *Candida* isolated from the respiratory tract is rarely indicative of invasive infection and does not require treatment unless it is in a lung transplant patient or anastomotic tracheobronchitis is a concern.[29] Diagnosis of *Candida* tracheobronchitis is based on visual inspection and histologic confirmation.

PARASITIC INFECTIONS

- Parasitic infections remain the most under-recognized of all infections in organ transplantation, with only limited studies and most treatment recommendations based on expert opinion only.
- Parasitic disease can occur as a result of reactivation of latent infection in the recipient, new infection, or transmission from the organ donor.
- Coinfection is a common feature. CMV has been associated with increased risk of invasive parasitic disease, but disseminated bacterial infections are also common coinfections.
- The incidence of parasitic infection is expected to increase, in part due to the decreased use of cyclosporine-based immunosuppressive regimens in favor of other regimens that lack the antiparasitic effect of cyclosporine.[32]

STRONGYLOIDES

GENERAL PRINCIPLES

- *Strongyloides stercoralis* infects 80 to 100 million people worldwide and is endemic to the tropics and subtropics, including the southeastern United States.[32]
- The parasite is found in the soil, where filariform larvae penetrate through intact skin and travel to the intestinal lumen, migrate through the mucosa, and travel to the lung and the duodenal mucosa, where they mature into adults.
- The adults release eggs into the stool that can infect the same host to perpetuate the cycle. The rate of autoinfection is regulated by the immune status of the host, with

maturation into filariform larvae accelerated with immunosuppression, increasing the rate of autoinfection.
- Manifestations of disease are related to damage inflicted by larvae as they penetrate through tissue, and severity of disease correlates with worm burden.
- Strongyloidiasis has mainly been described in renal transplant recipients with activation of latent infection and in pancreas and intestine transplants from donor infection.
- Risk factors for **hyperinfection syndrome and disseminated disease** include severe immunosuppression and corticosteroid use and are most likely to occur in the initial months posttransplant with the highest level of immunosuppression. Cyclosporine-sparing therapies, including the T-cell depletion regimens, have also been implicated.
- Mortality for hyperinfection syndrome is almost 50%, and around 70% in disseminated disease.[32]

DIAGNOSIS

- Clinical syndromes include acute or chronic infection, hyperinfection syndrome, and disseminated disease.
- Acute or chronic infection includes pulmonary involvement; bacterial sepsis or bacterial meningitis from intestinal flora exposed by larval damage; or acute and severe abdominal disease with bloody diarrhea, ileus, intestinal obstruction, or hemorrhage.
- Definitive diagnosis is made by identifying larvae in clinical specimens, but ELISA and gelatin particle indirect agglutination assays are also highly sensitive and specific.
- Eosinophilia can be found during acute infection but may not be present with chronic or severe disease.

TREATMENT

- The drug of choice is **ivermectin**, with length of treatment dependent upon severity.[32]
- Albendazole can be used as an alternative treatment option.

INFECTIOUS COMPLICATIONS ASSOCIATED WITH IMMUNOMODULATING BIOLOGIC AGENTS

- Technical advancements in the last decade have led to the creation of many novel biologics that have the ability to modulate the immune system.
- **Antilymphocyte therapies**, which include the following:
  - T-lymphocyte-depleting agents, ATGs, and alemtuzumab
  - Nondepleting costimulatory blockade therapies such as the interleukin (IL)-2 receptor antagonists basiliximab and daclizumab and the cytotoxic T-lymphocyte antigen (CTLA)-4 antagonists belatacept and abatacept
  - B-cell-depleting agents such as rituximab
- **Tumor necrosis factor (TNF)-α inhibitors** that treat chronic inflammatory conditions such as rheumatoid arthritis, Crohn disease, sarcoidosis, psoriasis, and

ankylosing spondylitis. These include monoclonal antibodies such as infliximab, adalimumab, and certolizumab pegol and the soluble TNF-α receptor etanercept.

- While these agents carry fewer infectious risks than traditional nontargeted immunosuppression with corticosteroids or azathioprine, **susceptibility to infection remains elevated**, and clinicians must continue to be vigilant.

T-LYMPHOCYTE-DEPLETING AGENTS

- Anti-T-lymphocyte therapies result in a dose-dependent depletion of T cells. The administration of T-cell-depleting agents such as ATG or alemtuzumab is most commonly used to treat or prevent allograft rejection and GVHD.
- **ATGs** are polyclonal antibodies generated from immunization of rabbits or horses with human thymocytes or T cells.
  - o ATGs induce T- and B-cell depletion and interfere with dendritic cells and NK cell function. Impaired T-cell reconstitution often persists for more than 1 year after administration. During this time period, a wide array of infections can occur.
  - o Most commonly, bacterial infections including urinary tract infections, pneumonia, bloodstream infections, and surgical site infections are seen. Infections with higher order bacteria such as *Nocardia* and mycobacteria are occasionally seen.[33]
  - o Viral infections, including viruses capable of latency and reactivation, are common. CMV reactivation, for example, can be triggered by ATG activation of nuclear factor-κB (NF-κB), which subsequently binds to the promoter region of the CMV immediate-early genes, thereby promoting viral replication.[33] Likewise, EBV-associated PTLD and BK virus–induced nephropathy are encountered.
  - o Fungal infections, including *Pneumocystis, Candida, Aspergillus,* other molds, *Cryptococcus*, and endemic mycoses, occur with relative frequency.
- **Alemtuzumab** is a humanized monoclonal antibody directed against CD52, a membrane glycoprotein of T and B cells, monocytes and macrophages, and NK cells.
  - o Alemtuzumab is indicated for induction and graft rejection therapy; use leads to profound T-cell depletion that persists for at least 9 months. A wide range of infections can occur, particularly herpesvirus infections, incident viral infections, and IFIs.
  - o In the absence of appropriate antiviral prophylaxis, herpesvirus (e.g., HSV, VZV, and CMV) reactivation is common, and severe illness can occur.[33]
  - o Respiratory viral infections (e.g., influenza, parainfluenza, RSV, and adenovirus) can progress from upper tract to lower tract disease and carry significant mortality risks.
  - o Mycobacterial infections have been reported.
  - o Fungal infections including *Pneumocystis, Candida, Aspergillus,* other molds, *Cryptococcus*, and endemic mycoses occur with relative frequency.
- The profound and long-standing immunosuppression associated with ATG and alemtuzumab use necessitates anti-infective prophylaxis. **Trimethoprim-sulfamethoxazole, dapsone, or atovaquone should be provided for *Pneumocystis* prophylaxis**. Seropositivity to herpesviruses should be determined, and relevant **antiviral preventive measures should be instituted**.[33] Antifungal prophylaxis is controversial since universal azole administration can breed resistance; definitive studies are needed.

INTERLEUKIN-2 RECEPTOR ANTAGONISTS

- **Basiliximab and daclizumab** are monoclonal antibodies against CD25, part of the IL-2 receptor expressed on the surface of progenitor T and B cells and activated mature T and B cells; resting lymphocytes are spared. CD25 participates in lymphocyte activation, differentiation, and proliferation.
- These agents are used for induction and maintenance of immunosuppression, not acute graft rejection.
- Basiliximab is a chimeric murine–human monoclonal antibody with selectivity for the IL-2 receptor (IL-2R). Induction therapy results in complete IL-2R saturation and suppression for at least 4 to 6 weeks.
- Daclizumab is a humanized IL-2R antagonist. Induction therapy saturates the IL-2R on circulating lymphocytes for at least 3 months after use.
- **Clinical data suggest infectious complications are reduced compared with other induction therapies.**[33]
- In general, daclizumab and basiliximab have not been found to be associated with increased infection risk in solid organ transplant recipients.
- High infection rates were reported in allogeneic stem cell transplant recipients with steroid-refractory GVHD receiving daclizumab; however, the risk attributable to daclizumab is unknown, given the high incidence of infections in this patient population.

CYTOTOXIC T-LYMPHOCYTE ANTIGEN-4 ANTAGONISTS

- These agents (belatacept and abatacept) are fusion proteins comprised of the Fc fragments of human IgG1 connected to the extracellular domain of CTLA-4.
- They block T-cell costimulation, thereby preventing T-cell activation.
- There are very little data on these agents, but in renal transplant recipients, PTLD has been reported with belatacept use.[33]

RITUXIMAB

- Rituximab is a humanized chimeric monoclonal antibody against CD20, a transmembrane protein on pre-B and mature cells, but not plasma cells. Administration results in rapid depletion of these cells for 6 to 9 months.
- It is used in induction therapy and in the treatment of graft rejection.
- Infection risk is especially elevated among individuals receiving repeated courses of rituximab, patients treated with other immunosuppressive medications, and individuals with low serum immunoglobulin levels.
- **Reactivation of HBV** is well-documented with rituximab administration; screening for occult infection should be performed prior to starting rituximab, and either periodic monitoring for reactivation or administration of antiviral agents such as tenofovir, entecavir, or lamivudine should be done for infected patients.[34,35]
- Rituximab maintenance therapy significantly increases the risk of infection and neutropenia in patients with lymphoma and other hematologic malignancies.[34,35]
- SOT recipients receiving rituximab in combination with intense immunosuppression experience increased incidence of severe and opportunistic infections.
- Progressive multifocal leukoencephalopathy (PML) has been reported to occur among patients treated with rituximab. PML should be considered in patients who present with new cognitive or neurologic defects, and an adequate workup should be performed.[34,35]

- *Pneumocystis* pneumonia is more frequently found among patients receiving rituximab plus CHOP (i.e., cyclophosphamide, hydroxydaunorubicin, oncovin [vincristine], and prednisone) chemotherapy versus CHOP alone.[34,35]

ANTITUMOR NECROSIS-α THERAPIES

- **Infliximab** is a chimeric protein composed of human IgG1 constant region fused to the murine variable region; **adalimumab** has human IgG1 constant and variable regions; **certolizumab pegol** is a pegylated humanized Fab fragment.
- **Etanercept** is a soluble TNF-α receptor and is composed of two extracellular domains of human TNF receptor 2 fused to the Fc fragment of human IgG1 and, therefore, binds TNF as well as related cytokines.
- These agents are approved for treatment of various autoimmune diseases.
- TNF-α is required for differentiation of monocytes into macrophages, macrophage activation, and recruitment of neutrophils and macrophages for granuloma formation.
- Important differences exist between these two classes of TNF-α antagonists with regard to risk of infection, especially tuberculosis (TB).
- **Infliximab and adalimumab are associated with greater risks (two- to twelvefold) of TB, coccidioidomycosis, and histoplasmosis**, shorter time to onset of TB, and a higher proportion of disseminated or extrapulmonary TB when compared with etanercept.[36]
- **Certolizumab has TB rates up to 8.5 to 12.5 times higher than placebo.**[36]
- **Screening for latent TB infection must be done** among prospective anti-TNF-α recipients, and treatment should be instituted if warranted. Concurrent TNF-α blockade does not interfere with treatment of latent TB.
- Patients who develop TB while on anti-TNF-α therapy should have TNF blocker therapy stopped until response to anti-infectives is observed. Stopping anti-TNF-α therapy, however, can lead to a paradoxical reaction wherein patients develop worsening inflammation, as a result of immune reconstitution. This usually occurs with disseminated or extrapulmonary disease and resolves with reinstitution of the TNF blockade.[36]
- There are few studies examining the effect of TNF blockade on other types of infections, but it appears that a small increased risk of herpes zoster reactivation exists with treatment with the monoclonal antibodies but not etanercept.[36]
- Furthermore, reactivation of HBV, but not HCV, infection has been noted in case reports and may be prevented with the use of antiviral therapy.[36]

REFERENCES

1. O'Grady NP, Barie PS, Bartlett JG, et al. Guidelines for evaluation of new fever in critically ill adult patients: 2008 update from the American College of Critical Care Medicine and the Infectious Diseases Society of America. *Crit Care Med.* 2008;36:1330-1349.
2. Freifeld AG, Bow EJ, Sepkowitz KA, et al. Clinical practice guidelines for the use of antimicrobial agents in neutropenic patients with cancer: 2010 update by the Infectious Diseases Society of America. *Clin Infect Dis.* 2011;52:e56-e93.
3. Talcott JA, Finberg R, Mayer RJ, et al. The medical course of cancer patients with fever and neutropenia. Clinical identification of a low-risk subgroup at presentation. *Arch Intern Med.* 1988;148:2561-2568.

4. Tomblyn M, Chiller T, Einsele H, et al. Guidelines for preventing infectious complications among hematopoietic cell transplantation recipients: a global perspective. *Biol Blood Marrow Transplant.* 2009;15:1143-1238.

5. Boechk M. The challenge of respiratory virus infections in hematopoietic cell transplant recipients. *Br J Haematol.* 2008;143:455-467.

6. Kontoyiannis DP, Marr KA, Park BJ, et al. Prospective surveillance for invasive fungal infections in hematopoietic stem cell transplant recipients, 2001–2006: overview of the Transplant-Associated Infection Surveillance Network (TRANSNET) Database. *Clin Infect Dis.* 2010;50:1091-1100.

7. Slavin MA, Osborne B, Adams R, et al. Efficacy and safety of fluconazole prophylaxis for fungal infections after marrow transplantation—a prospective, randomized, double-blind study. *J Infect Dis.* 1995;171:1545-1552.

8. Marr KA, Seidel K, Slavin MA. Prolonged fluconazole prophylaxis is associated with persistent protection against candidiasis-related death in allogeneic marrow transplant recipients: long-term follow-up of a randomized, placebo-controlled trial. *Blood.* 2000;96:2055-2061.

9. Robenshtok E, Gafter-Gvili A, Goldberg E, et al. Antifungal prophylaxis in cancer patients after chemotherapy or hematopoietic stem-cell transplantation: systematic review and meta-analysis. *J Clin Oncol.* 2007;25:5471-5489.

10. Pfeiffer CD, Fine JP, Safdar N. Diagnosis of invasive aspergillosis using a galactomannan assay: a meta-analysis. *Clin Infect Dis.* 2006;42:1417-1427.

11. D'Haese J, Theunissen K, Vermeulen E, et al. Detection of galactomannan in bronchoalveolar lavage fluid samples of patients at risk for invasive pulmonary aspergillosis: analytical and clinical validity. *J Clin Microbiol.* 2012;50:1258-1263.

12. Walsh TJ, Anaissie EJ, Denning DW, et al. Treatment of aspergillosis: clinical practice guidelines of the Infectious Diseases Society of America. *Clin Infect Dis.* 2008;46:327-360.

13. Lanternier F, Sun HY, Ribaud P, et al. Mucormycosis in organ and stem cell transplant recipients. *Clin Infect Dis.* 2012;54:1-8.

14. Chamilos G, Marom EM, Lewis RE, et al. Predictors of pulmonary zygomycosis versus invasive pulmonary aspergillosis in patients with cancer. *Clin Infect Dis.* 2005;41:60-66.

15. Nucci M, Anaissie E. Fusarium infections in immunocompromised patients. *Clin Microbiol Rev.* 2007;20:695-704.

16. Perfect JR, Marr KA, Walsh TJ, et al. Voriconazole treatment for less-common, emerging, or refractory fungal infections. *Clin Infect Dis.* 2003;36:1122-1131.

17. Zuckerman R, Wald A; the AST Infectious Disease Community of Practice. Herpes simplex virus infections in solid organ transplant patients. *Am J Transplant.* 2009;9:S104-S107.

18. Humar A, Snydman D; the AST Infectious Disease Community of Practice. Cytomegalovirus in solid organ transplant recipients. *Am J Transplant.* 2009;9:S78-S86.

19. Allen U, Preiksaitis J; the AST Infectious Disease Community of Practice. Epstein-Barr virus in posttransplant lymphoproliferative disorder in solid organ transplant recipients. *Am J Transplant.* 2009;9:S87-S96.

20. Tsai DE, Hardy CL, Tomaszewski JE, et al. Reduction in immunosuppression as initial therapy for posttransplant lymphoproliferative disorder: analysis of prognostic variables and long-term follow-up of 42 adult patients. *Transplantation.* 2001;71:1076-1088.

21. Oertel SH, Verschuuren E, Reinke P, et al. Effect of anti-CD 20 antibody rituximab in patients with post-transplant lymphoproliferative disorder (PTLD). *Am J Transplant.* 2005;5:2901-2906.

22. González-Barca E, Domingo-Domenech E, Capote FJ, et al. Prospective phase II trial of extended treatment with rituximab in patients with B-cell post-transplant lymphoproliferative disease. *Haematologica.* 2007;92:1489-1494.

23. Pergan SA, Limaye AP; the AST Infectious Disease Community of Practice. Varicella zoster virus in solid organ transplant recipients. *Am J Transplant.* 2009;9:S108-S115.

24. Hirsch HH, Randhawa P; the AST Infectious Disease Community of Practice. BK virus in solid organ transplant recipients. *Am J Transplant.* 2009;9:S136-S146.

25. Saad ER, Bresnahan BA, Cohen EP, et al. Successful treatment of BK viremia using reduction in immunosuppression without antiviral therapy. *Transplantation.* 2008;85:850-854.

26. Kuypers DR, Bammens B, Claes K, et al. A single-centre study of adjuvant cidofovir therapy for BK virus interstitial nephritis (BKVIN) in renal allograft recipients. *J Antimicrob Chemother.* 2009;63:417-419.
27. Liu X, Ling Z, Li L, Ruan B. Invasive fungal infections in liver transplantation. *Int J Infect Dis.* 2011;15:e298-e304.
28. Singh N, Forrest G, the AST Infectious Disease Community of Practice. Cryptococcosis in solid organ transplant recipients. *Am J Transplant.* 2009;9:S192-S198.
29. Pappas PG, Silveira FP; the AST Infectious Disease Community of Practice. Candida in solid organ transplant recipients. *Am J Transplant.* 2009;9:S173-S179.
30. Ostrosky-Zeichner L, Alexander BD, Kett DH, et al. Multicenter clinical evaluation of the (1-->3) beta-D-glucan assay as an aid to diagnosis of fungal infections in humans. *Clin Infect Dis.* 2005;41:654-659.
31. Pappas PG, Kauffman CA, Andes D, et al. Clinical practice guidelines for the management of candidiasis: 2009 update by the Infectious Diseases Society of America. *Clin Infect Dis.* 2009;48:503-535.
32. Kotton CN, Lattes R; the AST Infectious Disease Community of Practice. Parasitic infections in solid organ transplant recipients. *Am J Transplant.* 2009;9:S234-S261.
33. Issa NC, Fishman JA. Infectious complications of antilymphocyte therapies in solid organ transplantation. *Clin Infect Dis.* 2009;48:772-786.
34. Gea-Banacloche JC. Rituximab-associated infections. *Semin Hematol.* 2010;47:187-198.
35. Kelesidis T, Daikos G, Boumpas D, Tsiodras S. Does rituximab increase the incidence of infectious complications? A narrative review. *Int J Infect Dis.* 2011;15:e2-e16.
36. Wallis RS. Infectious complications of tumor necrosis factor blockade. *Curr Opin Infect Dis.* 2009; 22:403-409.

Endemic Mycoses

15

Brent W. Wieland and Keith F. Woeltje

- The endemic mycoses are a group of fungi that have a specific environmental niche and are able to cause infection in healthy individuals. They are dimorphic, meaning they exist in mold form at environmental temperatures and in yeast forms (or spherules, for coccidioidomycosis) at body temperatures.
- Although the endemic mycoses may cause disease in healthy individuals, immunocompromised individuals are at greater risk of severe or disseminated disease.
- The specific pathogens covered in this chapter include *Blastomyces dermatitidis*, *Coccidioides* spp., *Histoplasma capsulatum*, *Paracoccidioides brasiliensis*, and *Sporothrix schenckii*. Infections caused by *Candida* spp., *Aspergillus* spp., *Cryptococcus* spp., dermatophytes, and invasive molds are covered in Chapters 13 and 14.

BLASTOMYCOSIS

GENERAL PRINCIPLES

- *B. dermatitidis* is a dimorphic fungus that is endemic in the Ohio and Mississippi River valleys and to a lesser extent the Missouri and Arkansas River basins. It has also been found throughout North America and even in the Mediterranean basin.
- The primary habitat is thought to be soil and decaying wood.
- The usual route of entry is via inhalation of the conidia of the mold form. Much less commonly it may be directly inoculated by skin puncture. Once inhaled, the organisms change to the yeast form and multiply by budding. Infection can then disseminate hematogenously to affect other organs or tissues.
- Infection with *B. dermatitidis* is no more common in immunocompromised hosts than in immunocompetent hosts; however, infection tends to be more severe and dissemination and central nervous system (CNS) involvement is more common.

DIAGNOSIS

Clinical Presentation

- *B. dermatitidis* **most commonly causes pneumonia**. Initial infection varies from asymptomatic infection, to self-limited pneumonia, to severe infection with potential for dissemination of disease.
- Infection may present as an atypical pneumonia that does not respond to usual antibacterial treatment.
- Pneumonia may present acutely or as a subacute or chronic pneumonia.

- Chest radiography may reveal a lobar infiltrate and frequently may have a mass-like or cavitary lesion. Atypical presentations may be confused with lung cancer, tuberculosis, or other fungal infections.
- Occasionally pneumonia may be severe and can result in adult respiratory distress syndrome.
- **Skin lesions** are the second most common manifestation of blastomycosis. Usually skin manifestations follow subclinical pulmonary infection with hematogenous dissemination. Rarely, infection may occur as a result of direct inoculation from breaks in the skin. Skin lesions are typically well-circumscribed nonpainful papules or nodules; however, appearance may vary.
- Additional manifestations of blastomycosis include osteomyelitis, septic arthritis, infections of the genitourinary tract, meningitis, or less commonly ocular infection, intercranial abscesses, and oral or laryngeal infection.

Diagnostic Testing

- Definitive diagnosis of *B. dermatitidis* is via growth of the organism in culture of a clinical specimen such as sputum, bronchoalveolar lavage (BAL), or tissue biopsy. **Cultures may take up to several weeks to grow**.
- Rapid diagnosis can be achieved by **visualizing the organism in a tissue sample or clinical specimen**. Organisms can be identified from sputum or pus samples using a KOH wet prep, Papanicolaou stain, or calcofluor white smear. The former is cheap and readily available, while the latter requires a fluorescent microscope, but may be useful to detect smaller quantities of organisms.
- Organisms can be seen in tissue samples stained with the Gomori methenamine silver (GMS) stain or periodic acid–Schiff (PAS) stain.
- *B. dermatitidis* is easily identified by its classic morphology described as **broad-based budding yeast**.
- Serologic antibody assays are available; however, they are neither sensitive nor specific. Cross-reactivity with other fungal organisms exists. Due to these features, serology is rarely useful and should not be routinely performed. Newer enzyme immunoassays are available, which have shown increased sensitivity, but clinical data are limited.
- Antigen testing is available for testing serum, urine, and sputum. In limited studies, the antigen test is more sensitive than the available serologic tests, but cross-reactivity exists with other fungal organisms, specifically *H. capsulatum*. The current role of antigen testing for blastomycosis is not well defined.

TREATMENT

- For moderately severe to severe pneumonia, severe disseminated disease, CNS disease, or disease in the immunocompromised host, initial treatment should be with a **lipid formulation of amphotericin B**, 5 mg/kg IV daily (Table 15-1).[1] Once clinically improved, oral itraconazole may be substituted.
- Less severe infection may be treated with oral **itraconazole** suspension 200 mg three times daily for 3 days, followed by once or twice daily for 6 to 12 months.
- Due to inconsistent absorption, itraconazole levels should be monitored.
- Chronic lifelong suppression may be indicated for immunocompromised hosts.
- The new azole antifungal agents posaconazole and voriconazole have activity in

TABLE 15-1	TREATMENT OF BLASTOMYCOSIS		
Manifestation	**Treatment**	**Duration**	**Notes**
Nonmeningeal disease; mild to moderate disease; immunocompetent	Itraconazole 200 tid × 3 d followed by itraconazole 200–400 mg/day PO	6–12 mo	Itraconazole levels must be followed
Acute dissemination; severe disease; immunocompromised; meningitis	Lipid formulation of amphotericin B, 3–5 mg/kg/d IV until clinically improved, then itraconazole 200 tid × 3 d followed by once or twice daily	6–12 mo	Lifelong suppression should be considered in the immunocompromised

Adapted from Chapman SW, Dismukes WE, Proia LA, et al. Clinical practice guidelines for the management of blastomycosis: 2008 update by the Infectious Diseases Society of America. *Clin Infect Dis.* 2008;46:1801-1812.

vitro and in vivo against *B. dermatitidis*, but there is less clinical experience with their use; further investigation into their use is warranted.
- The echinocandins (e.g., caspofungin, anidulafungin, and micafungin) have variable activity and should not be used for *B. dermatitidis* infection.

COCCIDIOIDOMYCOSIS

GENERAL PRINCIPLES

Epidemiology
- *Coccidioides* spp. are dimorphic fungi that are endemic to the soil in the desert southwest of the United States and northern Mexico. Two species have been identified, *Coccidioides immitis* and *Coccidioides posadasii*. They are the causative agents of "valley fever."
- *Coccidioides* spp. exist either in the mycelial form or as unique spherules. Infection occurs by inhalation of arthroconidia of the mycelial form. In the lungs, the arthroconidia transform into spherules. These spherules form internal endospores. Upon rupture, hundreds of endospores are released, each of which is capable of maturing into viable fungi.
- The incidence of infection has been rising over recent decades due to an increase in the population of cities in the U.S. southwest. There have been reports of outbreaks associated with disruption of soil, such as occurs with excavations, earthquakes, or dust storms.
- Extrapulmonary disease is caused by hematogenous dissemination. Cutaneous inoculation has been reported but is exceedingly rare.

DIAGNOSIS

Clinical Manifestations

- The majority of *Coccidioides* exposures result in subclinical disease. Some patients develop pulmonary infection indistinguishable from community-acquired pneumonia. Pneumonia may be associated with fevers, rash, headache, and migratory polyarthralgia without actual dissemination of infection.
- Diffuse pneumonia is usually seen in immunocompromised patients or due to a large infectious inoculum. Diffuse pneumonia usually indicates the presence of fungemia.
- Approximately 4% of lung infections due to *Coccidioides* result in the formation of pulmonary nodules or cavities. These frequently have no associated symptoms, but may be indistinguishable from lung cancers or other infections such as tuberculosis. Cavities may rupture, resulting in hydropneumothorax.
- Chronic fibrocavitary pneumonia is characterized by pulmonary cavitation and interstitial fibrosis. This is more common among diabetics and patients with underlying lung disease.
- Extrapulmonary or disseminated disease is rare, but is seen more frequently in certain ethnic groups. People of Filipino or African ancestry seem to have a risk of disseminated disease that is several-fold higher than the Caucasian population. Extrapulmonary disease is often not associated with any pulmonary symptom and chest radiograph may be normal. The most common sites of extrapulmonary involvement include skin, bones, and joints.
- The least common, but most severe manifestation of coccidioidomycosis is meningitis, which is almost always fatal if not treated. Complications of *Coccidioides* meningitis include CNS vasculitis and hydrocephalus.

Diagnostic Testing

- Definitive diagnosis of *Coccidioides* infection is by **growth of the organisms in culture** of tissue or body fluid. Cultures usually grow within 5 to 7 days of incubation in anaerobic conditions. Once growth is evident, samples should only be handled in an appropriate biocontainment cabinet as the mycelial form is highly contagious.
- *Coccidioides* spp. may also be identified by direct **visualization of the organisms in clinical specimen or tissue**. Human-to-human transmission has not been reported and samples can be handled without specific precautions. Sputum and respiratory secretions may be examined with KOH prep or calcofluor white smear. Organisms can be identified in tissue stained with hematoxylin and eosin (H&E), GMS, or PAS stains.
- Unlike blastomycosis, **serologic testing for *Coccidioides* spp. is sensitive and specific**. Latex agglutination tests and complement fixation are useful screening tools. Complement fixation titers higher than 1:16 may indicate disseminated disease.
- CSF findings in *Coccidioides* meningitis are similar to bacterial meningitis. Cultures of CSF are frequently negative for *Coccidioides*, so a high index of suspicion and confirmation with serologic tests are required.

TREATMENT

- Treatment of acute pulmonary infection is controversial. Some experts advocate treatment of all symptomatic patients. Others advocate watchful waiting for otherwise healthy individuals. Immunosuppressed, pregnant, severely ill patients, as well as those with underlying diabetes, heart, or lung disease should receive treatment. The initial treatment of choice is usually **amphotericin B lipid formulation** (Table 15-2).[2] After initial improvement, therapy can be continued with an oral azole antifungal for a duration of 3 to 6 months. Fluconazole, itraconazole, and ketoconazole are the approved azole antifungal agents for *Coccidioides* infection.
- Asymptomatic pulmonary nodules or cavities likely do not require treatment with antifungal medications. Patients with symptoms such as pain, superinfection, or hemoptysis may benefit from treatment, although recurrence may occur once medications are stopped. For severe symptoms or cavity rupture, surgical evaluation with thoracotomy, lobectomy, and decortication may be required.
- Chronic fibrocavitary pneumonia requires treatment with oral azole antifungal agents for a duration of at least 1 year. If not improved on azoles, amphotericin B is the alternative treatment.
- Nonmeningeal extrapulmonary infection is usually treated with itraconazole or fluconazole. Amphotericin B is an alternative for pregnant patients or for patients with infection in a critical area, such as the axial skeleton. Surgical debridement

TABLE 15-2	TREATMENT OF COCCIDIOIDOMYCOSIS		
Manifestation	**Treatment**	**Duration**	**Notes**
Nonmeningeal disease	Itraconazole 200 mg PO bid or fluconazole 400 mg PO daily	12 mo Lifelong suppression if disseminated	Follow serum titers after treatment. Rising titers suggest recurrence.
Meningitis	Fluconazole 400–800 mg IV/PO q24h. Intrathecal amphotericin B 0.1–1.5 mg qd to qwk may be added for severe meningeal disease	Chronic lifelong suppression recommended	For pulmonary nodules and asymptomatic cavitary disease, no therapy indicated. Consider surgery if cavitary disease persists >2 y, progresses >1 y, or is located near pleura
Chronic fibrocavitary pneumonia	Fluconazole 400 mg PO daily or itraconazole 200 mg PO bid	12 mo	Amphotericin B is an alternative. Goal serum itraconazole level >1 µg/mL

or drainage may be an important aspect of treatment depending upon the location of infection.

- *Coccidioides* meningitis is treated with fluconazole at doses of 400 mg or higher. Some experts propose combination with intrathecal amphotericin B for initial treatment. Fluconazole should be continued for life, if tolerated. Hydrocephalus almost always requires shunt placement for decompression.
- The newer azole antifungals, voriconazole and posaconazole, show some promise in the treatment of *Coccidioides* infection. Echinocandins are also potential treatment options, although more studies are needed.

HISTOPLASMOSIS

GENERAL PRINCIPLES

- *H. capsulatum* is a dimorphic fungus that grows in soil. The fungus is endemic to several regions of North and South America, as well as areas in Asia and Africa. In the United States, it is most commonly found in the Mississippi and Ohio River valleys. *Histoplasma* is most abundant in soil contaminated with pigeon or bat excretions, as this accelerates sporulation.
- *H. capsulatum* exists as a mold in the environment and converts into its yeast form at body temperature. Entry into the body is by inhalation of microconidia. In the alveoli, these microconidia are phagocytosed by macrophages and neutrophils where they may disseminate, first to the hilar and mediastinal lymph nodes, followed by the reticuloendothelial system.
- **Infection is extremely common in endemic areas and most residents of these areas have been exposed by the time they reach adulthood.** Disease can occur in anyone, but immunosuppressed individuals are far more likely to experience severe or disseminated forms of disease.

DIAGNOSIS

Clinical Manifestations

- **Pneumonia is the most common manifestation** of infection with *H. capsulatum*. Most commonly, patients are asymptomatic or experience mild, subclinical infection. Patients exposed to a massive inoculum of *H. capsulatum* or the immunosuppressed may experience severe or life-threatening pneumonia.
- Complications of pulmonary histoplasmosis include pericarditis, mediastinal lymphadenitis, mediastinal granuloma, mediastinal fibrosis, arthralgias, erythema nodosum, and erythema multiforme.
- Chronic pulmonary histoplasmosis and cavitary histoplasmosis also occur, most commonly in older patients with underlying chronic lung disease such as emphysema.
- **Progressive disseminated histoplasmosis** (PDH) most commonly occurs in immunosuppressed individuals, such as those with AIDS and hematologic malignancy, recipients of organ transplantation, and patients receiving antitumor necrosis factor α medications.
  - Disseminated disease occurs from hematogenous spread of the organism and can affect almost any organ.

○ Signs and symptoms may include fevers, chills, weight loss, dyspnea, abdominal pain, diarrhea, hypotension, acute respiratory distress syndrome (ARDS), anemia, thrombocytopenia, hepatosplenomegaly, elevated liver enzymes, disseminated intravascular coagulation, Addisonian crisis, or meningitis.

○ There are acute, subacute, and chronic forms of PDH, which are distinguished by decreasing severity and increasing duration of symptoms.

Diagnostic Testing

• Definitive diagnosis of *H. capsulatum* infection is by **growth of the organisms in culture of tissue or body fluid**. Cultures can take up to several weeks to grow. In disseminated disease, the organism is frequently cultured from blood or bone marrow samples.

• Rapid diagnosis can be achieved by **visualizing the organism in a tissue sample or clinical specimen**. Organisms can be identified from tissue samples using GMS or PAS fungal stains. Unlike *Blastomyces*, the organisms are not generally identified by direct examination of a sputum or BAL fluid. The organism can be detected on Wright-Giemsa stain of peripheral blood in up to 40% of PDH cases.

• Antigen detection is a useful tool in the diagnosis of histoplasmosis. Antigen concentrates in the urine and **detection of antigen in the urine** is more sensitive than in the serum. Urinary antigen is detected in over 90% of cases of PDH, but is not as sensitive for pulmonary disease.[3] Titers of urine *Histoplasma* antigen can be used to monitor treatment.

• Serology testing is available for the detection of antibodies against *H. capsulatum*. A fourfold rise in acute and convalescent antibody titers by complement fixation is useful for the retrospective diagnosis of acute pulmonary histoplasmosis. Serology testing is not as useful for the diagnosis of chronic or disseminated disease.

TREATMENT

• Treatment is not required for the vast majority of patients with **acute pulmonary histoplasmosis**. For severe disease with hypoxia, or persistent infection (symptoms >1 month duration), oral **itraconazole** 200 mg tid for 3 days followed by bid for 6 to 12 weeks may be used. Alternatively, intravenous **lipid formulation of amphotericin B** may be used for more severe infections. When itraconazole is used, it is important to check serum itraconazole levels with a goal of >1 μg/mL to ensure absorption. Treatment recommendations are summarized in Table 15-3.[4]

• Antifungal treatment is usually not indicated for hilar or mediastinal lymphadenitis, granuloma, histoplasmoma, pericarditis, or arthralgias associated with acute infection. If symptoms are present, treatment is the same as acute pulmonary histoplasmosis. Surgery may be indicated if lymphadenopathy, granuloma, or histoplasmoma causes compressive symptoms in contiguous structures.

• Mediastinal fibrosis is not likely to respond to medical treatment. Intravascular stenting may be required if the pulmonary vessels are compressed. Surgery should be approached with great caution.

• Chronic or cavitary pulmonary histoplasmosis should be treated with itraconazole 200 mg tid for 3 days followed by once or twice daily for at least 1 year. Serum itraconazole levels should be checked with a goal of >1 μg/mL to ensure absorption.

• **PDH** should be treated initially with intravenous **lipid formulation of amphotericin B** 3 to 5 mg/kg/d for 2 weeks or until clinically improved, followed by itraconazole 200 mg bid × 12 months. Itraconazole should be continued in patients

TABLE 15-3   TREATMENT OF HISTOPLASMOSIS

Manifestation	Primary therapy	Duration	Notes
Acute pulmonary disease	Treatment likely not indicated. If symptoms persist >1 mo or severe pneumonia with hypoxia, treat with itraconazole 200 mg tid for 3 d followed by bid. Lipid amphotericin B 3–5 mg/kg/d is alternative in severe disease	6–12 wk	Goal serum itraconazole level >1 μg/mL
Acute dissemination; severe disease; immuno-compromised	Lipid amphotericin B, 3–5 mg/kg/d IV for 2 wk or until clinically improved, then itraconazole 200 mg PO bid	12 mo followed by long-term suppression for immunosuppressed; if HIV/AIDS, until CD4 count >200 for 6 mo	Goal serum itraconazole level >1 μg/mL
CNS histoplasmosis	Lipid amphotericin B 5 mg/kg/d for 4–6 wk followed by itraconazole 200 mg PO 2–3× daily	Minimum 6 mo followed by lifelong suppression in the immunocompromised	Goal serum itraconazole level >1 μg/mL
Chronic or cavitary pulmonary histoplasmosis	Itraconazole 200 mg PO once or twice daily	Minimum 12 mo	Goal serum itraconazole level >1 μg/mL
Mediastinal fibrosis	Antifungal therapy likely of no benefit		

CNS, central nervous system

Adapted from Wheat LJ, Freifeld AG, Kleiman MB, et al. Clinical practice guidelines for the management of patients with histoplasmosis: 2007 update by the Infectious Diseases Society of America. *Clin Infect Dis.* 2007;45:807-825.

with HIV/AIDS until CD4 count is >200 cells/mm^3. Longer treatment or lifelong suppression should be considered in immunosuppressed patients. Serum itraconazole levels should be checked with a goal of >1 μg/mL to ensure absorption.

- **CNS histoplasmosis** should be treated with **lipid amphotericin B** 5 mg/kg/d for 4 to 6 weeks followed by itraconazole 200 mg PO bid for a minimum of 6 months. Serum itraconazole levels should be checked with a goal of >1 μg/mL to ensure absorption.
- Arthralgias and pericarditis should be treated with anti-inflammatory agents such as nonsteroidal anti-inflammatory drugs or corticosteroids.

PARACOCCIDIOIDOMYCOSIS

GENERAL PRINCIPLES

- *P. brasiliensis* is a thermally dimorphic fungus that is limited to Latin America, from Mexico to Central and South America. The highest incidence of disease is in Brazil, Venezuela, and Colombia.
- *P. brasiliensis* **disproportionately affects men over age 30** with a ratio of men to women of 15:1.
- Disease is characterized by long periods of latency. **Clinical disease can present up to 30 years after exposure**. Therefore, disease can be identified in patients who have moved away from an endemic region

DIAGNOSIS

Clinical Presentation

- Disease occurs by inhalation of microconidia into the lungs. Usually, initial disease is subclinical, with overt infection occurring later.
- After a period of latency, clinical disease may develop as **pneumonia or disseminated disease** characterized by **ulcerative lesions of the buccal, nasal, or gastrointestinal mucosa**. Lymphadenopathy is frequently detectable at diagnosis. Skin lesions are present in about a quarter of cases.
- Pneumonia from paracoccidioidomycosis is commonly diagnosed only after disease has progressed to severe, chronic lung disease with fibrosis and emphysematous changes.

Diagnostic Testing

- Definitive diagnosis of *P. brasiliensis* infection is by **growth of the organism in culture from a clinical sample**. Cultures are not always positive and can take up to 1 month to grow.
- Rapid identification can be achieved by **visualizing the organism in clinical specimens** such as sputum, pus, or tissue. A simple KOH prep has a relatively high yield. Tissues can be stained with GMS to identify the organisms. In clinical specimens, the yeast are described as small, with thick walls and with multiple buds.
- Multiple **serologic tests** are available for antibody detection. Complement fixation can be used for diagnosis as well as for follow-up of response to treatment.
- Antigen detection can be more useful in immunocompromised individuals.

TREATMENT

- The treatment of choice for paracoccidioidomycosis is an **azole antifungal such as ketoconazole, itraconazole, or voriconazole**.[5,6] Treatment should be continued for 6 to 18 months to prevent relapse.
- Treatment of severe disease may include **amphotericin B**.
- Paracoccidioidomycosis is **the only endemic mycosis that can be treated with sulfonamides**, although the duration of treatment is usually longer when using these agents.

PENICILLIOSIS

GENERAL PRINCIPLES

- *Penicillium marneffei* is a thermally dimorphic fungus found in Southeast Asia. Disease from *P. marneffei* was exceedingly rare before the advent of the HIV/AIDS epidemic.
- Disease from *P. marneffei* **should be considered in immunocompromised individuals residing in, or in visitors to, the endemic region of Southeast Asia**.
- *P. marneffei* infection occurs after inhalation of the microconidia into the lungs.
- Although much more common in immunosuppressed individuals, disease has been described in children and otherwise healthy patients.

DIAGNOSIS

Clinical Presentation
- Disease usually presents with fevers, malaise, weight loss, and skin lesions.
- Other symptoms are myriad and may include cough, hemoptysis, diarrhea, subcutaneous nodules, lymphadenopathy, and mucosal lesions.
- In HIV-infected individuals, the skin lesions may be umbilicated and confused with molluscum contagiosum.

Diagnostic Testing
- *P. marneffei* can be diagnosed by **growth of the mold in culture of clinical specimen**.
- The organism can also be identified on smear or histopathologic studies.
- Serological testing is currently in the developmental stages.

TREATMENT

- Initial treatment is usually with **amphotericin B, with or without flucytosine**, followed by treatment with an azole antifungal.[7]
- Treatment with **itraconazole and voriconazole** has also been successful. Treatment is usually continued for at least 10 weeks.
- Patients with AIDS should be continued on prophylactic antifungal agents until antiretroviral therapy has resulted in CD4 lymphocyte counts greater than 100 cells/μL.

SPOROTRICHOSIS

GENERAL PRINCIPLES

- *S. schenckii* is a dimorphic fungus that exists in its hyphal form in the environment and as an oval- or cigar-shaped yeast at body temperature. *S. schenckii* lives in soil and has been isolated throughout the world, but it is most common in tropical or subtropical regions of the Americas.
- Unlike the other endemic mycoses, sporotrichosis infection is usually introduced by **direct inoculation into the skin or soft tissue**. This usually occurs after minor trauma and contact with soil or decaying plant matter.
- Pulmonary sporotrichosis is rare, but can occur after inhalation of microconidia. Pulmonary infection is more common among individuals with underlying lung disease and alcoholics.

DIAGNOSIS

Clinical Presentation

- Sporotrichosis is **predominately a cutaneous disease**. Following inoculation, the organism spreads via lymphatic channels.
- The primary lesion develops at the site of inoculation. A papule initially develops, which later ulcerates. The ulcer may or may not be painful. After lymphatic spread, nodules may form and then ulcerate in the lymphatic distribution. Infection may rarely spread to bones and joints, most frequently in alcoholics.
- **Pneumonia** from *S. schenckii* presents with fevers, night sweats, weight loss, fatigue, and cough. Nodular and cavitary lesions may be seen on chest radiograph. Presentation may mimic that of reactivation tuberculosis.
- Multifocal extracutaneous disease and meningitis have been described, but are exceedingly rare. Disseminated disease may be more common among the severely immunocompromised, such as patients with advanced AIDS.

Diagnostic Testing

- Definitive diagnosis of sporotrichosis is by **growth in culture from clinical specimens**. Material may be obtained from aspiration of a lesion or tissue biopsy. The organism usually grows within a week at room temperature.
- Histopathologic examination is less reliable and has a lower yield. The organism may be seen as tiny oval- or cigar-shaped yeasts with multiple buds.
- Serologic testing for sporotrichosis is not available.

TREATMENT

- Treatment of cutaneous or lymphocutaneous sporotrichosis is with **itraconazole** 200 mg daily for 2 to 4 weeks after all lesions have resolved, usually a total of 3 to 6 months.[8]
- Treatment of osteoarticular sporotrichosis is with itraconazole 200 mg twice daily for 12 months. Alternatively, amphotericin B may be used for initial therapy, followed by oral itraconazole.

- For pulmonary, meningeal, and disseminated sporotrichosis, initial therapy should be with IV **amphotericin B** followed by itraconazole for at least 12 months.[8]
- Patients with AIDS or other severely immunocompromised individuals should continue prophylactic itraconazole until immune recovery.

REFERENCES

1. Chapman SW, Dismukes WE, Proia LA, et al. Clinical practice guidelines for the management of blastomycosis: 2008 update by the Infectious Diseases Society of America. *Clin Infect Dis.* 2008;46:1801-1812.
2. Galgiani JN, Ampel NM, Blair JE, et al. Coccidioidomycosis. *Clin Infect Dis.* 2005;41:1217-1223.
3. Hage CA, Ribes JA, Wengenack NL, et al. A multicenter evaluation of tests for diagnosis of histoplasmosis. *Clin Infect Dis.* 2011;53:448-454.
4. Wheat LJ, Freifeld AG, Kleiman MB, et al. Clinical practice guidelines for the management of patients with histoplasmosis: 2007 update by the Infectious Diseases Society of America. *Clin Infect Dis.* 2007;45:807-825.
5. Queiroz-Telles F, Goldani LZ, Schlamm HT, et al. An open-label comparative pilot study of oral voriconazole and itraconazole for long-term treatment of paracoccidioidomycosis. *Clin Infect Dis.* 2007;45:1462-1469.
6. Shikanai-Yasuda MA, Benard G, Higaki Y, et al. Randomized trial with itraconazole, ketoconazole and sulfadiazine in paracoccidioidomycosis. *Med Mycol.* 2002;40:411-417.
7. Kaplan JE, Benson C, Holmes KH, et al. Guidelines for prevention and treatment of opportunistic infections in HIV-infected adults and adolescents: recommendations from CDC, the National Institutes of Health, and the HIV Medicine Association of the Infectious Diseases Society of America. *MMWR Recomm Rep.* 2009;58(RR-4):1-207.
8. Kauffman CA, Bustamante B, Chapman SW, Pappas PG. Clinical practice guidelines for the management of sporotrichosis: 2007 update by the Infectious Diseases Society of America. *Clin Infect Dis.* 2007;45:1255-1265.

Zoonotic Infections and Ectoparasites

16

José E. Hagan and Steven J. Lawrence

- Zoonoses are a broad group of over 200 diseases that are acquired from nonhuman animal reservoirs; human disease can form an occasional part of the life cycle of the pathogen or may represent a dead-end event.
- Ectoparasites are arthropods or helminths that infest the skin or hair of mammals. They feed on the blood and tissue of their hosts; disease is the result of tissue necrosis or hypersensitivity to substances injected as part of the feeding process.
- Zoonotic diseases make up the majority of emerging infections caused by the intersection of human and animal habitats and arthropod vectors. This can be due to natural phenomena, as well as human behavior such as migration, rapid urbanization, and recreational or occupational activities.
- Infection in humans occurs by a variety of routes: direct contact via broken skin or animal bites, ingestion of contaminated food or water, inhalation, or via an arthropod vector. Human-to-human transmission is possible with some infections in unusual circumstances, such as blood transfusion.
- A high index of suspicion and awareness of risk factors are important in diagnosis, as laboratory diagnosis is often difficult, requiring paired sera in many cases. An appropriate history should include attention to travel and location of residence, occupation and hobbies, pets and other animal exposures, arthropod exposure, and food history. High-risk occupations and hobbies include abattoir workers, farmers, veterinarians, pet store employees, and hunters.
- Included in this category are several highly fatal and easily produced microorganisms that have the potential to be used as agents of bioterrorism and produce substantial illness in large populations via an aerosol route of exposure.
- A bioterrorism-related outbreak should be considered if an unusually large number of patients present simultaneously with a respiratory, gastrointestinal (GI), or febrile rash syndrome; if several otherwise healthy patients present with unusually severe disease; or if an unusual pathogen for the region is isolated.

ANIMAL AND HUMAN BITE WOUNDS

GENERAL PRINCIPLES

Epidemiology
- Bite wounds are common, but most do not require treatment.
- Those who do receive treatment account for 300,000 emergency room (ER) visits, 10,000 hospitalizations (1% of all admissions originating within the ER), and approximately 20 deaths annually in the United States.[1]
- Infection is the most common complication of bites.

363

Etiology

- **Dog bites** are the most common of animal bites, accounting for 80% to 90% of cases. Half of the patients are bitten on the hand. **Cat bites** are 5% to 15% of bite wound injuries, which occur on the upper extremity in approximately two-thirds of cases.
- Cellulitis occurring within 24 hours after a dog or cat bite is **likely to be secondary to *Pasteurella multocida*,** a facultative anaerobic gram-negative bacillus. This organism can cause severe infections of soft tissues, bones, and joints.[1]
- The next most common bacteria causing infection associated with both cat and dog bites are *Streptococcus, Staphylococcus, Moraxella, Corynebacterium,* and *Neisseria. Capnocytophaga* species are facultative anaerobes that are normal flora of cat and dog saliva and may cause fulminant sepsis in immunocompromised or asplenic patients.[1,2] Numerous other organisms have been found to cause infection following animal bites, and polymicrobial infection is common.
- **Humans are the third most common cause of bite wounds**. The microbiology of human bite infections is complex. **Human bites develop infection more frequently than animal bites**. Most infections are polymicrobial and involve anaerobes that are commonly β-lactamase producers and penicillin resistant. *Streptococcus viridans* is the most frequent organism reported. *Staphylococcus aureus* is reported in up to 40% of wounds and may have a particular association with a patient's attempts at self-debridement.
- Most infections after venomous **snake bites** are caused by organisms that colonize the devitalized tissue that results from local envenomation. Enteric gram-negatives must also be considered when evaluating the patient with an infection secondary to snake bite, as the prey of snakes often defecate in their mouths during ingestion.

DIAGNOSIS

Clinical Presentation

- Immediately after a bite, the primary concern is crush injury. It is more common with bites induced by animals with teeth designed for grinding (e.g., dogs). After this, the concern for infectious complications arises. Deep puncture wounds such as those caused by cat bites are more likely to cause anaerobic abscesses. Additionally, occult inoculation of deep structures such as tendon and bone is possible with this kind of bite, as bites can be significantly deeper than is apparent from the surface injury.
- Complications include **cellulitis, tenosynovitis, local abscess formation, septic arthritis, osteomyelitis, and occasionally sepsis, endocarditis, meningitis, and brain abscess**. Concerning symptoms include fever, lymphangitis, lymphadenopathy, and decreased range of motion in or tenderness over a joint, tendon, or muscle in the proximity of the bite.
- **Human bites** are best divided into two categories.
  - ○ **Occlusive bite wounds** are those that occur when the teeth are closed forcibly and break the skin. The affected anatomic site varies by gender: In men, human bites typically occur on the hand, arm, and shoulder, whereas women are more often bitten on the breast, genitals, leg, and arm. Complications arise more frequently after occlusive bites to the hand than to any other site.
  - ○ **Clenched-fist injuries** account for the remainder of human bite wounds. These result when one person hits another person in the mouth, typically causing a

break in the skin overlying the third metacarpophalangeal (MCP) joint. This is the most serious type of human bite infection, as the metacarpal joint capsule is frequently perforated and often becomes involved in a septic arthritis. Cellulitis, tendonitis, and, rarely, nerve laceration or bone fracture are other possible complications of clenched-fist injuries.

History
When evaluating a bite wound, a careful history should include an assessment of the source of the bite, rabies vaccination status of the animal and any evidence of rabid behavior, as well as the patient's vaccination history, with attention to rabies vaccination and tetanus booster status.

Physical Examination
- Consider the possibility of a human bite wound or closed fist injury when examining any injury over the MCPs, as these wounds are often minimized by patients.
- Careful examination under local anesthesia should evaluate for damage to tendon sheath, fascia, joint capsule, or bone.

Diagnostic Testing

- When patients present with an infected bite wound or any associated infectious complication, data obtained from blood and wound cultures should be used to guide the choice of antimicrobial agents.
- Plain radiographs should be obtained to evaluate for foreign body retention or bone/joint involvement, especially in the case of cat bites and other deep puncture wounds.

TREATMENT

- The treatment of bite wounds centers on aggressive local wound cleaning with povidone iodine solution, pressure irrigation with sterile saline solution, debridement of devitalized tissue, and antibiotic therapy, if appropriate.
- **Closure of open wounds should be considered carefully**. In general, bite wounds, especially cat or human bites, should be closed by secondary intention unless there is significant concern for cosmetic outcome. In particular, bite wounds should not be closed unless they are clinically uninfected, are less than 12 hours old (24 hours on the face), and are located in a cosmetically sensitive area. Wounds on the hands or feet should not be closed by primary intention.
- **Prophylactic antibiotics should be given to all patients who present with a bite that penetrates the skin of the hand, face, or genitals or is in close proximity to bone, tendon, or muscle. All clenched-fist injuries should receive prophylaxis. Cat bites generally require prophylaxis** because of the higher risk of infection due to the puncture wounds. Length of prophylactic therapy is generally 7 days. Patients should be evaluated for need for antitetanus or rabies postexposure prophylaxis.[1]

Medications

- **Empiric treatment with amoxicillin plus clavulanate** orally or ampicillin plus sulbactam IV is usually indicated for infected bite wounds or any bite that perforates the skin of the hand or is in close proximity to bone, tendon, or muscle. Moxifloxacin or doxycycline are alternatives for penicillin-allergic patients. These drugs are generally the first choice for prophylactic treatment as well.

Definitive treatment should be directed by microbiologic data. A tetanus (Td) booster should also be given if appropriate.
- **Rabies** postexposure prophylaxis is detailed below.

RABIES

GENERAL PRINCIPLES

- Rabies is rare in the United States, and in the majority of recently reported cases, no history of animal bite or high-risk exposure could be elicited.
- **Undetected bites from bats may be the most common source of infection in the United States.**[3,4]

DIAGNOSIS

- After an extremely variable incubation period of days to months, determined in part by the location of inoculation, patients may present with a prodrome of fever, headache, malaise, and personality changes lasting 1 week. This is followed by agitated delirium, hydrophobia, and seizure ("furious rabies", 80%) or a meningitis syndrome with ascending paralysis ("paralytic rabies", 20%). This is rapidly followed by coma and death.
- Cerebrospinal fluid (CSF) may show a lymphocytic pleocytosis.
- Diagnosis is best made by direct fluorescent antibody of a skin biopsy specimen taken from the nape of the neck above the hairline, polymerase chain reaction (PCR) of tissue or saliva, or serology. Sensitivity of all tests increases with time after symptom onset.

TREATMENT

- **Preexposure rabies prophylaxis** is indicated for persons at high risk, such as travelers to endemic areas, spelunkers, or animal handlers. Vaccination should include three weekly doses of 1 mL administered IM or intradermally. Booster doses should be administered at 2- to 3-year intervals if still at risk.
- **Postexposure rabies prophylaxis** should be immediately given to any person who reports a nondomestic dog bite, a scratch, bite, or contact with mucous membranes of skunks or raccoons. Additionally, prophylaxis is warranted for any person who comes in contact with a bat and cannot rule out a bite: this includes situations in which a bat is found in the room of an infant or a sleeping person. Prophylaxis is not indicated if the bat is captured and tests negative for rabies. Further consultation may be required to determine the risk of exposure. **Routine domestic dog and cat bites in the United States do not warrant immediate rabies prophylaxis unless the animal was displaying unusual behavior or signs of hydrophobia.** Instead, it is recommended that the local health department be contacted immediately; the pet is observed for 10 days for the development of signs of rabies.[4,5]
  - Soap solution and povidone iodine wound irrigation reduces the risk of rabies by 90%. Early suturing may increase the risk of rabies.
  - Prophylaxis against rabies includes both passive and active immunization.

- If the patient **has not had a rabies vaccination within the last 3 years**, rabies immune globulin (RIG) 20 IU/kg should be administered, injected as much as possible around the wound site, with the rest given IM. Rabies vaccine should be administered 1 mL in the deltoid or thigh (away from the site of RIG injection) at days 0, 3, 7, and 14. Immunocompromised patients should receive an additional dose at day 28.
- If the patient **has been previously vaccinated within the last 3 years**, booster should be administered at days 0 and 3 only, without administration of RIG.
- Rabies is uniformly fatal, with one reported exception of a patient with symptomatic rabies who received a regimen of vaccination, induced coma, and ribavirin.[6] An active clinical trial for treatment of suspected cases of symptomatic rabies may be ongoing.

TICK-BORNE ILLNESSES

- Several human diseases are transmitted or caused by ticks. Two families of tick species can transmit human disease: *Ixodidae* (hard ticks) and *Argasidae* (soft ticks). All tick species have complex life cycles that involve progression from eggs to larvae (commonly known as seed ticks) to nymphs to adults. Blood meals are required for progression from stage to stage. Larvae, nymphs, and adults can all serve as vectors of infection while feeding on mammals, including humans. The soft ticks can survive for years in the adult form without taking blood meals.
- Diagnosis can be challenging, as <50% of the patients who are diagnosed with tick-borne illnesses recall having been bitten by a tick. A high level of clinical suspicion is thus necessary for patients living in or traveling to tick-endemic areas who present with compatible symptoms during warmer months. In most cases, serologic tests must be carefully used in the correct context of clinical presentation and epidemiologic information. **Coinfection with more than one tick-borne illness can occur** and can confuse the clinical presentation.
- **Prevention of tick bites is the most important preventative intervention**. This includes wearing light-colored, long-sleeved clothing, tucking pant legs into socks, application of DEET to skin and permethrin to clothing, and performing full-body tick checks after exposure to tick-infested areas.

LYME DISEASE

GENERAL PRINCIPLES

Epidemiology

- Lyme disease is the most frequently reported vector-borne disease in the United States, with 20,000 cases yearly. Most cases are reported between May and October.
- It is caused by the spirochete ***Borrelia burgdorferi***, which is endemic in >15 states but mostly occurs in three foci in the United States: the Northeast, upper Midwest (Wisconsin and Minnesota), and the West (California and Oregon). It is also endemic in Eurasia.
- The principal vector in the United States is the deer tick *Ixodes scapularis;* in Western regions, the primary vector is the black legged tick *Ixodes pacificus*. The infection is

usually transmitted by the nymph stage, which is very small and consequently often unnoticed. In most cases, prolonged attachment (>36 h) is required for transmission of the infection. The overall risk of Lyme disease after a deer tick bite is 3.2% in areas of highest prevalence.[7,8]

DIAGNOSIS

Clinical Presentation

- Lyme disease has three distinct stages.
- In the **early localized stage**, Lyme disease manifests with a rash (erythema migrans, EM) at the site of the tick bite in 70% to 80% of patients.[9] The most common sites are the thighs, groin, and axilla. There is significant variation in the final size and shape, but classically this begins as a nontender, red macule or papule that slowly expands to a final median diameter of about 15 cm. Central clearing occurs in larger lesions, causing the stereotypic "bulls-eye" appearance. This is frequently accompanied by influenza-like symptoms and regional lymphadenopathy. Headache and meningismus can sometimes be seen. Within 3 to 4 weeks, EM spontaneously resolves (range, 1 to 14 months).
- Within weeks to months after inoculation, multiple annular EM-like skin lesions may herald **early disseminated infection**, associated with more prominent fever and systemic symptoms. Malar rash, conjunctivitis, mild hepatitis, and migratory arthralgia without arthritis may also be seen. The most commonly involved end organs include the central nervous system (CNS) and the cardiovascular system.
  - **Neuroborreliosis** occurs in 10% to 15% of untreated patients with early disseminated disease.[10] This can include cranial neuritis (most commonly unilateral or bilateral facial nerve palsy), lymphocytic meningitis, mononeuritis multiplex, motor and sensory radiculopathy, myositis, and cerebellar ataxia. These symptoms can occur in various combinations, are usually fluctuating, and may be accompanied by CSF abnormalities (lymphocytic pleocytosis and increased protein). Symptoms commonly improve within weeks to months, even in untreated patients.
  - **Cardiac involvement** occurs in 4% to 10% of untreated patients with early disseminated disease.[11] The most common abnormality is atrioventricular block (first-degree, Wenckebach, or transient complete heart block); rarely, diffuse myocardial involvement consistent with myopericarditis can occur.
- **Late persistent infection** most prominently affects the joints and CNS. Chronic skin manifestations of late Lyme disease are seen in Europe but not in the United States, except in immigrants. Late persistent symptoms develop months to years after untreated primary disease and are largely related to the immune response to borrelial surface proteins. As a result, the response to antibiotics is varied, and symptoms occasionally persist after successful eradication of the organism with antibiotic therapy.
  - **Lyme arthritis** occurs in approximately 60% of untreated patients, months after the onset of illness in the context of strong cellular and humoral immune responses to *B. burgdorferi*.[12] Patients may experience intermittent attacks of oligoarticular joint swelling, especially involving the knee. Attacks of arthritis last from a few weeks to months, with periods of remission between episodes. Joint fluid white blood cell counts (WBCs) range from 50,000 to 110,000 and are predominantly polymorphonuclear. *B. burgdorferi* PCR is positive in the synovial fluid or tissue. Chronic Lyme arthritis generally resolves spontaneously within several years; permanent joint damage is uncommon. Because of molecular mimicry with synovial

tissue proteins, a minority of patients have persistent chronic arthritis (≥1 year of continuous joint inflammation) despite an adequate course of antibiotic therapy and clearance of the organism.

○ Untreated patients may progress to develop **chronic neuroborreliosis**, causing a chronic axonal polyneuropathy, with spinal radicular pain, or distal paresthesias. Lyme encephalopathy manifests as subtle cognitive defects and problems in mood, memory, or sleep. CSF inflammation is typically absent. Unlike Lyme arthritis, chronic neurologic Lyme can persist for >10 years if not treated.

• A small subset of patients continues to have subjective symptoms—mainly musculoskeletal pain, fatigue, and cognitive difficulties—which is referred to as "**post–Lyme disease syndrome.**" These symptoms do not respond to additional or prolonged antibiotic therapy.

Diagnostic Testing

• Diagnosis of Lyme disease is difficult and relies on a combination of clinical presentation, epidemiology, and serologic studies. **While Lyme should never be diagnosed based on subjective symptoms alone, the physical finding of EM in the appropriate geographic setting is pathognomonic for early Lyme disease.** *Borrelia* can be detected by PCR from a tissue biopsy of EM. Blood, joint, and CSF cultures are very insensitive and should not be used.

• Suspected cases of late disease must be supported with serology because clinical findings are often nonspecific. Enzyme-linked immunosorbent assay (ELISA) is used to detect IgG and IgM antibodies, followed by confirmation by Western blot. Pretest probability based on clinical syndrome, epidemiologic considerations, and physical findings is an important consideration.

○ IgM begins to rise at 2 weeks after infection and declines after 2 months. However, IgM should not be used to diagnose disease beyond 1 month of symptoms because of an unacceptably high rate of false positivity.

○ IgG rises at 6 to 8 weeks after infection and persists for life. A negative IgG titer rules out late disease. Early antibiotic treatment blocks the rise of antibody titers.

• Neuroborreliosis can be specifically confirmed by reference laboratories by demonstrating a CSF Lyme antibody to serum Lyme antibody ratio of >1. In Lyme arthritis, PCR of the joint fluid is often positive. Repeat PCR for test of cure is not recommended, as *Borrelia* DNA can often be detected after successful treatment.

TREATMENT

• Tick avoidance and removal of an embedded tick within 36 hours are the most important steps in prevention.

• Postexposure prophylaxis with a single dose of doxycycline 200 mg PO is 87% effective in preventing Lyme disease after a tick bite in hyperendemic areas.[8]

Medications

• The preferred oral regimen for treatment of most stages in nonpregnant adults is **doxycycline** 100 mg PO q12h, in part because it can also treat other potentially cotransmitted infections (e.g., ehrlichiosis, anaplasmosis, or Rocky Mountain spotted fever). Alternatives include azithromycin 500 mg PO daily, amoxicillin 500 mg PO q8h, or cefuroxime 500 mg PO q12h.

• Preferred parenteral regimens include ceftriaxone 2 g IV daily or penicillin G 3 to 4 million units q4h.

Treatment of Specific Syndromes
- **Early disease** with EM: oral regimen for 14 days.
- **Isolated cranial nerve palsy** without CSF abnormality: oral regimen for 14 days.
- **Neuroborreliosis or high-degree atrioventricular block**: parenteral regimen for 14 to 28 days.
- **Late arthritis**: oral regimen for 28 days. An oral or parenteral regimen may be repeated once in the case of recurrent arthritis after completed treatment. Chronic arthritis after treatment may require anti-inflammatory medications or surgical synovectomy.
- **Post–Lyme disease syndrome.** Chronic subjective symptoms after appropriate antibiotic treatment **do not respond to further antibiotic therapy** as compared with placebo. These patients should be treated symptomatically rather than with prolonged courses of antibiotics.

SPECIAL CONSIDERATIONS

- A syndrome (STARI, southern tick-associated rash illness) resembling early Lyme disease has been associated with Lone Star tick bites (*Amblyomma americanum*), but no causative agent has been identified.
- The rash resembles EM, except the central clearing is more prominent and the major symptom is fatigue.
- Lone Star ticks are distributed across the Southern and Eastern United States. Patients with a compatible syndrome and epidemiologic exposure can be treated as per early Lyme disease recommendations.

ROCKY MOUNTAIN SPOTTED FEVER

GENERAL PRINCIPLES

- Rocky Mountain Spotted Fever (RMSF) is the most common rickettsial disease in the United States, caused by an obligate intracellular gram-negative bacterium *Rickettsia rickettsii*.
- The disease manifests itself as a diffuse vasculitis and if untreated can be fulminant and fatal.
- The endemic areas are east of the Rocky Mountains, most commonly in the Carolinas, Maryland, Oklahoma, and Virginia. The principal vectors are the dog tick (*Dermacentor variabilis*) in the eastern states and wood tick (*Dermacentor andersoni*) in the western states. Approximately 600 to 1,200 cases occur throughout the United States each year, with peak incidence in April through September, although winter cases can be seen in southern states.

DIAGNOSIS

Clinical Presentation
- The presentation can be very nonspecific and is easily mistaken for a viral syndrome, drug allergy, or meningococcemia. About 60% of cases recall a history of tick bite.[13]
- After incubation of 2 to 14 days, initial symptoms are acute, including fever, malaise, myalgia, headache, nausea, diarrhea, and abdominal pain.

- Approximately 2 to 7 days after symptom onset, the classic rash begins as red macules that initially have a centripetal distribution on the extremities, including the palms of the hands and soles of the feet. The rash then spreads centrally, and the macules can fuse to form petechiae or purpura. About 10% of cases can occur without the classic rash, particularly among African Americans and the elderly.[14,15]
- As the disease progresses, conjunctivitis, lymphadenopathy, and hepatosplenomegaly are common physical examination findings. Severe disease can progress to include aseptic meningitis, renal failure, myocarditis, acute respiratory distress syndrome, and digital ischemia. Those at higher risk for these complications include men, the elderly, alcoholics, and patients with glucose-6-phosphate dehydrogenase deficiency.

Diagnostic Testing

- The diagnosis can be made pathologically by immunofluorescence staining or PCR of skin biopsies.
- Retrospective serological diagnosis of RMSF requires demonstration of a fourfold convalescent rise in antibodies against the rickettsial organisms by latex agglutination or immunofluorescence.
- Routine laboratory findings are varied and nonspecific, including hyponatremia, elevated creatinine, elevated transaminases and bilirubin, anemia, thrombocytopenia, and coagulopathy. The peripheral WBC can vary widely.

TREATMENT

- In heavily endemic areas, there should be a low threshold for empiric treatment because of the high potential for rapid lethality. Mortality is 22% without treatment and 6% with appropriate treatment.[16]
- **The drug of choice is doxycycline**, 100 mg PO q12h for 7 days, or until 3 days after fever resolution. IV doxycycline should be used for severe disease.[16] Doxycycline has the advantage of covering unrecognized tick-borne coinfections such as ehrlichiosis, anaplasmosis, and Lyme disease. Ciprofloxacin is a second-line agent.
- Pediatric cases should be treated with doxycycline because of the potential for rapid lethality and the low likelihood of tooth staining with a 7-day course of doxycycline.
- Tetracyclines are generally contraindicated in pregnancy; however, they may be considered for severe RMSF. IV chloramphenicol (50 to 100 mg/kg/d in four divided doses) is an alternative option for severe disease, although chloramphenicol may be associated with the gray baby syndrome if given during the third trimester. Oral chloramphenicol (500 mg q6h) is not available in the United States.
- No vaccine is available, and there is no consensus on postexposure prophylaxis for RMSF after a tick bite.

HUMAN EHRLICHIOSIS: MONOCYTIC AND GRANULOCYTIC

GENERAL PRINCIPLES

- Human ehrlichiosis is a syndrome of severe multisystem disease caused by small intracellular gram-negative rods: **Human monocytic ehrlichiosis (HME)**, caused by monocyte infection with *Ehrlichia chaffeensis*, and **human granulocytic anaplasmosis (HGA)**, caused by granulocyte infection with

Anaplasma phagocytophilum. Ehrlichia ewingii is an unusual cause of ehrlichiosis usually limited to immunocompromised patients.
- Small mammals are the natural reservoir for both organisms; geographic distribution follows that of their tick vectors. *Ehrlichia chafeensis* is transmitted by *A. americanum* (Lone Star tick) and may also be occasionally transmitted by other tick vectors such as *D. variabilis* (dog tick). *A. phagocytophilum* is transmitted by the same vectors as Lyme disease: on the East Coast the deer tick (*I. scapularis*) and on the West Coast the western blacklegged tick (*I. pacificus*).

DIAGNOSIS

Clinical Presentation
- Definitive diagnosis can be difficult and may involve significant delay. The recognition of a compatible clinical syndrome in a patient from an endemic region during the spring or summer should provide the basis for initiating empiric therapy while awaiting laboratory confirmation.
- **HME and HGA are nearly identical in their clinical presentation**. Initial symptoms typically include fever, severe headache, and myalgias. Nausea and vomiting are frequently seen; abdominal pain is rare. Cough and arthralgias are also frequently seen.
- Severe disease, especially seen in patients with compromised immunity, can manifest with mental status changes, renal failure, respiratory failure, heart failure, or disseminated intravascular coagulation.
- A faint maculopapular rash can be seen in approximately 30% of HME cases but is very unusual in HGA. Petechiae are uncommon unless they are a result of thrombocytopenia or disseminated intravascular coagulation (DIC). Rash is much more common in children, occurring in approximately two-thirds of infections.[16]
- Hepatomegaly and lymphadenopathy are rare physical findings. Physical examination is otherwise unremarkable.

Diagnostic Testing
- Diagnosis is typically made by PCR of the blood or serology (a single indirect fluorescent antibody titer of >1:256 or fourfold convalescent rise after 14 days from the onset of symptoms).
- Examination of the buffy coat can allow direct observation of morulae in the cytoplasm of monocytes in HME or granulocytes in HGA, which is diagnostic. **Direct observation of morulae is common in HGA but unusual in HME**. Culture is extremely low yield.
- Routine laboratory findings are nonspecific and similar to those of other tick-borne illnesses. However, characteristic laboratory findings include **leukopenia and thrombocytopenia without anemia and mildly elevated transaminases**.
- If clinically compatible findings are present and epidemiologically appropriate, coinfection with other tick-borne illnesses should be considered and the appropriate testing performed.

TREATMENT

- **Doxycycline** 100 mg PO or IV q12h is the drug of choice for HGA and HME, even in children.[7,16,17] This also provides treatment for RMSF, which presents similarly, and could potentially be cotransmitted by a dog tick. Treatment should be continued for 10 days or at least 3 days after defervescence.

- Rifampin and chloramphenicol should be considered second line in patients who cannot receive doxycycline. In pregnancy, rifampin can be used for mild cases of ehrlichiosis; however, as for RMSF, doxycycline should still be strongly considered to treat life-threatening infections.

BABESIOSIS

GENERAL PRINCIPLES

- Infection by protozoa of the genus *Babesia* (primarily *B. microti* in the United States and *B. divergens* in Europe) is transmitted during the summer and fall months. This intraerythrocytic infection causes a febrile malaria-like syndrome with hemolysis.
- The primary tick vectors are ixodid ticks; therefore, coinfection with Lyme disease or HGA is possible and should be considered when evaluating a patient with an atypical presentation in the appropriate epidemiologic setting.

DIAGNOSIS

Clinical Presentation

- Clinical presentation of *B. microti* ranges from an asymptomatic infection to severe and life-threatening disease with high parasitemia. Incubation typically ranges from 1 to 6 weeks after inoculation by a feeding tick. *B. divergens* tends to present as fulminant life-threatening illness.
- **Mild illness** is characterized by gradual onset of high fever, fatigue, and malaise. Other associated symptoms can include headache, myalgia, arthralgia, cough, neck stiffness, nausea, vomiting, or diarrhea.
- **Severe illness** is usually seen in older patients, those with splenectomy or immuno-compromise, and patients who are coinfected with *B. burgdorferi*. Potential complications of severe disease include disseminated intravascular coagulation, acute respiratory distress syndrome, renal failure, and splenic infarction.
- Physical examination will reveal high fever in most patients, which can be intermittent or constant. Hepatosplenomegaly may be noted in some patients. Other findings such as jaundice and splinter hemorrhages are unusual except in severe cases. Rash is unusual and should prompt evaluation for Lyme coinfection.

Diagnostic Testing

- Diagnostic testing should include routine blood chemistries, blood counts, and examination of the peripheral smear. Routine urinalysis may reveal hemoglobinuria. Liver enzymes are typically elevated, as with most tick-borne illnesses.
- Common hematologic findings include variable WBC, thrombocytopenia, and evidence of hemolytic anemia, with low hematocrit, low haptoglobin, high total bilirubin, and reticulocytosis. Peripheral smear may reveal parasitemia as high as 80% in asplenic patients. Severe disease manifestations correlate with severe anemia (<10 mg/dL) and high parasitemia (>10%), although the level of parasitemia does not predict the severity of anemia.
- Laboratory confirmation is made by PCR-based detection of parasitemia or by microscopic examination of Wright- or Giemsa-stained thin blood smears by experienced

personnel. Some *Babesia* forms, especially the ring forms of *B. microti*, can appear similar in appearance to those of *Plasmodium falciparum*; attention to distinguishing features, such as the absence of schizonts and gametocytes, and the characteristic appearance of merozoite "Maltese Cross" tetrads help to confirm *Babesia*. Serology using indirect immunofluorescence with a titer ≥1:64 can be useful to confirm the diagnosis after clearance of parasitemia. Concurrent testing for Lyme disease or HGA should also be considered if the epidemiologic setting is appropriate.

TREATMENT

- Treatment is indicated for patients who have parasitemia detected by PCR or direct microscopy and should not be administered for seropositivity alone.
- Treatment of *B. microti* requires combination therapy with **atovaquone** 750 mg PO q12h plus **azithromycin** 250 mg PO daily after 500 mg to 1 g oral loading dose on day 1 (mild disease) or quinine 650 mg PO q6-8h plus clindamycin 300 to 600 mg IV q6h or 600 mg PO q8h (mild or severe disease). Immunocompromised patients with mild disease should receive atovaquone and high-dose azithromycin 500 mg to 1 g/d. *B. divergens* should be treated as for severe disease.[7]
- Mild disease should be treated for 7 to 10 days. Severe disease should be treated for 2 weeks beyond clearance of parasitemia. Refractory or relapsing disease and immunocompromised patients should be treated for at least 6 weeks, including 2 weeks beyond clearance of parasitemia.
- While treating severe disease, daily examination of hematocrit and peripheral smear should be performed to follow response to therapy.
- Severe disease with high-grade parasitemia (>10%), severe anemia (<10 mg/dL), or evidence of organ failure should be treated with partial or complete exchange transfusion.
- Symptoms that persist 3 months after completion of treatment should be evaluated by repeat PCR and thin smear examination to rule out relapsing or persistent infection. This typically occurs in asplenic or immunocompromised patients.

OTHER TICK-BORNE ILLNESSES

- **Tick-borne relapsing fever** is caused by many species of the spirochete *Borrelia* transmitted in remote areas of the western United States.
  - A 2- to 3-mm eschar develops at the site of the tick bite, and high fever begins after an incubation period of approximately 1 week. The febrile period lasts 3 to 6 days and is followed by a rapid defervescence.
  - Rash develops as the fever resolves in up to half of the patients.
  - If untreated, patients will relapse after an afebrile period of approximately 8 days, with an average of three to five relapses.
  - Diagnosis is by blood culture or by Giemsa- or Wright-stained thick and thin blood smears.
  - Treatment of mild cases is 10 days of tetracycline or erythromycin. CNS symptoms should be treated with parenteral PCN or ceftriaxone for 14 to 28 days.
- **Tick paralysis** is a noninfectious, rapidly ascending paralysis caused by a neurotoxin that affects acetylcholine transmission at the neuromuscular junction and that is secreted into the bloodstream by an actively feeding, engorged *Dermacentor* tick.

- o The illness is rapid in onset, within hours of the first tick exposure.
- o Additional symptoms include ataxia, loss of tendon reflexes, and late-stage cranial nerve and diaphragmatic muscle weakness.
- o Mortality is approximately 10%, and children are more often and more severely affected.
- o Tick paralysis is often confused with Guillain-Barré syndrome; however, the rapid course of the paralysis and the concomitant ataxia differentiate it from Guillain-Barré syndrome and other acute paralytic illnesses.
- o The potentially fatal illness can be completely cured within hours by removal of the offending tick.
- o A variant caused by *Ixodes holocyclus* in Australia should be treated with antitoxin prior to removal to avoid transient worsening of symptoms after removal.

BARTONELLOSIS

GENERAL PRINCIPLES

- Bartonellosis is caused by six species of *Bartonella*, a small fastidious intracellular Gram-negative bacillus. *Bartonella henselae* and *Bartonella quintana* cause most human diseases in the United States.
- Children are the primary risk group for **cat scratch disease** (CSD). Special populations include the homeless, who can develop louse-borne **urban trench fever**, and patients with advanced HIV, who can develop complications such as **bacillary angiomatosis and peliosis hepatis**.
- Cats are the major reservoir for *B. henselae*.
- Transmission occurs by scratches (especially by kittens) and bites, as well as bites from lice, fleas, and ticks.
- *B. quintana* is transmitted by the body louse. Humans are the primary reservoir of this pathogen, which disproportionally affects socially vulnerable populations such as the urban homeless.

DIAGNOSIS

Clinical Presentation

- *B. henselae* primarily causes CSD. This usually begins as a single or few vesicular, papular, or pustular lesions, appearing 3 to 10 days after a cat bite or scratch. This is followed by painful regional lymphadenitis (usually a single fluctuant cervical or axillary node) and mild constitutional symptoms, including fever. Hepatosplenomegaly is sometimes seen. CSD is a common cause of prolonged **fever of unknown origin** (FUO) in children. In patients with systemic disease or prolonged fever, lymphadenopathy is less common.
- *B. quintana* is the cause of "urban trench fever," an undifferentiated febrile illness with headache, body pain, and conjunctival injection. This can be a single self-limited episode or, classically, a chronic debilitating relapsing illness with episodes that last around 5 days each.
- Unusual manifestations of *Bartonella* infection may occur in 5% to 10% of cases, which can include "culture-negative" endocarditis, oculoglandular infections (especially uveitis), arthritis, and neurological syndromes.

- Endocarditis and bacteremia may be associated with conjunctival injection, maculopapular rash, lymphadenopathy, or hepatosplenomegaly. Leukocytosis and thrombocytopenia may be present. Native valves are most commonly affected.
- Neurological deficits are uncommon, but can carry significant morbidity. Encephalopathy can manifest with headache, mental status changes, seizure, and focal or generalized neurological deficits including hemiplegia and ataxia. Other unusual sequelae are retinal neuritis and transverse myelitis.
- Patients with advanced HIV can develop unusual forms of disseminated bartonellosis. **Bacillary angiomatosis** is characterized by dark violaceous subcutaneous vascular nodules, which may be numerous. These **can be easily mistaken for the lesions of Kaposi sarcoma**. Visceral, neurologic, and bone involvement of bacillary angiomatosis can be seen. Peliosis hepatis is a visceral manifestation of disseminated bartonellosis that presents as vomiting, diarrhea, hepatosplenomegaly, and fever.

Diagnostic Testing

- **PCR** of tissue is very sensitive and specific. It is of particular use on heart valve tissue to diagnose culture-negative endocarditis due to *Bartonella* species, as it is not affected by prior use of antibiotics.
- **Serology** can be very useful for diagnosis of CSD. Positive IgM ($\geq$1:16) or high IgG titer (>1:256) suggests current *Bartonella* infection. Decrease in antibody titer should follow 10 to 14 days after antibiotic treatment. An IgG titer of >1:800 suggests chronic infection.
- Cross-reactivity occurs between *Bartonella*, *Chlamydia*, and *Coxiella* species. This can lead to confusion between inguinal cat scratch and lymphogranuloma venereum, for example.
- False negatives may occur in patients who are immunocompromised.
- Culture is difficult and low yield, requiring special media and growth conditions, and can take 2 to 6 weeks. It is therefore not useful in the diagnosis of routine CSD; however, it may play a role in the diagnosis of other clinical manifestations, such as FUO, encephalitis, endocarditis, peliosis, or bacillary angiomatosis. Lysis-centrifugation (isolator) tubes can increase the yield of blood cultures. In vitro antibiotic susceptibility does not correlate well to clinical response.
- Tissue biopsy can be helpful. Lymph node biopsy can reveal granulomata with stellate necrosis, and the organism can be seen with silver stains. Bacillary angiomatosis and peliosis hepatis have characteristic patterns of blood vessel proliferation on pathological examination.

TREATMENT

- CSD is almost always self-limited; however, symptoms can last several weeks. Treatment with antibiotics is reserved for patients with extensive or painful lymphadenopathy. The drug of choice for limited CSD is **azithromycin** 500 mg PO daily on day 1 followed by 4 days of 250 mg PO daily. Alternative medications include erythromycin, doxycycline, trimethoprim–sulfamethoxazole (TMP-SMX), or a fluoroquinolone.[18]
- Disseminated CSD or trench fever requires at least 4 weeks of therapy. Peliosis hepatis and bacillary angiomatosis require 3 to 4 months of therapy. Retinitis is treated for 4 to 6 weeks with a combination of rifampin and doxycycline or azithromycin.[18]
- Endocarditis is treated with ceftriaxone and gentamicin and/or doxycycline for 6 weeks. Valve replacement is often required.[18]

BRUCELLOSIS

GENERAL PRINCIPLES

- Human brucellosis is caused by a group of small, aerobic, nonmotile, non–spore-forming, intracellular gram-negative coccobacilli belonging to the genus *Brucella*. The most important animal reservoirs are ruminant animals such as cattle and goats.
- Transmission occurs by exposure to infected animals (especially placental tissue and vaginal secretions) or consumption of contaminated dairy products.
- Human disease in the United States is typically diagnosed in Latin American migrant workers or travelers who consume **unpasteurized cheese and milk products**. **Abattoir workers, farmers, and veterinarians** are also at increased risk.
- Endemic disease is found in the Mediterranean, Middle East, and Latin American regions.

DIAGNOSIS

Clinical Presentation

- The clinical manifestations can vary significantly, from an undulant undifferentiated febrile illness to focal complications of large joints, genitourinary, neurologic, cardiac, and hepatosplenic systems.
- Subacute and chronic infection can present months to >1 year after infection without treatment.
- Manifestations can be seen in any organ system; however, most patients with acute disease report sudden or gradual onset of malaise, high fever, chills, sweats, fatigue, weakness, arthralgias, and myalgias. Symptoms of extreme fatigue and depression are classically associated with this disease, can be severe, and can persist after successful treatment.
- Physical examination may include splenomegaly and lymphadenopathy (usually axillary, cervical, and supraclavicular). Osteoarticular complaints are common, and sacroiliitis or arthritis of large weight-bearing joints is characteristic. Orchitis may also occur in infected men.

Diagnostic Testing

- Laboratory findings are nonspecific, but can include anemia, thrombocytopenia, and elevated liver enzymes. WBCs can vary significantly.
- **Culture is considered the gold standard, but is difficult** and yield decreases with duration of infection. Cultures must be observed for ≥4 weeks. Culture of bone marrow aspirate and use of lysis-centrifugation tubes can improve yield. Special laboratory precautions are required to prevent aerosol infection of laboratory workers.
- **Serology** is an insensitive method of detection; agglutination titer of >1:160 or fourfold change in titer indicates infection. ELISA is more sensitive but must be confirmed by agglutination assay. Relapse can be detected by demonstrating a rise in agglutination titer.

TREATMENT

- Treatment requires combination antibiotic therapy that can achieve good intracellular penetration. The best clinical outcomes are seen with **doxycycline** 100 mg PO q12h **plus rifampin** 600 to 900 mg PO daily for 6 weeks, **plus gentamicin** 5 mg/kg daily for 7 days.[19,20]

- TMP-SMX plus an aminoglycoside is the preferred treatment for children aged <8. Pregnant women have been successfully treated with rifampin 900 mg PO daily, as monotherapy.

TULAREMIA

GENERAL PRINCIPLES

- The small gram-negative coccobacillus *Francisella tularensis* is enzootic in rabbits and other small rodent reservoirs in the United States.
- It can be transmitted to humans in a variety of ways: contact with infected animal tissues (e.g., skinning rabbits), inhalation of aerosolized particles, contact with contaminated food or water, and bites of infected ticks, mammals, mosquitoes, or deer flies.
- Approximately 50% of cases are attributed to the bite of the *A. americanum*, *D. andersoni*, and *D. variabilis* ticks.
- Incidence is declining in the United States. Most cases are reported in the midwestern United States, particularly Oklahoma, Missouri, and Arkansas.
- Inadvertent spread can occur in the microbiology laboratory setting. Person-to-person transmission does not occur.

DIAGNOSIS

Clinical Presentation

- The clinical manifestations of tularemia depend on the route of inoculation. In general, initial systemic manifestations include fever, chills, and low back pain. Temperature-pulse dissociation is a classic finding. Multiple symptom complexes may occur simultaneously.
- **Ulceroglandular**. Regional lymphadenopathy and necrotic, painful, erythematous ulcers occur at the site of inoculation.
- **Typhoidal/systemic**. A more severe febrile illness that manifests with chills, headache, myalgias, sore throat, anorexia, nausea, vomiting, diarrhea, abdominal pain, and cough. Pulmonary involvement is common. Severe cases can progress to hyponatremia, rhabdomyolysis, renal failure, and sepsis. Lymphadenopathy and skin involvement are absent.
- **Glandular**. Tender, localized lymphadenopathy without skin or mucosal involvement.
- **Pharyngeal**. Sore throat, cervical and retropharyngeal lymphadenopathy, and, rarely, a mild pseudomembranous pharyngitis result from direct pharyngeal contact with contaminated food, water, or droplets.
- **Oculoglandular**. Painful conjunctivitis with preauricular, submandibular, or cervical lymphadenopathy secondary to conjunctival inoculation by contaminated fingers, splashes, or aerosols. Vision loss is rare.
- **GI**. Persistent, fulminant diarrhea secondary to consumption of contaminated food or water; can be fatal.
- **Pneumonic**. Lobar or diffuse pneumonia secondary to inhalation of the organism (very rare) or hematologic spread of any of the above forms, especially ulceroglandular or typhoidal.

Diagnostic Testing

- Diagnosis is usually made serologically with any one titer of >1:160 or a fourfold increase in convalescent titers.
- *F. tularensis* can be grown from a number of different specimens but is difficult to culture and is rarely seen on Gram stain. Moreover, the laboratory should be fore-warned when tularemia is suspected, as the organism can be transmitted to labora-tory workers by aerosol from actively growing cultures.

TREATMENT

- **The treatment of choice is streptomycin**, 15 mg/kg IM q12h for 10 days. Gentamicin 5 mg/kg IV daily is nearly as effective. Other aminoglycosides are also excellent therapeutic choices.[21]
- **Fluoroquinolones** are rapidly being accepted as good alternative therapies.
- Relapses are more common after treatment with tetracyclines and chloramphenicol. Cephalosporins are ineffective.
- Tularemia meningitis should be treated with an aminoglycoside plus IV chloramphenicol.

LEPTOSPIROSIS

GENERAL PRINCIPLES

- Leptospirosis is **presumed to be the most ubiquitous zoonosis worldwide**. Most disease is observed in the tropical developing world, especially in the Americas and in Asia.
- Infected animal reservoirs, particularly rats, livestock, and dogs, become infected with spirochetes of the genus *Leptospira* and shed the organism in urine, where it is highly concentrated. Direct contact with infected animals or contaminated water or soil leads to human infection.
- This disease is endemic in rural subsistence farmers and seasonal epidemics can be seen in urban slum environments as a result of flooding and poor sanitation. In the developed world, risk groups include farmers, abattoir workers, and veterinarians. Additionally, recreational exposure to contaminated water can cause sporadic or clus-tered disease. Sporadic cases are also reported in the urban poor in the United States.
- Most U.S. cases are found in Hawaii.

DIAGNOSIS

Clinical Presentation

- Clinical presentation after a 5- to 14-day incubation period ranges from subclinical or undifferentiated febrile illness to life-threatening disease with multiorgan failure. This disease is characteristically biphasic, with an early nonspecific febrile phase, followed by progression to severe late manifestations in a minority of patients.
- **Early-phase** symptoms typically begin with abrupt onset of high fever, severe myal-gias, and frontal headache. Other associated symptoms may include abdominal pain, nausea, vomiting, diarrhea, or cough.

- **Late-phase** disease occurs in 5% to 15% of patients and can include life-threatening complications such as shock, severe hemorrhage, respiratory failure, myocarditis, and severe nonoliguric renal failure associated with electrolyte wasting. **Weil disease** is a severe form of late-phase disease that is characterized by a triad of jaundice, acute renal failure, and hemorrhage. Acute respiratory distress syndrome and leptospirosis pulmonary hemorrhage syndrome, characterized by massive pulmonary hemorrhage and respiratory failure, are increasingly recognized complications. Anicteric late-phase disease is milder and self-limited, typically characterized by abrupt fever, myalgias, and intense headache with or without aseptic meningitis.
- Physical examination may reveal hepatosplenomegaly or lymphadenopathy in a minority of patients. The finding of **conjunctival suffusion** (i.e., hyperemia of the conjunctival vessels and chemosis) is a pathognomonic finding that is seen in 30% of cases.[22] Jaundice is a poor prognostic sign and should prompt observation for development of acute renal failure and hemorrhage.

Diagnostic Testing

- Routine diagnostic testing in early-phase illness is nonspecific.
- In late-phase disease, laboratory studies may reveal severe thrombocytopenia and anemia, but minimally abnormal coagulation studies, even in the case of severe hemorrhage. WBCs are variable. Chemistry studies may reveal severe renal failure, as well as hypokalemia and other electrolyte derangements. Total bilirubin is typically elevated out of proportion to serum transaminases and alkaline phosphatase.
- Laboratory confirmation is challenging, in most settings requiring a fourfold rise in **antibody titers by microagglutination testing** (MAT) **or culture of the organism** from blood, urine, or CSF. Both of these methods provide only retrospective confirmation, as culture is difficult and can take several weeks.
- A single acute-phase MAT titer of >1:100 is indicative of infection; however, it may reflect prior infection in endemic settings.
- Detection of IgM or IgA by ELISA or immunofluorescence testing can also provide supportive evidence of acute infection.
- PCR is highly sensitive, especially during early infection, but is not widely available.

TREATMENT

- Management should include aggressive supportive care and vigilance for severe complications. Severe disease requires hospitalization, and icteric leptospirosis requires intensive care unit management with cardiac monitoring. Daily or continuous dialysis is an important component of management when renal failure occurs.
- Mild leptospirosis can be treated orally with **doxycycline** 100 mg q12h or amoxicillin 500 mg q8h.[23]
- Severe leptospirosis should be treated with IV **penicillin** 1.5 million units q6h or **ceftriaxone** 1 g daily.[24] Jarisch-Herxheimer reaction can occur but is typically mild.
- Chemoprophylaxis with doxycycline offers an alternative prevention strategy for persons with exposure to high-risk areas of endemic disease.[25]

PLAGUE

GENERAL PRINCIPLES

- Plague is caused by the gram-negative bacillus *Yersinia pestis.*
- Naturally acquired plague occurs rarely in the southwestern United States after exposure to infected animals.

DIAGNOSIS

- Plague takes one of three forms:
  - **Bubonic**. Local painful lymphadenitis (bubo) and fever (15% case fatality ratio)
  - **Septicemic** disease. Can cause peripheral necrosis and DIC (i.e., "black death"). Usually from progression of bubonic disease (30% to 50% case fatality ratio)
  - **Pneumonic**. Severe pneumonia with hemoptysis preceded by initial influenza-like illness (50% case fatality ratio, nearing 100% when treatment is delayed). Pneumonic disease can be transmitted from person to person and would be expected after inhalation of aerosolized *Y. pestis*
- Diagnosis is confirmed by isolation of *Y. pestis* from blood, sputum, or CSF. Notify local infection control and public health departments immediately.

TREATMENT

- Treatment should start at first suspicion of plague because rapid initiation of antibiotics improves survival.
- Agents of choice are **streptomycin** 1 g IM q12h; **gentamicin**, 5 mg/kg IV/IM daily or a 2 mg/kg loading dose, then 1.7 mg/kg IV/IM q8h, with appropriate monitoring of drug levels; or **doxycycline**, 100 mg PO/IV bid.[26]
- Alternatives include ciprofloxacin and chloramphenicol.
- Oral therapy can be started after clinical improvement, for a total course of 10 to 14 days.
- **Postexposure prophylaxis is doxycycline**, 100 mg PO bid, or ciprofloxacin, 500 mg PO bid, for 7 days after exposure.

ANTHRAX

GENERAL PRINCIPLES

- Spores from the gram-positive *Bacillus anthracis* germinate at the site of entry into the body, causing inhalational, cutaneous, or GI anthrax.
- Natural transmission can occur through butchering and eating infected animals, usually leading to cutaneous ("Woolsorter's disease") and GI disease.

DIAGNOSIS

- Inhalational anthrax (45% case fatality rate) presents initially with influenza-like illness, GI symptoms, or both, followed by fulminant respiratory distress and multiorgan failure.

- Cutaneous anthrax is characterized by a painless black eschar with surrounding edema.
- Diagnosis of inhalational disease is suggested by a widened mediastinum without infiltrates on chest radiography and confirmed by blood culture. Cutaneous and GI disease are also diagnosed by culture of blood or tissue. Notify local infection control and public health officials immediately for confirmed cases.

TREATMENT

- Treatment with immediate antibiotic initiation on first suspicion of inhalational anthrax reduces mortality.
- Empiric therapy should be either **ciprofloxacin** 400 mg IV bid or **doxycycline** 100 mg IV q12h **plus two other antibiotics that are active against *B. anthracis*** (e.g., penicillin, clindamycin, and vancomycin).[27]
- Oral therapy with ciprofloxacin 500 mg PO bid or doxycycline 100 mg PO bid and one other active agent should be started after improvement and continued for 60 days to reduce the risk of delayed spore germination.
- Uncomplicated cutaneous anthrax can be treated with oral ciprofloxacin, 500 mg bid, or doxycycline, 100 mg bid, for the same duration.
- **Postexposure prophylaxis** consists of oral ciprofloxacin, 500 mg q12h for 60 days after exposure. Doxycycline or amoxicillin is an alternative if the strain proves susceptible.

Q FEVER

GENERAL PRINCIPLES

- Q fever is caused by *Coxiella burnetii*, an obligate intracellular gram-negative bacillus found in the feces and body fluids of infected animals, most commonly ruminant animals. Placental tissue has especially high concentrations of the organism.
- Infection is uncommon in the United States but is widespread throughout the world.
- Infection typically occurs via inhalation of infected material, such as dust contaminated by infected fluids or tissue. Risk groups include farmers, veterinarians, and abattoir workers.

DIAGNOSIS

Clinical Presentation
- **Acute Q fever** is characterized by abrupt onset of high fever, severe headache, and influenza-like symptoms. Chest pain and GI distress are also seen. Liver function abnormalities and pneumonia are common sequelae of acute Q fever. **Most acute infections will resolve spontaneously**.
- **Chronic Q fever** can occur long after the initial infection, often years. *C. burnetii* endocarditis is a cause of **"culture-negative" endocarditis** and most commonly affects patients with prosthetic or otherwise abnormal heart valves or patients with

compromised immunity. Other forms of chronic Q fever include pneumonia, hepatitis, chronic fatigue, and hepatitis. **Chronic Q fever carries high morbidity and mortality**.

Diagnostic Testing

- Diagnosis is made by **serology** to detect one of two antigenic phases. Antibodies directed against phase II antigens appear rapidly and high antibody levels indicate acute Q fever. Phase I antibodies indicate continuous exposure to *C. burnetii* antigens and are highest in chronic Q fever. Both phase I and phase II antibodies persist long after the initial infection.
- Notify local infection control and the public health department immediately for confirmed cases.

TREATMENT

- Treatment for acute Q fever with **doxycycline** 100 mg PO q12h for 2 to 3 weeks is most effective if initiated within the first days of illness. Ciprofloxacin and a macrolide with or without rifampin are alternatives. Treatment should be restarted if symptoms relapse.[28]
- Chronic Q fever requires prolonged therapy with **doxycycline and chloroquine** 200 mg PO q8h for at least 18 months, until phase I IgG titer falls to below 1:200. This may require 3 years of therapy or more.[29]

SCABIES

GENERAL PRINCIPLES

- Scabies is caused by the human mite *Sarcoptes scabiei*.
- Symptoms are caused by host hypersensitivity to the eggs and excreta of gravid females creating linear burrows into the skin.
- Transmission of scabies results from close person-to-person contact. The mite does not survive >24 hours without a host; therefore, transmission by sharing contaminated clothing or bedding does occur but is not efficient.
- Although scabies is more common in persons living in crowded conditions and poverty, it is not limited to this population; outbreaks occur in households, hospitals, nursing homes, and day care centers.

DIAGNOSIS

- The clinical presentation is characterized by an **intensely pruritic rash**. Small excoriated papular lesions are typically found in the finger webs, wrists, elbows, and along skin folds. **Burrows may be noted, particularly in the finger webs**. Pruritus is typically worse at night or after a hot shower or bath. In the immunocompromised, a severe form called "Norwegian scabies" can occur.
- Diagnosis requires identification of the organisms or their eggs and fecal pellets. This is best accomplished by placing a drop of mineral oil on a lesion, scraping it with a scalpel, and examining the specimen under a microscope. Burrows may be

identified by applying dark ink from a felt-tip or fountain pen. After cleansing with an alcohol pad, the ink may be partially retained in the burrows.

TREATMENT

- **Treatment** of choice for all patients older than 2 months is **5% permethrin cream**, which should be applied from the chin to the toes and washed off after 8 hours. This should be repeated within 1 to 2 weeks.[30]
- Washing all bedding and potentially infected clothes in hot water can prevent reinfection.
- A single dose of **ivermectin** 200 μg/kg PO is also effective and may be helpful in refractory infestations or for immunocompromised patients with severe manifestations. A second dose can be repeated in 10 days.[30]

PEDICULOSIS

GENERAL PRINCIPLES

- Pediculosis is the term given to infestation by lice of the genus *Pediculus* or *Phthirus*. There are three species in these two genera that are specifically important: *Pediculus humanus corporis* (the body louse), *Pediculus humanus capitis* (the head louse), and *Phthirus pubis* (the crab louse).
- Lice are wingless insects with three pairs of legs, each terminating with a curved claw. Lice grasp the clothes or hairs of their hosts and obtain a blood meal. The bite is painless; symptoms are caused by hypersensitivity to the insects' saliva. Sensitization and development of symptoms occur approximately 1 month after the initial infestation.
- Transmission of lice also results from close person-to-person contact; certain populations are more affected by each of these organisms (e.g., body lice in those with poor hygiene, head lice in school children, and pubic lice in sexually active individuals).

DIAGNOSIS

- The clinical presentation depends on the site of infection; on the head, it is characterized by localized pruritus and crusted lesions. Body lice and pubic lice result in discrete areas of erythematous or bluish maculopapular rash.
- Diagnosis of pediculosis is made by identifying the eggs, or "nits," at the sites of the lesions. The use of a magnifying glass may be helpful in differentiating the nits from other artifacts, such as dandruff, dried hair spray, or casts of sebum from the hair follicle.

TREATMENT

- The treatment of choice for pediculosis is **1% permethrin cream** to affected areas. Alternative therapies include 0.5% malathion and 1% lindane; however, these agents are less effective and more toxic.[30]

- Oral **ivermectin** can also be used for severe or refractory cases as for scabies (see above).[30]
- Combs and brushes should be sterilized with hot water (65°C [149°F]) for 5 to 15 minutes. Clothing and bedding should also be sterilized with hot water and drying (54°C [129.2°F]) for 30 to 45 minutes.

REFERENCES

1. Goldstein EJC. Bite wounds and infection. *Clin Infect Dis.* 1992;14:633-638.
2. Abrahamian FM, Goldstein EJ. Microbiology of animal bite wound infections. *Clin Microbiol Rev.* 2011;24:231-246.
3. Noah DL, Drenzek CL, Smith JS, et al. Epidemiology of human rabies in the United States, 1980 to 1996. *Ann Intern Med.* 1998;128:922-930.
4. Manning SE, Rupprecht CE, Fishbein D, et al. Human rabies prevention—United States, 2008: recommendations of the Advisory Committee on Immunization Practices. *MMWR Recomm Rep.* 2008;57(RR-3):1-28.
5. Rupprecht CE, Briggs D, Brown CM, et al. Use of a reduced (4-dose) vaccine schedule for postexposure prophylaxis to prevent human rabies: recommendations of the Advisory Committee on Immunization Practices. *MMWR Recomm Rep.* 2010;59(rRR-2):1-9.
6. Willoughby RE, Tieves KS, Hoffman GM, et al. Survival after treatment of rabies with induction of coma. *N Engl J Med.* 2005;352:2508-2514.
7. Wormser GP, Dattwyler RJ, Shapiro ED, et al. The clinical assessment, treatment, and prevention of Lyme disease, human granulocytic anaplasmosis, and babesiosis: clinical practice guidelines by the Infectious Diseases Society of America. *Clin Infect Dis.* 2006;43:1089-1134.
8. Nadelman RB, Nowakowski J, Fish D, et al. Prophylaxis with single-dose doxycycline for the prevention of Lyme disease after an *Ixodes scapularis* tick bite. *N Engl J Med.* 2001;345:79-84.
9. Steere AC, Sikand VK. The presenting manifestations of Lyme disease and outcomes of treatment. *N Engl J Med.* 2003;348:2472-2474.
10. Halperin JJ. Nervous system Lyme disease. *Infect Dis Clin North Am.* 2008;22:261-274.
11. Fish AF, Pride YB, Pinto DS. Lyme carditis. *Infect Dis Clin North Am.* 2008;22:275-288.
12. Steere AC, Schoen RT, Taylor E. The clinical evolution of Lyme arthritis. *Ann Intern Med.* 1987;107:725-731.
13. Dalton MJ, Clarke MJ, Holman RC, et al. National surveillance for Rocky Mountain spotted fever, 1981-1992: epidemiologic summary and evaluation of risk factors for fatal outcome. *Am J Trop Med Hyg.* 1995;52:405-413.
14. Helmick CG, Bernard KW, D'Angelo LJ. Rocky Mountain spotted fever: clinical, laboratory, and epidemiological features of 262 cases. *J Infect Dis.* 1984;150:480-488.
15. Sexton DJ, Corey GR. Rocky Mountain "spotless" and "almost spotless" fever: a wolf in sheep's clothing. *Clin Infect Dis.* 1992;15:439-448.
16. Chapman AS, Bakken JS, Folk SM, et al. Diagnosis and management of tickborne rickettsial diseases: Rocky Mountain spotted fever, ehrlichiosis, and anaplasmosis—United States: a practical guide for physicians and other health-care and public health professionals. *MMWR Recomm Rep.* 2006;55(RR-4):1-27.
17. Thomas RJ, Dumler JS, Carlyon JA. Current management of human granulocytic anaplasmosis, human monocytic ehrlichiosis and *Ehrlichia ewingii* ehrlichiosis. *Expert Rev Anti Infect Ther.* 2009;7:709-722.
18. Rolain JM, Brouqui P, Koehler JE, et al. Recommendations for treatment of human infections caused by *Bartonella* species. *Antimicrob Agents Chemother.* 2004;48:1921-1933.
19. Franco MP, Mulder M, Gilman RH, Smits HL. Human brucellosis. *Lancet Infect Dis.* 2007;7:775-786.
20. Skalsky K, Yahav D, Bishara J, et al. Treatment of human brucellosis: systematic review and meta-analysis of randomised controlled trials. *BMJ.* 2008;336:701-704.

21. Nigrovic LE, Wingerter SL. Tularemia. *Infect Dis Clin North Am.* 2008;22:489-504.

22. Katz AR, Ansdell VE, Effler PV, et al. Assessment of the clinical presentation and treatment of 353 cases of laboratory-confirmed leptospirosis in Hawaii, 1974-1998. *Clin Infect Dis.* 2001;33:1834-1841.

23. McClain JB, Ballou WR, Harrison SM, Steinweg DL. Doxycycline therapy for leptospirosis. *Ann Intern Med.* 1984;100:696-698.

24. Suputtamongkol Y, Niwattayakul K, Suttinont C, et al. An open, randomized, controlled trial of penicillin, doxycycline, and cefotaxime for patients with severe leptospirosis. *Clin Infect Dis.* 2004;39:1417-1424.

25. Sehgal SC, Sugunan AP, Murhekar MV, et al. Randomized controlled trial of doxycycline prophylaxis against leptospirosis in an endemic area. *Int J Antimicrob Agents.* 2000;13:249-255.

26. Inglesby TV, Dennis DT, Henderson DA, et al. Plague as a biological weapon: medical and public health management. *JAMA.* 2000;283:2281-2290.

27. Inglesby TV, Henderson DA, Bartlett JG, et al. Anthrax as a biological weapon: medical and public health management. *JAMA.* 1999;281:1735-1745.

28. Gikas A, Kokkini S, Tsioutis C. Q fever: clinical manifestations and treatment. *Expert Rev Anti Infect Ther.* 2010;8:529-539.

29. Karakousis PC, Trucksis M, Dumler JS. Chronic Q fever in the United States. *J Clin Microbiol.* 2006;44:2283-2287.

30. Diaz JH. The epidemiology, diagnosis, management, and prevention of ectoparasitic diseases in travelers. *J Travel Med.* 2006;13:100-111.

Protozoal Infection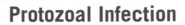

Luis A. Marcos and F. Matthew Kuhlmann

- Protozoa are unicellular organisms infecting billions of people globally. Most cases occur in developing countries while travel and migration lead to cases anywhere in the world.
- Table 17-1 provides a brief description of most protozoal infections.

TABLE 17-1	SUMMARY OF PROTOZOA INFECTIONS		
Protozoa (disease)	**Clinical manifestations**	**Diagnosis**	**Treatment**
	Vector-borne protozoa		
Plasmodium spp. (malaria)	Fever, prostration, anemia	Blood smear, rapid antigen testing	See text
Toxoplasma gondii (toxoplasmosis)	Fever, lymph-adenopathy, severe manifestations in immunocompromised or pregnant patients	Direct parasite detection, serology, or PCR	See text
Babesia spp. (babesiosis)	Fever, anemia, malaise	Direct detection of parasite on blood smear	See text
Leishmania spp. (cutaneous or mucocutaneous leishmaniasis)	Ulcer with heaped border	Direct parasite detection on skin biopsy	See text
Leishmania spp. (visceral leishmaniasis)	Fever, hepatosplenomegaly	Direct parasite detection or serology	See text
Trypanosoma cruzi (Chagas' disease)	Acute cellulitis followed by cardiomegaly, megacolon, or megaesophagus years later	Direct detection of parasites in acute phases, serology in chronic phases	See text
Trypanosoma brucei rhodesiense (East African sleeping sickness)	Acute onset of fever, lymphadenopathy, and mental status changes	Direct detection of parasites in blood or CSF	Suramin for acute disease.

(continued)

TABLE 17-5 (CONTINUED)

			Melarsoprol for CNS disease
Trypanosoma brucei gambiense (West African sleeping sickness)	Fevers, lymphadenopathy, and pruritus in the acute stage Progressive mental status changes over months to years (chronic)	Direct detection of parasites in blood or CSF	Pentamidine for acute disease Eflornithine or melarsoprol for CNS disease
Free-living ameba			
Acanthamoeba spp.	Granulomatous amebic encephalitis, keratitis	Biopsy and/or culture	Propamidine and surgical debridement (keratitis)
Balamuthia mandrillaris	Meningoencephalitis	Biopsy or postmortem	Amphotericin
Naegleria fowleri	Meningoencephalitis	CSF analysis for trophozoites	Amphotericin and rifampin or azoles
Intestinal protozoa			
Entamoeba spp. (amebiasis)	Bloody diarrhea, abdominal pain, liver abscess	Microscopic stool examination Antibody detection by EIA	See text
Endolimax nana	Nonpathogenic	Stool microscopy	None
Iodamoeba bütschlii	Nonpathogenic swine protozoa	Stool microscopy	None
Blastocystis hominis	Controversial pathogen. May cause bloating, diarrhea, abdominal pain	Microscopic stool examination	Controversial, metronidazole or TMP-SMX may be tried
Giardia lamblia (synonymous with *Giardia intestinalis*) (giardiasis)	Bloating, diarrhea, abdominal pain, malabsorption, nausea	Microscopic stool examination Fecal immunoassays	See text

Dientamoeba fragilis	Diarrhea, abdominal pain	Stool microscopy	Iodoquinol
Cryptosporidium spp. (cryptosporidiosis)	Watery diarrhea and abdominal pain, especially immunocompromised (e.g., AIDS)	Microscopic stool examination using acid-fast staining, smaller; DFA; enzyme immunoassays to detect antigens in stools	Self-limiting; nitazoxanide in AIDS
Cyclospora cayetanensis	Chronic diarrhea, abdominal pain, bloating	Stool microscopy with acid-fast staining, larger	TMP-SMX
Isospora belli	Watery diarrhea and abdominal pain (life-threatening in AIDS)	Microscopic stool examination using acid-fast staining, ovoid	TMP-SMX
Enterocytozoon hieneusi	Chronic, watery diarrhea and abdominal pain, especially in HIV	Microscopic stool examination, electron microscopy of small bowel biopsy	Albendazole
Encephalitozoon spp.	Rare cause of persistent diarrhea	Stool microscopy	Albendazole

PCR, polymerase chain reaction; CSF, cerebrospinal fluid; CNS, central nervous system; EIA, enzyme immunoassay; TMP-SMX, trimethoprim–sulfamethoxazole; DFA, direct fluorescent antibody.

MALARIA

GENERAL PRINCIPLES

Epidemiology

- An estimated 150 to 275 million infections occurred worldwide, resulting in 537,000 to 907,000 deaths in 2010.[1] Most deaths occur in children living in sub-Saharan Africa.
- Each species inhabits distinct geographical regions, each with unique clinical characteristics and treatments.
- A detailed map of malarious regions can be found in the website of the CDC (www.cdc.gov/travel, last accessed May 15, 2012) or in their travel reference called the "Yellow Book."

Etiology

- Five species of malaria can cause disease in humans:
  - *Plasmodium falciparum*: Worldwide distribution, high mortality
  - *Plasmodium vivax*: Most common in Asia, Central and South America, Oceania and India
  - *Plasmodium ovale*: Mainly in West Africa
  - *Plasmodium malariae*: Rare cause of disease, mostly in Africa
  - *Plasmodium knowlesi*: Simian malaria rarely causing infections in Southeast Asia

Pathophysiology

- Transmission is via bites from female *Anopheles* mosquitoes. Less common means include blood transfusion, transplantation, shared needle use, or congenital transmission.
- Life cycles
  - Sexual stages (sporogony) occur in the mosquito.
  - Asexual stages (schizogony) occur in the mammalian host as briefly described below:
    - Sporozoites are injected by the mosquito and infect hepatocytes. After 1 to 3 weeks, hepatocytes rupture, releasing merozoites into the bloodstream, which invade red blood cells (RBCs). Dormant liver stages (hypnozoites) form with *P. ovale* and *P. vivax* infections.
    - Intraerythrocytic ring forms replicate, releasing additional merozoites and causing RBC lysis.
    - Merozoites infect additional RBCs or are taken up by biting mosquitoes to complete the life cycle.
- Host consequences
  - RBC lysis generates many symptoms.
    - Cytokines, induced by released glycolipids, cause many symptoms including fever.
    - RBC lysis is cyclical, leading to classical descriptions of quotidian fever (occurring daily as with *P. falciparum*) or tertian fever (every other day for *P. vivax* and *P. ovale*).
  - RBC lysis and decreased production contribute to profound anemia.
  - Microvascular sequestration causes renal failure, tissue hypoxia, and central nervous system (CNS) pathology.
  - Severity of symptoms depends in part on the type of RBC infected.
    - *P. falciparum*: Infects any RBC, causes severe infection
    - *P. vivax*: Reticulocytes only, less severe infection
    - *P. malariae*: Mature RBCs, mild chronic infection

Risk Factors

- Indigenous patients at risk for severe malaria include pregnant women and nonimmune children; sickle cell disease or thalassemia may be protective.
- Travelers at high risk for severe malaria are pregnant, older than 50, or indigenous persons returning home.

Prevention

- Prevention of malaria depends upon types of exposures and risk of acquiring disease.
- For patients living in endemic regions:
  - Insecticide-impregnated bed nets prevent malaria and other vector-borne diseases.
  - Intermittent treatment during pregnancy reduces the risk of placental disease.

- For travelers to endemic regions:
  - Risk appropriate chemoprophylaxis is indicated.
  - Wearing protective clothing should be encouraged.
  - Use of bed nets when accommodations place one at risk.
  - Insect repellents; several are available and beyond the scope of this discussion.

DIAGNOSIS

Clinical Presentation

History
- Malaria presents with nonspecific symptoms including fever and prostration.
- Any patient returning from or residing in endemic regions should be evaluated for malaria.
- The type of prophylaxis and adherence to the prophylactic regimen help determine risk of malaria.
- Usual presentation is 1 to 2 weeks after exposure; longer incubation times or recrudescence (*P. vivax* or *P. ovale*) can occur.
- Factors indicative of severe malaria include mental status changes, changes in urine color, or palpitations.

Physical Examination
- Pallor, jaundice, tachycardia, systolic murmurs, or shortness of breath may indicate hemolytic anemia.
- Signs of severe malaria include dark urine, pulmonary rales, disorientation, altered mental status, focal neurological deficits, or papilledema.

Diagnostic Criteria

Severe or complicated malaria includes any of the following:
- Cerebral malaria with coma, encephalopathy, seizures, focal neurological deficits, or altered consciousness
- Acute renal failure with acute tubular necrosis or macroscopic hemoglobinuria (blackwater fever)
- Acute pulmonary edema with acute respiratory distress syndrome (ARDS), which may occur up to 2 to 3 days after starting therapy
- Hypoglycemia
- Severe anemia (hemoglobin <5 g/dL)
- Spontaneous bleeding, thrombocytopenia (<100,000/mm^3)
- Metabolic acidosis
- Shock
- Hyperparasitemia (>5%)

Differential Diagnosis

The differential is quite broad; other common illnesses include dengue fever, leptospirosis, meningococcal sepsis, or typhoid fever.

Diagnostic Testing

- Complete blood counts and comprehensive metabolic panels should be obtained.
- **Blood thick and thin smears are the gold standard**; obtain multiple samples, especially during fever.

- **Intraerythrocytic ring forms or schizonts** on microscopy confirm the diagnosis and can identify the plasmodial species.
- Rapid diagnostic tests identify plasmodial antigens in the blood (FDA approved), which may soon replace microscopy.[1,2]
  - A positive test is highly specific and can identify *P. falciparum*.
  - A false negative may occur with low parasitemia and the test may need repeating.
- Polymerase chain reaction (PCR) identifies malaria to a species level but is not yet available.
- A lumbar puncture may be needed to rule out meningoencephalitis; spinal fluid in cerebral malaria is benign, usually with elevated protein.

TREATMENT

- Therapy must be initiated as soon as possible.
- Infectious disease consultation should be considered in severe malaria.

Medications

- Treatment of uncomplicated malaria due to *P. falciparum*.[2,3]
  - For chloroquine-sensitive areas: Chloroquine 600 mg base orally followed by 300 mg base at 6, 24, and 48 hours.
  - For chloroquine-resistant areas (oral treatment):
    - Atovaquone–proguanil (250 mg atovaquone/100 mg proguanil) four tablets daily for 3 days
    - Artemether–lumefantrine (20 mg artemether, 120 mg lumefantrine), for weight ≥35 kg, four tablets at 0 and 8 hours followed by four tablets twice daily for 2 days
    - Quinine (542 mg base) three times daily for 3 to 7 days PLUS one of the following:
      - Tetracycline 250 mg four times daily for 7 days
      - Doxycycline 100 mg twice daily for 7 days
      - Clindamycin 20 mg base/kg/d divided into three doses daily × 7 days sulfadoxine–pyrimethamine (25/1.25 mg base/kg) one dose
      - Side effects of quinine are tinnitus, hearing loss, confusion, other CNS effects, thrombocytopenia, hypotension, and cardiotoxicity
    - As a third-line agent, mefloquine can be used in combination with artesunate or doxycycline
- Malaria due to *P. vivax* or *P. ovale*: Chloroquine or atovaquone–proguanil PLUS primaquine 30 mg base daily for 14 days in patients with normal glucose-6-phosphate dehydrogenase (screen before treatment).
- Complicated malaria:
  - Quinidine gluconate 6.25 mg base/kg loading dose IV over 1 to 2 hours, then 0.0125 mg base/kg/min continuous infusion for at least 24 hours, plus doxycycline, tetracycline, or clindamycin as above.
  - Artesunate 2.4 mg/kg at 0, 12, and 24 hours followed by daily treatment.
- Prophylaxis in travelers: Chemoprophylaxis for malaria depends on the presence of chloroquine resistance (more details can be found in the CDC website). In general, the drugs used for prophylaxis are as follows:
  - Atovaquone/proguanil to start 1 to 2 days before traveling and 7 days after returning. Side effects are uncommon, usually mild gastrointestinal (GI) discomfort.

Contraindicated in women who are pregnant or breast-feeding a child weighing less than 5 kg.
○ Chloroquine 300 mg once weekly, to start 1 week before traveling and to continue 4 weeks after returning. Used in pregnancy but only in chloroquine-sensitive malaria.
○ Doxycycline 100 mg PO daily, started 1 day before travel and continued for 4 weeks after returning. Photosensitivity may limit use. Cannot be used in pregnant women and children less than age 8.
○ Mefloquine 250 mg PO weekly, started 2 weeks prior and to continue 4 weeks after traveling. Use with caution in people with psychiatric and seizure disorders.

REFERRAL

The CDC Malaria Hotline can be reached at (770) 488-7788 and http://www.cdc.gov/MALARIA/ (last accessed May 16, 2012).

BABESIOSIS

GENERAL PRINCIPLES

Epidemiology
- Babesiosis is a zoonotic tick-borne infection caused by *Babesia* spp., which infects RBCs.
- Babesiosis occurs both in Europe and in North America; European infections tend to be more severe.
- North American infections:
  ○ Are caused by *Babesia microti* and is frequently asymptomatic
  ○ Shares *Ixodes* tick vector with *Borrelia burgdorferi*, making coinfections common

Pathophysiology
- Transmission occurs after *Ixodes* tick bites, rarely through blood transfusions or congenital transmission.
- Massive RBC lysis leads to hemolytic anemia resulting in hyperbilirubinemia, hemoglobinuria, and acute tubular necrosis.
- Thrombocytopenia, pulmonary edema, and ARDS can also be seen.
- Severe disease occurs in the elderly, immunocompromised, or asplenic patients.
- The only effective means of prevention is tick avoidance by using insect repellants and covering exposed areas of skin.

DIAGNOSIS

Clinical Presentation
History
- Fever, chills, sweats, headache, body aches, loss of appetite, nausea, or fatigue occur 1 to 3 weeks after exposure.
- A history of tick bite in an endemic region is helpful but not necessary.

- A history of splenectomy or immunodeficiency suggests the potential for severe infection.

Physical Examination
- Fever, hepatomegaly, splenomegaly, and evidence of anemia are potential findings.
- In severe disease, findings of acute respiratory distress or congestive heart failure may be present.

Differential Diagnosis
- Malaria, leptospirosis, viral hepatitis, and other tick-borne diseases should be considered.
- Intraerythrocytic *Babesia* organisms are frequently confused with *P. falciparum*.

Diagnostic Testing
- Complete blood cell count may reveal mild to severe anemia, thrombocytopenia, atypical lymphocytes, leukopenia, or leukocytosis.
- Haptoglobin and reticulocyte count may be decreased.
- Transaminitis and indirect hyperbilirubinemia may be present.
- Hemoglobinuria or proteinuria may be present.
- The gold standard for diagnosis is **identification of intraerythrocytic parasites on blood smear**.
  ○ The percent parasitemia can be as high as 80% in splenectomized patients but may not correlate directly with disease severity.
  ○ Classically, "Maltese cross" forms are identified but may be absent on microscopy.
  ○ Serodiagnosis using indirect fluorescence antibody tests (IFATs); titers above 1:64 are usually diagnostic.

TREATMENT

- *B. microti* infections tend to be subclinical and treatment may not be indicated.
- In cases of prolonged symptoms, **atovaquone** (750 mg orally twice daily for 7 to 10 days) **PLUS azithromycin** (500 mg orally on day 1 followed by 250 mg daily for 6 days) OR **quinine** (650 mg orally three times daily for 7 days) **PLUS clindamycin** (600 mg orally three times daily for 7 days) may be given.[4]
- In severe cases, exchange transfusion may be indicated.

TOXOPLASMOSIS

GENERAL PRINCIPLES

- *Toxoplasma gondii* causes toxoplasmosis.
- Toxoplasmosis is usually a self-limiting disease, but reactivates or disseminates in HIV-positive patients or organ transplant recipients.
- Primary infection in nonimmune mothers causes severe congenital disease of the fetus.

Epidemiology
- Toxoplasmosis occurs worldwide, especially where raw or undercooked meats are consumed.

- In the United States, approximately 1% of domestic cats shed *Toxoplasma* cysts while 11% to 31% of humans are seropositive.

Pathophysiology

- Transmission occurs by ingesting cysts in undercooked meat, ingesting food contaminated with sporocysts, congenitally, or through transplantation.
- Life cycle:
  ○ Sporocysts are shed in cat feces.
  ○ Tachyzoites are actively replicating parasites forming cysts in host tissues, dormant stages are referred to as bradyzoites.

Prevention

- Cook food to appropriate temperatures.
- Wash fruits and vegetables before eating.
- Freeze meat for several days before cooking.
- Do not feed cats raw or undercooked meat.
- Wear gloves when gardening or during contact with soil.
- Pregnant women should avoid changing litter boxes as well as adopting kittens

DIAGNOSIS

Clinical Presentation

- Primary infection in immunocompetent hosts is usually asymptomatic. Some patients may note fever, fatigue, or lymphadenopathy. Symptoms of primary infection are similar to infectious mononucleosis.[5]
- Reactivation in AIDS patients presents as fever, headache, worsening mental status, and focal neurological deficits in patients with CD4 <100 cells/mL. As disease progresses, other organ systems may be involved.
- Ocular toxoplasmosis presents as a sudden blurring of vision.
- The risk of congenital infection increases with gestational age but since infection is asymptomatic, most disease goes unnoticed until after delivery. Severe manifestations occur in <10% of maternal infections and include hydrocephalus, mental retardation, and even death. Infected infants may develop ocular disease later in life.

Differential Diagnosis

CNS reactivation can be confused with brain abscess, metastasis, lymphoma, and tuberculosis.

Diagnostic Testing

- For acute infection
  ○ The detection of IgM antibodies or isolation of *T. gondii* from body fluids suggests acute infection.
  ○ Cysts may be present in the tissue of chronically infected individuals.
- Reactivation in HIV is diagnosed by the following:
  ○ A compatible clinical syndrome with consistent lesions on radiography and response to empirical therapy
  ○ Demonstration of the parasite by biopsy or cerebrospinal fluid PCR
- Risk of congenital infection is determined by positive maternal IgM testing or positive PCR of amniotic fluid.

TREATMENT

- The standard treatment consists of **pyrimethamine, sulfadiazine, and supplementation with folinic acid** to avoid bone marrow toxicity. In immunocompetent hosts, treatment of acute infection does not alter outcomes.
- Pregnant women should be treated with spiramycin (3 g/day) throughout pregnancy. If fetal infection has been detected, further therapy with sulfadiazine and pyrimethamine is indicated.
- In AIDS patients, therapy is similar to standard therapy in immunocopetent hosts, but should be continued until CD4 counts have increased.
- Ocular disease requires consultation with an ophthalmologist.

LEISHMANIASIS

GENERAL PRINCIPLES

- The three main types of disease are as follows:
  - Cutaneous leishmaniasis (the most common form) resulting in ulcerative skin lesions
  - Visceral leishmaniasis causing severe disease of the reticuloendothelial system
  - Mucocutaneous leishmaniasis in which severe ulcerative lesions of the mucosa develop
- Living or traveling to an endemic region is the essential risk factor.
- Protective clothing and insect repellants are the only means of prevention.

Epidemiology
- Cutaneous leishmaniasis
  - Occurs in the Middle East, Africa, and Central and South America; caused by several *Leishmania* species
  - Recent epidemics in Afghanistan due to *Leishmania major* have been reported[6]
  - Disease occurs in travelers to endemic countries and military personnel
- Visceral leishmaniasis
  - Frequently caused by *Leishmania donovani* or *Leishmania infantum/tropica*
  - **Untreated symptomatic disease is frequently fatal and is a major cause of death, especially in children**
  - Occurs in India, Bangladesh, Sudan, Brazil, and the Mediterranean coast
- Mucocutaneous leishmaniasis: Occurs primarily in South America; usually caused by *L. brasiliensis*
- Various mammals provide an animal reservoir for most *Leishmania* spp. (e.g., dogs or rodents)

Pathophysiology
- Transmission occurs primarily through the bites of **female sandflies**, rarely by blood transfusion or needle sharing.
- Life cycle: Sandflies inject infectious metacyclic promastigotes that differentiate into intracellular amastigotes residing within host macrophages.
- Host consequences
  - The immune response is central to the development of pathology within the mammalian host.

■ Th2 responses generally lead to symptomatic disease or nonhealing lesions.

■ Th1 responses result in spontaneous cure.

○ Disease resolution leads to lifelong immunity, but reactivation can occur in the setting of immunosuppression.

○ Secondary bacterial infections are a frequent cause of death in visceral leishmaniasis.

DIAGNOSIS

Clinical Presentation

History

• Cutaneous disease: Patients notice a papule that appears weeks to months after the bite, which eventually ulcerates.

• Mucocutaneous disease

○ Patients present with a cutaneous lesion that heals spontaneously.

○ Mucosal lesions develop weeks to years after exposure.

• Visceral disease

○ Patients present with fever, weight loss, massive hepatosplenomegaly, and pancytopenia.

○ Hyperpigmentation of the skin may occur, leading to the term *kala-azar*, or "black fever."

Physical Examination

• Cutaneous disease

○ Shallow painless ulcers with a heaped-up border occur on exposed extremities or face.

○ Mucosal evaluation is important in patients from Central and South America.

○ Satellite lesions and lymphadenopathy can also occur.

• Visceral disease: Hepatosplenomegaly is a hallmark of the disease.

Differential Diagnosis

• Cutaneous disease: various fungal, bacterial, or malignant conditions should be considered.

• Visceral disease: typhoid fever, miliary tuberculosis, brucellosis, malaria, and acute schistosomiasis are all possibilities.

Diagnostic Testing

• Visceral disease may be associated with hypergammaglobulinemia, leukopenia, anemia, thrombocytopenia, and/or hypoalbuminemia.

• The gold standard for diagnosis is **culture of parasites** from ulcers (cutaneous or mucocutaneous) or bone marrow/splenic aspirates (visceral).

• Serologic tests, leishmanin skin tests, PCR testing, or demonstration of parasites on histopathology provide adjunctive diagnostic confirmation.

• Immunodiagnostics

○ Cutaneous disease: Delayed-type hypersensitivity testing using leishmanin skin testing can be used; 15 mm of induration on leishmanin testing is considered positive.

○ Visceral disease: Antibody detection using enzyme-linked immunosorbent assay (ELISA), IFAT, or recombinant kinesin antigen (rK39) dipstick are used.[7]

TREATMENT

- Cutaneous disease
  - Since spontaneous resolution of cutaneous ulcers frequently occurs, treatment may not be necessary.
  - In all cases, lesions affecting function or cosmetics (such as the face) should be treated to prevent further disfiguration.
- Visceral and mucocutaneous disease: Treatment is indicated in all symptomatic patients.
- Treatment options[8]
  - Antimonials: Pentavalent antimonials have been the mainstay of therapy for many years. Their use is limited by multiple toxicities and widespread resistance. In the United States, **sodium stibogluconate** (Pentostam) is considered first-line treatment and is available from the CDC.
  - Miltefosine: Has become the first-line agent for visceral leishmaniasis in India and has been used in South American leishmaniasis.
  - Amphotericin B: Recent demonstration of the efficacy of single-dose liposomal amphotericin B suggests that it may become standard therapy.
- Treatment failures occur in patients with HIV or other immunosuppression.
- Mucocutaneous leishmaniasis is difficult to treat, with relapses being common.

AMERICAN TRYPANOSOMIASIS

GENERAL PRINCIPLES

- American trypanosomiasis (Chagas' disease) is a protozoan infection caused by *Trypanosoma cruzi*.
- Disease is divided into two main phases
  - Acute disease, in which cutaneous manifestations of disease predominate with minimal mortality
  - Chronic disease, in which symptoms of end-stage organ failure develop with high mortality rates

Epidemiology
- Chagas' disease affects 10 to 12 million people in Central and South America.
- Immigrant populations are commonly infected with *T. cruzi*.
- The seroprevalence in blood donation varies by region of the county, the highest rates being in California (1:8,300) and Florida (1:3,800). The values are derived from 14 million blood donations in 2007 and 2008. The overall seroprevalence was 1:27,500.[9]

Pathophysiology
- Transmission
  - Primarily vector-borne through bites of reduviid bugs, also called **kissing bugs** (*Triatoma* **spp.**).
  - Other transmission sources include blood donors, transplantation, and congenital transmission.

- o Oral transmission from food contaminated by triatome feces is increasingly recognized as a source of transmission.
- o Various mammals including dogs and rodents serve as reservoirs of infection.
- Life cycle
  - o Triatomines deposit infectious trypomastigotes in its feces near the site of a blood meal.
  - o Scratching or other behaviors help trypomastigotes enter the host through the puncture site.
  - o Trypomastigotes differentiate into intracellular amastigotes In various host tissues, primarily cardiac myocytes and GI smooth muscle cells.
- Host consequences
  - o Acute infection occurs days or weeks after exposure; local swelling, similar to cellulitis, is followed by malaise, fever, and anorexia.
  - o Chronic infection appears years after the latent stage.
  - o **The immune response to chronically infected tissues likely causes end-organ disease** such as cardiomegaly, megaesophagus, and megacolon. This occurs in 20% to 30% of infected patients.

Prevention

- Campaigns utilizing insecticide in homes and outbuildings have been highly effective.
- Bed nets prevent insects from biting, which mostly occurs at night.

DIAGNOSIS

Clinical Presentation

History
- A high level of suspicion based on epidemiological risk factors is necessary.
- In endemic regions, acute infection occurs in children.
- In chronic stages, adults may describe symptoms of heart failure, palpitations, severe constipation, vomiting after meals, dysphagia, or odynophagia.

Physical Examination
- Acute phase: Cutaneous swellings known as chagomas form at the initial site of parasite entry. **Facial swelling with periorbital edema and conjunctivitis is a specific manifestation of acute Chagas' disease**, also known as Romaña sign. Local lymphadenopathy or hepatosplenomegaly may also be present.
- Chronic infection: Physical examination findings depend on the specific organs affected.
  - o Cardiac disease may manifest as signs of heart failure or arrhythmias.
  - o GI disease may result in abdominal tenderness or distension.
  - o Reactivation of chronic disease occurs in immunocompromised patients in the form of meningoencephalitis with altered mental status.

Differential Diagnosis

- Acute infection: Infectious mononucleosis, acute HIV, periorbital cellulitis, allergic reaction to triatomine bites.
- Chronic infection: dilated cardiomyopathy by other causes, achalasia, congenital aganglionosis (Hirschsprung disease), hypothyroidism, or severe esophagitis.

Diagnostic Testing

- Acute infection: Parasites may be **directly visualized on thick blood smears**; PCR on blood remains investigational.
- Chronic infection
  - Xenodiagnosis: 10 to 20 sterile triatomine bugs are fed on patients; 3 weeks later, the insects are inspected for *T. cruzi*, a highly sensitive and specific but difficult method.
  - Serology: At least two distinct serological tests are required to diagnose Chagas' disease in the appropriate clinical setting.
  - PCR on infected tissues is experimental.
  - Direct visualization on biopsy of infected tissues is extremely insensitive but highly specific.
- ECG and echocardiogram may be indicated to evaluate for cardiac involvement.
- Barium swallow/enema may be done to identify abnormalities of the alimentary tract.

TREATMENT

- Treatment with **benznidazole** is highly effective in acute stages and can prevent complications of chronic Chagas' disease.[10]
- All serologically confirmed cases of chronic Chagas' disease should be offered treatment versus watchful waiting, with initiation of treatment at the first sign of end-organ damage.
- Benznidazole is the first-line treatment (5 to 7 mg/kg/d in two divided doses for 60 days); rash and dermatitis are frequent side effects.
- Nifurtimox (8 to 10 mg/kg/d in three divided doses for 90 days) has many toxicities including psychological disturbances and GI upset.
- Sequela of chronic Chagas' disease should be treated with medical or surgical approaches.
  - Cardiac disease: Antiarrhythmics should be administered in consultation with cardiology. Interestingly, amiodarone is under evaluation as a synergistic agent with posaconazole to treat Chagas' disease.[11]
  - GI disease: Conservative approaches and laxatives may provide symptomatic relief; surgical approaches may be indicated.

COMPLICATIONS

Complications of chronic disease include the following:
- Cardiac: ventricular arrhythmias, heart block, severe heart failure, and death from cardiac disease
- GI: constipation, aspiration, and inability to eat

MONITORING/FOLLOW-UP

Serological reversion occurring within 1 year for acute disease or several years for chronic disease suggests cure.

TRICHOMONIASIS

See "Trichomoniasis" in Chapter 11.

AMEBIASIS

GENERAL PRINCIPLES

Epidemiology

- *Entamoeba histolytica* causes intestinal amebiasis manifested by amebic dysentery or liver abscess.
- *E. histolytica* occurs in tropical countries or areas with poor sanitation worldwide.
- It affects around 500 million people worldwide, with an annual mortality of 40,000 to 100,000 persons.[12] Alternatively, many people may be colonized with nonpathogenic *Entamoeba dispar.*
- The prevalence in the United States is 1% to 2%.
- The main risk groups are travelers, immigrants, men who have sex with men, and institutionalized persons.
- Proper water treatment and sanitation dramatically reduces the incidence of disease.

Pathophysiology

- Transmission: *E. histolytica* is spread by the fecal–oral route when cysts are ingested.
- Life cycle
  - ○ Cysts are ingested and resist the acidic environment of the stomach.
  - ○ In the small intestine, trophozoites are released that mature and eventually form new cysts.
- Host consequences
  - ○ When trophozoites invade the bowel mucosa, they release enzymes that cause tissue lysis. Symptoms develop 2 to 6 weeks after cyst ingestion.
    - ■ Submucosal lesions enlarge and form "teardrop" ulcers.
    - ■ Dissemination occurs upon entry into the portal circulation.
  - ○ The most frequent site of systemic disease is the liver, where abscesses form, resembling anchovy paste.

DIAGNOSIS

Clinical Presentation

- Most disease is asymptomatic, patients become carriers, but most clear carriage within a year.
- Acute infection
  - ○ Crampy lower abdominal discomfort, flatulence, tenesmus, with bloody or mucoid diarrhea
  - ○ Some patients may develop an ameboma, a submucosal mass of granulation tissue often mistaken for malignancy

- Extra-intestinal manifestations
  - ○ Liver abscess
    - Most common extra-intestinal site of infection, occurs more commonly in adults
    - Amebic abscess of the liver is characterized by the abrupt onset of right upper quadrant pain, weight loss, high fever, and a tender, enlarged liver
  - ○ Rarely, *E. histolytica* may infect other tissues such as the lungs, brain, peritoneum, or pericardial space.

Differential Diagnosis

- Causes of dysentery include *Shigella*, *Escherichia coli*, *Salmonella*, *Campylobacter*, and some *Vibrio* species.
- Amebic liver abscess must be differentiated from pyogenic liver abscess, carcinoma, or echinococcal disease.

Diagnostic Testing

- The primary means of diagnosis is the **detection of *E. histolytica* trophozoites or cysts in the stool**. Samples must be examined within 30 minutes for detection of motile trophozoites or can be fixed for later staining. A minimum of three stool samples should be screened for parasites.
- *E. histolytica* is indistinguishable from *E. dispar* in stool; additional confirmatory tests such as ELISA or PCR are needed, but are frequently impractical.
- Serology may be negative in patients with acute disease and should be repeated in 5 to 7 days.
- Hepatic abscesses can be detected with either ultrasound or CT; aspiration may reveal material resembling anchovy paste.

TREATMENT

Medications

- **Iodoquinol or paromomycin** will eradicate **cysts** in asymptomatic carriers.
- **Metronidazole** 750 mg by mouth three times a day for 10 to 14 days should be followed by iodoquinol or paromomycin to eradicate cysts in patients with **colitis** or **liver abscess**.

Surgical Management

- Abscesses can be drained either surgically or by percutaneous intervention.
- Ruptured abscess or bacterial superinfection should be treated surgically.

GIARDIASIS

GENERAL PRINCIPLES

Epidemiology

- *Giardia lamblia* (also known as *Giardia intestinalis* and *Giardia duodenalis*) is the cause of giardiasis.
- It occurs worldwide, infecting mostly humans but also other mammals.

- Outbreaks in day care centers are common.
- Hikers and skiers in the Rocky Mountains are also at risk.

Pathophysiology

- Transmission occurs through fecal–oral routes.
- Life cycle
  - ○ Cysts are ingested from contaminated food or water and release trophozoites in the duodenum.
  - ○ The trophozoite then attaches to the GI tract wall causing disease manifestations.
- Host consequences
  - ○ Inflammation of the duodenal mucosa leads to malabsorption of protein and fat.
  - ○ Humoral immunity is thought to be important. Patients with hypogammaglobulinemia develop prolonged, severe infections that respond poorly to therapy.

Prevention

- The cysts persist for months in the environment.
- Chlorination does not kill the cysts, but they can be removed by filtration.

DIAGNOSIS

Clinical Presentation

- The majority of patients are asymptomatic carriers.
- Symptoms occur after an incubation period of 1 to 3 weeks. Commonly, patients complain of bloating, abdominal pain, nausea, flatulence, emesis, and diarrhea. Symptoms usually resolve spontaneously.
- Chronically infected children may have retarded growth and development

Differential Diagnosis

The differential diagnosis includes other parasitological causes of chronic diarrhea such as strongyloidiasis, cryptosporidiosis, cyclosporiasis, or microsporidiosis.

Diagnostic Testing

- The gold standard for diagnosis is **direct detection of parasites in the stool**.
- ELISA-based antigen detection is replacing microscopy, but suffers from poorer sensitivity; repeated testing is indicated.

TREATMENT

Metronidazole is the treatment of choice. Multiple alternative agents are available but difficult to find in the United States.[12]

REFERENCES

1. WHO Global Malaria Programme. *World Malaria Report: 2011.* Geneva: World Health Organization; 2011. http://www.who.int/malaria/world_malaria_report_2011/en/. Accessed May 15, 2012.
2. WHO. *Guidelines for the Treatment of Malaria.* 2nd ed. Geneva: World Health Organization; 2010. http://www.who.int/malaria/publications/atoz/9789241547925/en/index.html. Accessed May 15, 2012.

3. *Treatment of Malaria* (guideline for clinicians). Centers for Disease Control and Prevention. http://www.cdc.gov/malaria/diagnosis_treatment/treatment.html. Accessed May 15, 2012.

4. Vannier E, Gewurz BE, Krause PJ. Human babesiosis. *Infect Dis Clin North Am.* 2008;22:469-488.

5. Dubey JP, Jones JL. Toxoplasma gondii infection in humans and animals in the United States. *Int J Parasitol.* 2008;38:1257-1278.

6. van Thiel PP, Leenstra T, de Vries HJ, et al. Cutaneous leishmaniasis (*Leishmania major* infection) in Dutch troops deployed in northern Afghanistan: epidemiology, clinical aspects, and treatment. *Am J Top Med Hyg.* 2010;83:1295-1300.

7. Mandal J, Khurana S, Dubey ML, et al. Evaluation of direct agglutination test, rk39 Test, and ELISA for the diagnosis of visceral leishmaniasis. *Am J Trop Med Hyg.* 2008;79:76-78.

8. Murray HW. Leishmaniasis in the United States: treatment in 2012. *Am J Trop Med Hyg.* 2012;86:434-440.

9. Bern C, Montgomery SP, Katz L, et al. Chagas disease and the US blood supply. *Curr Opin Infect Dis.* 2008;21:476-482.

10. Bern C, Montgomery SP, Herwaldt BL, et al. Evaluation and treatment of Chagas disease in the United States: a systematic review. *JAMA.* 2007;298:2171-2181.

11. Serrano-Martín X, Payares G, De Lucca M, et al. Amiodarone and miltefosine act synergistically against *Leishmania mexicana* and can induce parasitological cure in a murine model of cutaneous leishmaniasis. *Antimicrob Agents Chemother.* 2009;53:5108-5113.

12. Stanley SL Jr. Amoebiasis. *Lancet.* 2003;361:1025-1034.

Helminthic Infections

18

Luis A. Marcos and F. Matthew Kuhlmann

- Helminths (Greek for "worms") are common in poorer regions of tropical and subtropical developing countries.
- Travel and immigration lead to cases in nonendemic countries such as North America and Europe. Additionally, some helminths remain endemic in temperate countries.
- In general, disease severity depends on extent of exposure as worms do not replicate within a host. The presence of eosinophilia generally relates to increased worm burden.
- Helminths are classified as follows:
  - **Nematodes** (roundworms):
    - Intestinal worms: *Ascaris lumbricoides*, *Trichuris trichiura* (whipworm), *Ancylostoma duodenale* (hookworm), *Necator americanus* (hookworm), *Strongyloides stercoralis*, and *Enterobius vermicularis* (pinworm) are a few examples
    - Tissue worms: *Trichinella spiralis*, filarial roundworms (e.g., *Onchocerca volvulus* and *Wuchereria bancrofti*), and *Toxocara* spp., among others
  - **Trematodes** (flukes): *Schistosoma* spp., *Clonorchis sinensis*, *Opisthorchis viverrini*, *Fasciola* spp., *Paragonimus* spp.
  - **Cestodes** (tapeworms):
    - Intestinal tapeworms: *Taenia* spp. and *Diphyllobothrium latum*
    - Larval tapeworms: *Taenia solium* (pork tapeworm) and *Echinococcus* spp.
- Helminth infections commonly occurring in adults the United States will be discussed. Additional helminths are briefly described in Table 18-1.

CYSTICERCOSIS

GENERAL PRINCIPLES

- The cestode *Taenia solium* has a complicated life cycle in that the human is host for both tapeworms and cysts, the only helminth infection in which this phenomenon occurs. The larval stage causes significant pathology while worms elicit minimal disease.
- Adult worm infections (taeniasis) are limited to the intestines.
- **Larval infections (cysticercosis)** cause disease primarily in the central nervous system (CNS), leading to significant morbidity and mortality or calcifications in muscle tissue.

Epidemiology

- High-prevalence areas of *T. solium* include Central and South America and Southeast Asia. Meat inspections and improved sanitation have eliminated the disease in many developed countries.
- In the United States, cases occur **primarily in immigrants from Central and South America**.

TABLE 18-1	OVERVIEW OF CLINICALLY IMPORTANT INFECTIONS CAUSED BY HELMINTHS			
Classification	Helminth disease	Clinical manifestations	Diagnosis	Treatment
Nematodes (Round worms) Soil-transmitted	Ascaris lumbricoides	Asymptomatic infections are common. Other symptoms include abdominal pain and intestinal obstruction. Pulmonary symptoms occur during larval migration, inducing asthma-like symptoms. Eosinophilia is present during larval migration through host tissues	Identify eggs in stools by microscopy	Albendazole 400 mg single dose
	Trichuris trichiura (whipworm)	Range from asymptomatic to abdominal pain, dysentery, and rectal prolapse. Anemia is common. Eosinophilia suggests coinfections	Identify eggs in stools by microscopy	Albendazole, dosing depends on severity of infection
	Ancylostoma duodenale and Necator americanus (hookworm)	Range from asymptomatic to severe, pulmonary symptoms may occur. Hallmark of infection is severe iron deficiency anemia, eosinophilia may occur	Identify eggs or larvae in stool by microscopy	Albendazole 400 mg single dose
	Toxocara canis (visceral larva migrans)	Abdominal pain and hepatomegaly, more details in text	Identify eggs on microscopy, serology may help	See text
	Strongyloides stercoralis	Symptoms include abdominal pain, pulmonary complaints, or other life-threatening disease in hyperinfection syndromes (see text)	Identify worms in feces or sputum. Serologies may help	Drug of choice is ivermectin

Soil-transmitted Nematodes	*Anisakis* and *Pseudoterranova* spp. (anisakiasis)	Intense abdominal pain after eating undercooked fish. Eosinophilia is rare	Identify worms on endoscopy, serology helps in chronic cases	Observation, worm removal by endoscopy or albendazole
	Ancylostoma braziliense (cutaneous larva migrans)	Pruritic serpiginous rash, usually of the lower extremities	Based on clinical suspicion	Albendazole or ivermectin
	Enterobius vermicularis (pinworm)	Perianal itching in children upon external egg deposition	Identify eggs in feces or perianal worms (at night)	Treat entire family with albendazole, multiple treatments may be necessary
Tissue Nematodes	*Trichinella spiralis* (trichinosis)	Classically described as myalgias, periorbital edema, and eosinophilia. Heavier disease burden associated with cachexia and CNS disease	Demonstration of larvae in muscle tissue or serology	Mebendazole and/or steroids
	Dracunculus medinensis (guinea worm)	Blisters form upon exposure to water followed by emergence of the worm	Identify worms in blisters or ulcers	Slow worm extraction
Nematodes-Filarial worms	*Wuchereria bancrofti Brugia malayi* Lymphatic filariasis	Extreme lymphatic swelling including elephantiasis of the lower extremities and hydrocele	Thin and thick blood smear to identify the microfilariae, serologies	Albendazole Ivermectin DEC
	Loa loa	Calabar swellings, transient cutaneous swelling, are the hallmark of infection. Worms frequently migrate across conjunctiva	Direct detection of worms or serology	DEC

(continued)

TABLE 18-1	(CONTINUED)			
Filarial worms (continued)	*Onchocerca volvulus* (onchocerciasis or river blindness)	Pruritic cutaneous swellings, occasionally with leopard skin. Blindness	Identify worms in skin snips or obtain serologies	Ivermectin—use with caution in *Loa loa* coinfections; Albendazole
Trematodes (Flukes)	*Schistosoma* spp. (schistosomiasis)	*Schistosoma hematobium*—hematuria, bladder cancer; Other *Schistosoma* spp.—hepatomegaly, fibrosis, liver failure	Identify eggs in stool or urine	See text
	Opisthorchis viverrini and *Clonorchis sinensis* (liver flukes)	Generally asymptomatic, increased risk of cholangiocarcinoma, hepatomegaly	Identify eggs on stool microscopy	Praziquantel
	Paragnonimus spp. (lung flukes)	Pulmonary effusions, transient cutaneous migrations	Direct detection of eggs or serologies	See text
	Fasciola hepatica and *Fasciola gigantica* Fascioliasis (liver flukes)	Symptoms range from asymptomatic infections to diarrhea, coughing, hepatomegaly, and right upper quadrant pain with eosinophilia	Serologies are quite helpful as egg detection in feces can be difficult	Triclabendazole 10 mg/kg orally single dose, may need repeating
Cestodes (Tape worms)	*Taenia solium*	*Taenia solium* (pork tapeworm) — Cysticercosis CNS and other tissue lesions, seizures	Clinical suspicion	See text
		Taeniasis, abdominal pain	Identify eggs or proglottids in feces	

Cestodes (Tape worms) (continued)			
Taenia sanginata	*Taenia sanginata*—beef tapeworm, abdominal pain	Identify eggs or proglottids in feces	Praziquantel
Echinococcus granulosus (cystic echinococcosis)	Disseminated infections involving the liver, lungs, spleen, heart, or other organs. Large cysts form leading to symptoms in the affected organ	Positive serologies with associated cysts on imaging	Observation versus surgical removal or nonsurgical drainage of cyst followed by albendazole
Echinococcus multilocularis (alveolar echinococcosis, exclusive to North America)	The liver is the primary organ infected	Serology C⁻ scan may help	Surgical removal of cyst and long-term albendazole
Diphyllobothrium latum (fish tapeworm)	Frequently asymptomatic, abdominal pain may be noted historically associated with vitamin B12 deficiency	Identify eggs or proglottids in feces	Praziquantel Niclosamide
Hymenolepis nana or *Hymenolepis diminuta*	Mild abdominal pain, diarrhea, and eosinophilia	Identify eggs in stool examination	Praziquantel Niclosamide

CNS, central nervous system; DEC, diethylcarbamazine.

Pathophysiology

- Transmission of *T. solium* occurs through two separate routes
  - Ingestion of infected meats containing **cysts** leads to taeniasis (intestinal tapeworm infection).
  - **Ingestion of proglottids or eggs through fecal–oral transmission leads to cysticercosis.**
- Life cycle
  - Ingested eggs of *T. solium* differentiate into larvae (oncospheres), which cross the gut mucosa and disseminate to other tissues forming cysts, termed cysticerci.
  - Ingestion of cysts from infected tissues allows for evagination of the worm and attachment of the tapeworm to the gut mucosa. The worm develops characteristic proglottids, the hermaphroditic reproductive segments of tapeworms, which release eggs in feces and complete the life cycle.
  - The human is the only known definitive host, that is, the only species that allows for development of the tapeworm and subsequent shedding of eggs.
- Effects on the host
  - Like most cestode infections, **taeniasis** results in long-term, chronic, asymptomatic infections allowing for prolonged shedding of eggs.
  - Cyst forms of cestode infections cause significant pathology. This includes ocular disease, meningitis, and brain and spinal cord lesions.
  - **Neurocysticercosis** is the most frequently diagnosed form of *T. solium* infections, presenting as space-occupying lesions. Cyst expansion results in CNS pathology, primarily seizures.

Risk Factors

- Pork consumption is a risk factor for taeniasis.
- Risk factors for cysticercosis include taeniasis, poor hygiene, and living in endemic regions. Risk increases with age.

Prevention

- Prevention strategies include the following:
  - Improved sanitation and meat inspections.
  - Avoiding consumption of undercooked pork prevents taeniasis.
  - Treatment of taeniasis reduces the risk of cysticercosis.
- No vaccines are available.

DIAGNOSIS

Clinical Presentation

History

- Taeniasis is generally asymptomatic; patients may pass proglottids in their stool.
- Cysticercosis may have protean manifestations ranging from vague neurological symptoms to seizures and rarely symptoms from other infected organs.
- The peak incidence of neurocysticercosis occurs between ages 30 and 40.

Physical Examination

- Various neurological processes may be found depending on the location of the CNS lesion.

- Rapid paralysis may occur with spinal lesions.
- Subcutaneous lesions may be identified.

Diagnostic Criteria
Guidelines are under development by the Infectious Diseases Society of America.

Differential Diagnosis
The differential includes any space-occupying brain lesion, subarachnoid hemorrhage, bacterial abscess, toxoplasmosis, nocardiosis, malignancy, and septic emboli.

Diagnostic Testing
Laboratories
- Peripheral eosinophilia is not present in cysticercosis or taeniasis.
- Cerebrospinal fluid analysis may reveal lymphocytic pleocytosis or eosinophils and elevated protein.
- Serological testing is frequently indicated.
  - **The immunoblot is highly specific but false negatives** occur in 30% of the cases with a single brain lesion.[1,2]
  - Enzyme-linked immunosorbent assay (ELISA) has cross-reactivity with both *Taenia saginata* (beef tapeworm) and *Echinococcus.*
- For taeniasis, at least three stool examinations are recommended to increase detection rate of eggs.

Imaging
- CT scan of the brain can show the typical lesions that are generally small or calcified with a bright central spot of the protoscolex.
- MRI provides more detail and may assist in identifying the etiology of CNS lesions.

TREATMENT

- Therapy remains highly controversial and infectious disease consultation is strongly recommended.[3,4]
- **Albendazole** has become the drug of first choice over praziquantel as it has better CNS penetration and does not interact with antiepileptics or steroids.
- Corticosteroids are recommended along with the antiparasitic therapy to reduce brain edema caused by the death of the parasite.
- Antiepileptics should be continued for at least 1 year or more.

STRONGYLOIDIASIS

GENERAL PRINCIPLES

- *S. stercoralis* and *Strongyloides fuelleborni* are intestinal nematodes causing strongyloidiasis.
- Unlike other nematodes, *Strongyloides* **replicates within the human host allowing for persistence of infection over several years**.
- Overwhelming **hyperinfection syndromes** occur in immunocompromised patients.

Epidemiology

- Strongyloidiasis affects 3 to 100 million people globally, mostly in tropical and subtropical regions.[5]
- It is uncommon in developed countries with adequate sanitation.
- It is frequently found in rural areas, institutional settings, and lower socioeconomic groups.
- The majority of cases in the United States are imported by travelers and immigrants. Kentucky and Tennessee have reported local cases of disease.

Pathophysiology

- Transmission: Filariform larvae penetrate skin from contaminated soil.
- Life cycle:
  ○ After skin penetration, larvae migrate (via the circulation and lungs where they eventually are swallowed) to the small bowel mucosa.
  ○ In the small bowel, female adult worms produce eggs that are either shed in the feces and complete an external life cycle or the eggs develop into filariform larvae within the intestines. **The internally developed filariform larvae penetrate the colonic mucosa and can repeat the life cycle (autoinfection).**
- Effects on the host:
  ○ The immune response to *Strongyloides* is quite broad, inducing both cell-mediated and humoral responses coinciding with eosinophilia.
  ○ Immunosuppression by steroids, malignancies, or drugs leads to hyperinfection syndromes where worms invade many other organ systems.
  ○ Gram-negative sepsis or meningitis is associated with *Strongyloides* infections due to gut epithelial disruption or dissemination of bacteria within the worms as they migrate through host tissues.
  ○ Pneumonia or other pulmonary manifestations may occur if worms become trapped and mature in the lungs.

Risk Factors

- For strongyloidiasis: walking barefoot or swimming in infected areas, contact with human waste or sewage
- For hyperinfection syndromes: various forms of immunodeficiency as well as coinfection with human T-lymphotropic virus (HTLV)-1. Advanced HIV disease itself does not appear to be a risk factor for disseminated disease

Prevention

- Improved sanitation reduces disease burden.
- Avoid walking barefoot or swimming in areas known to be infested with *Strongyloides* larvae.

DIAGNOSIS

Clinical Presentation

History

- Manifestations of strongyloidiasis can range from abdominal pain to pulmonary complaints.
- A pruritic lesion can develop at the sight of entry.
- Pulmonary symptoms occur shortly thereafter and resolve spontaneously.

- Chronic infections in immunocompetent hosts are rarely symptomatic. Patients may complain of perianal pruritus when autoinfection occurs with larvae penetrating skin.
- Mental status changes and gram-negative meningitis are associated with intestinal strongyloidiasis.

Physical Examination
- Signs of pneumonia may be observed.
- Recurrent rashes known as "larva currens" may occur. They present as a linear eruption that is intensely pruritic, lasting several hours before spontaneous resolution.

Differential Diagnosis
The differential includes chronic causes of diarrhea, duodenitis, and colitis.

Diagnostic Testing
Laboratories
- Peripheral eosinophilia varies throughout the course of infection.
- In immunocompromised hosts, eosinophilia may not be present and loss of eosinophilia portends a worse prognosis.
- Direct parasitological confirmation of larvae in the stool or lungs confirms the diagnosis. A minimum of three stool examinations are frequently required to make a diagnosis.
- Serological tests detect antibodies in suspected cases but are rather nonspecific.
- Screening for disease may be indicated in high-risk patients who will become immunosuppressed.

Imaging
Various abnormalities may be seen depending on the disease manifestation.
- Pulmonary infiltrates on chest radiograph
- Duodenitis on CT scan or esophagogastroduodenoscopy
- CNS infarcts in hyperinfection syndromes with dissemination

TREATMENT

- All disease should be treated.
- The drug of choice for uncomplicated disease is **ivermectin** (200 µg/kg for 2 to 3 days); hyperinfections require prolonged treatment courses and the advice of specialists.[6]
- Follow-up examinations for cure are recommended.
- Empiric treatment for high-risk patients who will undergo immunosuppression is frequently advised.

PARAGONIMIASIS

GENERAL PRINCIPLES

Epidemiology
- *Paragonimus* spp. are trematodes (lung flukes) causing paragonimiasis.
- *Paragonimus* species are present worldwide causing upward of 10 to 20 million cases; *Paragonimus westermani* is the most significant. They are most common in eastern Asia.

- While less recognized globally, *Paragonimus kellicotti* is increasingly recognized in North America. More than 10 cases have been diagnosed in Missouri from 2007 to 2010 associated with the consumption of raw crayfish; the vast majority of cases are in men.[7]

Pathophysiology

- Transmission
  - Humans acquire disease by eating **undercooked crustaceans** infected with metacercariae and by eating **wild boar**.
  - The major risk factor is consumption of raw or undercooked crayfish from endemic areas. Therefore, all crustaceans should be cooked thoroughly.
- Life cycle
  - After ingestion, metacercariae excyst in the stomach and juvenile larvae migrate through the lungs, where they mature into adult worms.
  - Eggs are expectorated or swallowed and excreted in the feces.
  - Once in water, the eggs (miracidia) hatch, penetrating snails. The snails release cercariae, which attach to the gills, muscle, or liver of crustaceans and mature to metacercariae.
- Effects on the host
  - Disease manifestations depend on the migration of larvae and inflammatory reaction to the worms or eggs.
  - Larvae reside and mature in the lungs. Rarely, disease may spread to cutaneous tissues, the brain, or the heart.

DIAGNOSIS

Clinical Presentation

History
- Pulmonary symptoms and peripheral or pulmonary eosinophilia should suggest paragonimiasis, even in North America.
- Initial infections are rarely symptomatic; patients may have abdominal pain or diarrhea. Other symptoms include chest pain, urticaria, or chills.
- Progressive shortness of breath is the primary complaint.

Physical Examination
- Pleural effusions may be detected on auscultation.
- Painless mobile lesions may be seen in the skin.
- Mental status changes may occur in the setting of CNS disease.

Differential Diagnosis

Chronic paragonimiasis may resemble pulmonary or pleural tuberculosis, malignancy, or vasculitis and is often misdiagnosed.

Diagnostic Testing

- Peripheral eosinophilia is common during the acute infection and the following 3 to 5 months.
- Pleural fluid analysis may reveal eosinophilia of ≥10%.
- **Detection of *Paragonimus* eggs in the sputum or stool** requires multiple examinations.

- For either acute or chronic infections, **serology** may be helpful.
- Imaging of the lungs by chest radiograph or CT is useful in identifying pulmonary disease, primarily effusions.
- MRI of the brain may reveal "soap bubble" ventricular swelling along with other significant calcifications.

TREATMENT

- The drug of choice is **praziquantel** (25 mg/kg orally three times daily for 2 to 3 days).[8]
- Other treatments are difficult to obtain or administer.
- Caution must be used when treating patients as increased inflammation may occur upon death of the parasite.

TOXOCARIASIS

GENERAL PRINCIPLES

Epidemiology

- *Toxocara canis* (dogs) and less frequently *Toxocara catis* (cats) are nematodes causing toxocariasis or visceral larva migrans (VLM).
- Young children are especially vulnerable due to dirt pica (geophagia), poor hygiene, or frequent contact with dogs.
- Treating infected dogs and cats reduces the number of eggs and the potential burden for humans.
- In the United States, the overall seroprevalence rate is about 14%, but many are asymptomatic.[9]
- Many puppies in the United States shed *Toxocara* eggs, potentiated by the ability of infections to spread vertically.

Pathophysiology

- Transmission: Ingestion of parasite eggs from contaminated soil causes infection.
- Life cycle: Eggs excyst and larvae migrate through the circulation to the pulmonary system where they migrate up the trachea and are swallowed. In dogs and cats, adult worms develop in the intestine and shed eggs in the stool, which contaminate the environment.
- Effects on the host
  ○ Humans are incidental hosts, meaning larvae are unable to mature into adult worms.
  ○ Larvae migrate but become trapped in host tissues, primarily the liver, where they are killed by granulomatous reactions from the host.

DIAGNOSIS

Clinical Presentation

- Most infected people are asymptomatic or symptoms are self-limited.
- Severity of symptoms depends on extent of exposure and resultant worm burden.
- Two clinical syndromes occur in children, VLM and ocular toxocariasis (OT).
  ○ VLM presents with episodes of fever, coughing and wheezing, anemia, eosinophilia, urticaria, and/or hepatomegaly.

  ○ OT presents as an inflamed tissue mass resembling a tumor. Patients present with loss of vision, strabismus, and/or retinal lesions.

Differential Diagnosis

- For VLM: infection with other helminths that migrate through tissues, asthma, and rheumatologic diseases
- For OT: retinoblastoma and other causes of chorioretinitis

Diagnostic Testing

- Leukocytosis with eosinophilia and hypergammaglobulinemia may be present.
- **The presence of larvae in infected tissues is diagnostic, but is very difficult to accomplish**.
- **Serologies fail to distinguish between current and prior infections** and cross-react with other helminths. Clinical suspicion, appropriate clinical findings, and positive serologies will lead to a diagnosis.
- Chest radiography may show nonspecific pulmonary infiltrates.
- Abdominal ultrasound may identify granulomas in the liver.

TREATMENT

- Most patients recover with supportive care and anti-inflammatory medications.
- Short courses of **albendazole** may be indicated.
- For OT, treatment may help prevent vision loss but damage is irreversible.

SCHISTOSOMIASIS

GENERAL PRINCIPLES

- Schistosomiasis, also known as bilharzia, is caused by trematodes (flukes) of the genus *Schistosoma.*
- *Schistosoma haematobium* affects the genitourinary system while *Schistosoma mansoni* causes disease of the liver.
- Swimmer's itch is a local dermatitis caused by penetration of the skin by avian schistosomes.

Epidemiology

- Approximately 200 million people globally are affected with 14,000 deaths annually.[10]
- Persons swimming in contaminated freshwater are at highest risk for disease. Exposed persons can vigorously dry off with a towel to reduce cercarial penetration.
- Distribution of their intermediate snail vector determines the *Schistosoma* spp. present.
  ○ *S. mansoni*: Africa, South America, and parts of the Caribbean
  ○ *Schistosoma haematobium*: Africa and the Middle East
  ○ *Schistosoma japonicum* and *Schistosoma mekongi*: Southeast Asia
- Appropriate snail hosts are not present in the United States. Cases are frequently diagnosed in travelers and immigrants.

Pathophysiology

- Transmission: Occurs when cercariae penetrate human skin.
- Life cycle
  - ○ Cercariae penetrate skin, migrate through host tissues, and develop into adult worms within host venules.
  - ○ Female adult worms are wrapped by male worms. The female worms then begin depositing eggs, which are released in the urine (*S. haematobium*) or feces (all other species).
  - ○ In freshwater, eggs develop into miracidia, which enter the snail intermediate host, eventually developing into cercariae.
- Effects on the host
  - ○ Host pathology develops due to the inflammatory response to adult worms and eggs within host tissues.
    - ■ *S. mansoni, S. japonicum,* and *S. mekongi* **reside within portal and mesenteric veins**, leading to portal fibrosis and liver failure that are exacerbated by coinfections with hepatitis viruses.
    - ■ *S. haematobium* resides within the **bladder wall**, leading to hematuria and bladder cancer.
    Patients may have recurrent *Salmonella* infections (either bacteremia or bacteriuria).

DIAGNOSIS

Clinical Presentation

- Manifestations of chronic disease depend on the infecting species.
- Severity of symptoms depends on extent of exposure and worm burden.

History

- Swimmer's itch is usually seen within a day of swimming in infected water. The rash is usually on the legs and is pruritic. Symptoms may last for over a week.
- Acute disease (Katayama fever) presents within weeks to 2 months after exposure as a self-limited febrile illness. Complaints can include fever, myalgias, arthralgias, headache, cough, and diarrhea.
- *S. haematobium* infection may be asymptomatic or cause hematuria, frequency, dysuria, and incontinence.
- Intestinal schistosomiasis may result in chronic abdominal pain and diarrhea.
- Hepatic schistosomiasis may present with symptoms of liver failure.

Physical Examination

- Rashes may occur with acute disease.
- Women with *S. haematobium* may have polyps on external genitalia.
- In intestinal schistosomiasis, hepatomegaly with splenomegaly and jaundice can be seen.
- For *S. japonicum*, CNS disease or pulmonary findings occur in a minority of patients.

Differential Diagnosis

Geography and exposure history provide useful clues, as other helminthic infections can present similarity.

Diagnostic Testing

- Eosinophilia is frequent; anemia may occur with chronic blood loss
- With *S. haematobium*, urinalysis may reveal hematuria
- Hyperbilirubinemia and thrombocytopenia may be present in liver failure
- Definitive diagnosis is made by identifying eggs of schistosomes in the stool or urine
- Serological tests are available but are unable to differentiate between acute and chronic infections. They may be useful in acute disease prior to maturation of adult worms
- Abdominal imaging may detect hepatomegaly, fibrosis, or portal hypertension
- Other imaging modalities for pulmonary or CNS disease

TREATMENT

- All patients with schistosomiasis should be offered therapy.
- **Praziquantel** is the drug of choice, which is administered for 1 to 2 days in all cases.[10]
- Corticosteroids can limit inflammation associated with killing of parasites upon treatment with praziquantel.
- Repeat screening examinations followed by repeat therapy with praziquantel may be indicated, as egg production is only temporarily inhibited.
- Management of hepatic complications should coincide with therapy.
- Infectious disease consultation is advised for management of cases in the United States.

REFERENCES

1. Garcia HH, Gonzalez AE, Evans CAW, Gilman RH. *Taenia solium* cysticercosis. *Lancet.* 2003;362:547-556.
2. Wilson M, Bryan RE, Fried JA, et al. Clinical evaluation of the cysticercosis enzyme-linked immunoelectrotransfer blot in patients with neurocysticercosis. *J Infect Dis.* 1991;164:1007-1009.
3. García HH, Evans CA, Nash TE, et al. Current consensus guidelines for treatment of neurocysticercosis. *Clin Microbiol Rev.* 2002;15:747-756.
4. Matthaiou DK, Panos G, Adamidi ES, Falagas ME. Albendazole versus praziquantel in the treatment of neurocysticercosis: a meta-analysis of comparative trials. I. 2008;2:e194.
5. Centers for Disease Control and Prevention. Strongyloidiasis. http://www.cdc.gov/parasites/strongyloides/epi.html. Accessed May 16, 2012.
6. Bisoffi Z, Buonfrate D, Angheben A, et al. Randomized clinical trial on ivermectin versus thiabendazole for the treatment of strongyloidiasis. *PLoS Negl Trop Dis.* 2001;5:e1254.
7. Lane, MA, Barsanti MC, Santos CA, et al. Human paragonimiasis in North America following ingestion of raw crayfish. *Clin Infect Dis.* 2009;49:e55-e61.
8. Udonsi JK. Clinical field trials of praziquantel in pulmonary paragonimiasis due to *Paragonimus uterobilateralis* in endemic populations of the Igwun Basin, Nigeria. *Trop Med Parasitol.* 1989;40:65-68.
9. Won KY, Kruszon-Moran D, Schantz PM, Jones JL. National seroprevalence and risk factors for zoonotic *Toxocara* spp. infection. *Am J Trop Med Hyg.* 2008;79:552-557.
10. Gryseels B, Polman K, Clerinx J, Kestens L. Human schistosomiasis. *Lancet.* 2006;368:1106-1118.

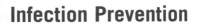

Infection Prevention

19

Hitoshi Honda and Hilary M. Babcock

INTRODUCTION

Decades of improvements in infection prevention science and implementation have resulted in significant decreases in health care–associated infections (HAIs); however, they remain a constant threat to hospitalized patients, resulting in significant morbidity and mortality and increases in health care costs. The Centers for Disease Control and Prevention (CDC) estimates that 5% to 10% of hospitalized patients develop a HAI, corresponding to approximately 2 million HAIs associated with nearly 100,000 deaths annually in US hospitals.[1,2] The emergence of new pathogens (e.g., severe acute respiratory syndrome coronavirus [SARS-CoV], avian influenza, epidemic influenza, HIV) and changes in existing pathogens (e.g., multidrug-resistant gram-negative organisms, methicillin-resistant *Staphylococcus aureus* [MRSA], *Clostridium difficile*) create an ongoing need for more efficient and effective infection prevention practices in both community and hospital settings.[3]

INFECTION PREVENTION STRATEGIES

Current infection prevention strategies consist of two main sets of precautions: **standard precautions and transmission-based precautions**.[3] Standard precautions should be used with all patients who are admitted to the hospital. Frequent hand-washing with good technique is the most important factor in effective control of horizontal transmission of most pathogens.[4-6] **Hand hygiene is recommended before and after all patient contacts**, when moving from a contaminated to a clean body site on a single patient, after contact with any potentially contaminated fluid or environmental surfaces, and after glove removal. Gloves are not a substitute for hand hygiene. Wearing gloves is required when health care workers (HCWs) anticipate contact with body substances, mucous membranes, and nonintact skin of patients. Additional precautions such as gowns and eye/face protection (i.e., masks and goggles) are indicated when splashes of body substances or blood are possible. Standard precautions were developed not only for the prevention of transmission of blood-borne pathogens (e.g., HIV, hepatitis B, and hepatitis C) through percutaneous and mucous membrane contacts but also to protect against exposure to other pathogens.[3]

Transmission-based precautions include contact precautions, droplet precautions, and airborne precautions.[3] These are designed to control the spread of infectious organisms not adequately controlled by standard precautions alone. **Contact precautions** are recommended for patients infected or colonized with epidemiologically significant organisms that are transmitted by direct patient contact or by contact with items in the patient environment. The elements of contact precautions include wearing gowns and gloves when in a patient's room, using dedicated equipment that stays in the patient's room, and private room assignment or cohorting patients if private rooms are unavailable. Contact precautions should be used for patients with

419

MRSA and other multidrug-resistant pathogens. **Droplet precautions** are indicated for infections that are spread by large respiratory droplets, such as *Neisseria meningitidis*, *Haemophilus influenza*, and influenza virus. HCWs should wear surgical/isolation masks when entering the room of a patient on droplet precautions. **Airborne precautions** are indicated for infections spread by small airborne particles. Since these infectious particles can remain in the air for prolonged periods of time, negative-pressure ventilation rooms are required and HCWs must wear an N95 mask that can filter the small particles. Tuberculosis, measles, and chicken pox (varicella zoster virus) are common pathogens requiring airborne precautions. The CDC-Healthcare Infection Control Practices Advisory Committee (HICPAC) maintains an updated guideline for isolation precautions in hospitals that includes an appendix listing the type and duration of precautions needed for selected infections and conditions.[3] The type of precautions indicated for select clinically important pathogens is shown in Table 19-1.[3,7]

TABLE 19-1	ISOLATION PRECAUTIONS FOR SELECTED INFECTIONS AND CONDITIONS	
Infection/condition	Type	Precautions duration
Multidrug-resistant pathogens (MRSA, MDR-GNR)	Contact	CN
Clostridium difficile infection	Contact	DI
Conjunctivitis, acute viral (acute hemorrhagic)	Contact	DI
Epiglottitis due to *Haemophilus influenza*	Droplet	U (24 h)
Hepatitis A virus, diapered or incontinent patients	Contact	F[a]
Herpes simplex virus		
Encephalitis	Standard	
Mucocutaneous, disseminated or primary, severe	Contact	DI
Influenza	Droplet	DI
Seasonal influenza	Airborne	F[b]
Avian (H5N1) influenza	Droplet	DI
Pandemic influenza (2009 H1N1)		
Measles (rubeola), all presentations	Airborne	DI
Meningitis		
Haemophilus influenzae, known or suspected	Droplet	U (24 h)
Neisseria meningitidis, known or suspected	Droplet	U (24 h)
Other diagnosed bacterial	Standard	
Meningococcal pneumonia	Droplet	U (24 h)
Meningococcemia (meningococcal sepsis)	Droplet	U (24 h)
Pneumococcal diseases	Standard	

Parvovirus B19	Droplet	F[c]
Pertussis (whooping cough)	Droplet	U (5 d)
Rabies	Standard	
Respiratory syncytial virus infection, infants, young children, or immunocompromised adults	Contact	DI
Streptococcal disease (group A streptococcus), skin, wound, or burn		
Major (no dressing or uncontained drainage)	Contact	U (24 h)
Minor or limited (contained drainage)	Standard	
Tuberculosis		
Extrapulmonary, draining lesion (including scrofula)	Standard	
Extrapulmonary, meningitis	Standard	
Pulmonary or laryngeal disease, confirmed or suspected	Airborne	F[d]
Skin test positive, without evidence of pulmonary disease	Standard	
Varicella zoster virus[e]		
Varicella (chickenpox)	Airborne and contact	F[f]
Zoster		
Localized in immunocompromised patient, disseminated	Airborne and contact	F[e]
Localized in normal patient	Standard	
Wound infections		
Major (no dressing or uncontained drainage)	Contact	DI
Minor or limited (contained drainage)	Standard	

---

[a]Maintain precautions in infants and children younger than age 3 for duration of hospitalization; in children ages 3–14, for 2 weeks after onset of symptoms; for children over age 14, for 1 week after onset of symptoms.

[h]See http://www.cdc.gov/flu/avianflu/ for current avian influenza guidance. Accessed May 22, 2012.

[c]Maintain precautions for duration of hospitalization when chronic disease occurs in an immunocompromised patient. For patients with transient aplastic crisis or red cell crisis, maintain precautions for 7 d. Duration of precautions for immunosuppressed patients with persistently positive polymerase chain reaction test not defined, but transmission has occurred.

[d]Discontinue precautions ONLY when patient is on effective therapy, is improving clinically, AND has three consecutive negative sputum smears collected on different days; or tuberculosis is ruled out.

(continued)

TABLE 19-1	(CONTINUED)

[e]Maintain precautions until all lesions are crusted.

[f]Persons susceptible to varicella are at risk for varicella when exposed to patients with herpes zoster lesions or varicella and should not enter the room.

MDR-GNR multidrug-resistant gram negative rod.

MRSA, methicillin-resistant *Staphylococcus aureus*. Duration of precautions: CN, until off antibiotics and culture negative; DI, duration of illness; U, until time specified after initiation of effective therapy; F, see footnote.

Adapted from Siegel JD, Rhinehart E, Jackson J, Chiarello L. *2007 Guideline for Isolation Precautions: Preventing Transmission of Infectious Agents in Healthcare Settings*. Atlanta, GA: Centers for Disease Control and Prevention; 2007.

COMMON HAIs AND PREVENTION STRATEGIES

An important aspect of hospital infection control is the development of preventive strategies to curtail the acquisition and transmission of HAIs. **HAIs are generally defined as infections occurring more than 48 hours after hospital admission** (the definition might be changed by the type of HAI and the incubation period of causative pathogens). The most common types of HAIs are **central line–associated bloodstream infections**,[8,9] **catheter-associated urinary tract infections**,[10,11] **surgical site infections**,[12,13] **ventilator-associated pneumonia**,[14,15] and *C. difficile* infection.[16] These infections result in significantly increased costs, morbidity, and even mortality. Prevention of HAIs is extremely important since these are frequently caused by multidrug-resistant pathogens such as MRSA, vancomycin-resistant enterococci, multidrug-resistant gram-negative organisms, and *C. difficile*.[17] Besides meticulous hand hygiene and implementation of proper isolation precautions, there are detailed preventive strategies for each of these HAIs that are published as guidelines.

OCCUPATIONAL HEALTH AND INFECTION PREVENTION

Occupational health is closely linked to infection prevention. HCWs are at risk for being exposed to various types of infections during patient care. Prompt action may be necessary for assessment of a HCW exposed to infectious pathogens.

The most important strategy to protect HCWs from potentially infectious pathogens is prevention of the exposure. This is achieved through adherence to all advised standard and transmission-based precautions as outlined above.[3] In addition, **vaccination against certain pathogens is a crucial component** of an occupational health program. Vaccinations recommended for HCWs include measles/mumps/rubella, varicella, hepatitis B, pertussis, and influenza. Influenza vaccination of HCWs is an important method to prevent transmission of influenza to patients, by creating herd immunity in the health care environment and reducing the risk of HCW infection. HCWs should receive annual influenza vaccination unless they have a medical contraindication.[18-20] Among pathogens commonly seen in the setting of occupational exposure, blood-borne pathogens including hepatitis B virus (HBV), hepatitis C virus (HCV), and HIV are particularly important.[21,22] The risks for a HCW acquiring infection after a contaminated percutaneous exposure to HBV,

TABLE 19-2   POSTEXPOSURE PROPHYLAXIS FOR SELECTED ORGANISMS OR INFECTION

Infection or condition	Postexposure prophylaxis	Comments
Hepatitis B (known HBsAg-positive source)		
Percutaneous injury:		
Unvaccinated health care worker	HBIG × 1 and HBV vaccine series	If HBIG is indicated, it should be administered as soon as possible (preferably within 24 h)
Previously vaccinated:		
Known responder	No treatment	
Known nonresponder	HBIG × 2 (previously revaccinated) OR HBIG × 1 and initiate revaccination (not previously revaccinated)	
Antibody response unknown	Test exposed person for anti-HBsAb. If adequate HBsAb response (≥10 mIU/mL), no treatment; if inadequate HBsAb response (<10 mIU/mL), HBIG × 1 and vaccine booster	
HIV body substance exposure		
HIV positive, class 1 (asymptomatic or low viral load, <1,500 copies/mL):		
Less severe exposure (e.g., solid needle or superficial injury)	Basic two-drug postexposure prophylaxis[a]	For details of regimens for postexposure prophylaxis, see the guidelines from the CDC[c]
More severe exposure (e.g., hollow needle recently in vessel)	Expanded three-drug postexposure prophylaxis[b]	
HIV positive, class 2 (symptomatic, AIDS, acute seroconversion, known high viral load):		
Less severe exposure (e.g., solid needle or superficial injury)	Expanded three-drug postexposure prophylaxis[b]	

(continued)

TABLE 19-2 (CONTINUED)

More severe exposure (e.g., hollow needle recently in vessel)	Expanded three-drug postexposure prophylaxis[b]
Hepatitis C body substance exposure	No evidence of benefit of therapy (e.g., immunoglobulin or antiviral therapy) for postexposure prophylaxis; consider early treatment if seroconversion
Influenza virus	Consider giving influenza vaccination and antiviral agents (e.g., oseltamivir and zanamivir)	Vaccination should be considered for exposed nonimmune health care worker
		Chemoprophylaxis may vary by location, season, and drug susceptibility
Bordetella pertussis	Azithromycin 500 mg PO daily × 5 d or erythromycin 40 mg/kg PO daily (maximum 2 g/d) in four divided doses for 14 d	Does not require work restriction for exposed, asymptomatic health care worker
	For nonimmune health care worker, Tdap should also be given	For infected health care worker, they may return to work after receiving effective therapy for at least 5 d
Varicella zoster virus	Consider varicella virus vaccine within 3 d after exposure	Day 8–21 after exposure, nonimmune health care worker must not work or must not have direct patient contact and must work only with immune persons away from patient care areas
	For nonimmune immunocompromised health care worker, consider giving VZIG within 96 h after exposure	For health care workers who received IVIG, restrict work until day 28
		Giving the vaccine does not change the work restriction

Measles virus	For health care workers who have not received two doses of measles vaccine, consider giving MMR vaccine within 3 d after exposure	Day 5–21 after the exposure, nonimmune health care worker must be excluded from work setting Giving vaccine after exposure does not change work restriction
Rubella virus	No prophylaxis is recommended	Rubella vaccine or immunoglobulin is not proven to prevent infection after exposure Day 7–21 after exposure, nonimmune health care worker must not work or must not have direct patient contact and must work only with immune persons away from patient care areas
Mumps virus	No prophylaxis is recommended	Vaccine or immunoglobulin is not proven to prevent infection after exposure Day 12–26 after exposure, health care worker must not work or must not have direct patient contact and must work only with immune persons away from patient care areas
Meningococcal disease	Ciprofloxacin 20 mg/kg (maximum 500 mg) PO single dose or rifampin 10 mg/kg (maximum 600 mg) PO q12 h for 2 d or ceftriaxone 250 mg IM in a single dose	For pregnant health care worker, IM ceftriaxone should be used Local antimicrobial susceptibility for *N. meningitidis* should be checked since ciprofloxacin-resistant strains have been reported in the United States.

(continued)

TABLE 19-2 (CONTINUED)

[a]Two nucleoside reverse transcriptase inhibitors (NRTIs) OR one NRTI and one nucleotide reverse transcriptase inhibitor (NtRTI).

[b]Two NRTIs PLUS a protease inhibitor (PI) OR one NRTI and one NtRTI PLUS PI.

[c]Panilio AL, Cardo DM, Grohskopf LA, et al. Updated U.S. Public Health Service guidelines for the management of occupational exposures to HIV and recommendations for postexposure prophylaxis. *MMWR Recomm Rep.* 2005;54(RR-9):1-17.

HBsAg, hepatitis B surface antigen; HBIG, hepatitis B immunoglobulin; HBV, hepatitis B virus; HBsAb, hepatitis B surface antibody; Tdap, tetanus, diphtheria, and acellular pertussis vaccination; VZIG, varicella zoster immunoglobulin; IVIG, intravenous immunoglobulin; MMR, measles/mumps/rubella vaccination.

HCV, or HIV are approximately 30% (for an unvaccinated HCW), 3%, and 0.3%, respectively. High-risk exposures include those from an infected source with high viremia or exposures involving a large-bore hollow needle, deep puncture, or large amount of visible blood. When exposures occur despite all efforts at prevention, for some infections **postexposure prophylaxis** is available. Postexposure prophylaxis can include vaccination (e.g., HBV), use of infused immunoglobulin (IVIG) (e.g., HBV, varicella), and/or chemoprophylaxis with antimicrobials and antiviral agents (e.g., pertussis and influenza). The pathogens that require postexposure prophylaxis and the type of postexposure prophylaxis are shown in Table 19-2.[22]

REFERENCES

1. Klevens RM, Edwards JR, Richard CL, et al. Estimating health care-associated infections and deaths in U.S. hospitals, 2002. *Public Health Rep.* 2007;122:160-166.
2. Centers for Disease Control and Prevention. Healthcare-associated infections. http://www.cdc.gov/hai/. Accessed May 22, 2012.
3. Siegel JD, Rhinehart E, Jackson J, Chiarello L. *2007 Guideline for Isolation Precautions: Preventing Transmission of Infectious Agents in Healthcare Settings.* Atlanta, GA: Centers for Disease Control and Prevention; 2007. http://www.cdc.gov/hicpac/2007IP/2007isolation Precautions.html. Accessed May 22, 2012.
4. Centers for Disease Control and Prevention. Guideline for hand hygiene in health-care settings. Recommendations of the Healthcare Infection Control Practices Advisory Committee and the HICPAC/SHEA/APIC/IDSA Hand Hygiene Task Force. *MMWR Recomm Rep.* 2002;51(RR-16):1-45.
5. *WHO Guidelines on Hand Hygiene for Health Care.* Geneva: World Health Organization; 2009. http://whqlibdoc.who.int/publications/2009/9789241597906_eng.pdf. Accessed May 22, 2012.
6. Centers for Disease Control and Prevention. Hand hygiene training tools. http://www.cdc.gov/handhygiene/training.html. Accessed May 22, 2012.
7. Centers for Disease Control and Prevention. Information on avian influenza. http://www.cdc.gov/flu/avianflu/. Accessed May 22, 2012.
8. Marschall J, Mermel LA, Classen D, et al. Strategies to prevent central line-associated bloodstream infection in acute care hospitals. *Infect Control Hosp Epidemiol.* 2008;29:S22-S30.
9. O'Grady NP, Alexander M, Burns LA, et al. *Guidelines for prevention of intravascular catheter-related infections, 2011.* Atlanta, GA: Centers for Disease Control and Prevention; 2011. http://www.cdc.gov/hicpac/BSI/BSI-guidelines-2011.html. Accessed May 22, 2012.
10. Lo E, Nicolle L, Classen D, et al. Strategies to prevent catheter-associated urinary tract infections in acute care hospitals. *Infect Control Hosp Epidemiol.* 2008;29:S41-S50.
11. Gould CV, Umscheid CA, Agarwal RK, et al. *Guideline for Prevention of Catheter-Associated Urinary Tract Infections 2009.* Atlanta, GA: Centers for Disease Control and Prevention; 2009. http://www.cdc.gov/hicpac/cauti/002_cauti_toc.html. Accessed May 22, 2012.
12. Anderson DJ, Kaye KS, Classen D, et al. Strategies to prevent surgical site infections in acute care hospitals. *Infect Control Hosp Epidemiol.* 2008;29:S51-S61.
13. Mangram AJ, Horan TC, Pearson ML, et al. *Guideline for Prevention of Surgical Site Infection, 1999.* Atlanta, GA: Centers for Disease Control and Prevention; 1999. http://www.cdc.gov/hicpac/SSI/001_SSI.html. Accessed May 22, 2012.
14. Coffin SE, Klompas M, Classen D, et al. Strategies to prevent ventilator-associated pneumonia in acute care hospitals. *Infect Control Hosp Epidemiol.* 2008;29:S31-S40.
15. Tablan OC, Anderson LJ, Besser R, et al. Guidelines for preventing health-care-associated pneumonia, 2003: recommendations of CDC and the Healthcare Infection Control Practices Advisory Committee. *MMWR Recomm Rep.* 2004;53(RR-3):1-36.
16. Dubberke ER, Gerding DN, Classen D, et al. Strategies to prevent *Clostridium difficile* infections in acute care hospitals. *Infect Control Hosp Epidemiol.* 2008;29:S81-S92.

17. Siegel JD, Rhinehart E, Jackson J, Chiarello L. *Management of Multidrug-Resistant Organisms in Healthcare Settings, 2006.* Atlanta, GA: Centers for Disease Control and Prevention; 2006. http://www.cdc.gov/hicpac/mdro/mdro_toc.html. Accessed May 22, 2012.

18. Centers for Disease Control and Prevention. Prevention strategies for seasonal influenza in healthcare settings. http://www.cdc.gov/flu/professionals/infectioncontrol/healthcaresettings.htm. Accessed May 22, 2012.

19. Smith NM, Bresee JS, Shay DK, et al. Prevention and control of influenza: recommendations of the Advisory Committee on Immunization Practices (ACIP). *MMWR Recomm Rep.* 2006;55(RR-10):1-42.

20. Talbot TR, Babcock H, Caplan AL, et al. Revised SHEA position paper: influenza vaccination of healthcare personnel. *Infect Control Hosp Epidemiol.* 2010;31:987-995.

21. U.S. Public Health Service. Updated U.S. Public Health Service guidelines for the management of occupational exposures to HBV, HCV, and HIV and recommendations for postexposure prophylaxis. *MMWR Recomm Rep.* 2001;50(RR-11):1-52.

22. Panlilio AL, Cardo DM, Grohskopf LA, et al. Updated U.S. Public Health Service guidelines for the management of occupational exposures to HIV and recommendations for postexposure prophylaxis. *MMWR Recomm Rep.* 2005;54(RR-9):1-17.

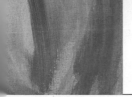

Antimicrobial Agents

20

David J. Ritchie and Nigar Kirmani

INTRODUCTION

This chapter highlights key information for antibacterials, antimycobacterials, antifungals, and antivirals and is intended to serve as a quick reference to assist prescribers in the clinical use and monitoring of the agents discussed. The content of this chapter is derived from numerous primary, secondary, and tertiary sources. Additional information on products mentioned in this chapter may be obtained from the American Hospital Formulary Service, the Physicians' Desk Reference, LexiDrugs PDA reference, The Pharmacological Basis of Therapeutics, relevant product package inserts, Drug Prescribing in Renal Failure: Dosing Guidelines for Adults and Children, Treatment Guidelines from the Medical Letter, and a variety of other print-based sources.[1-6]

Definitions used consistently throughout the chapter include CrCl, creatinine clearance; CVVHD, continuous venovenous hemodialysis; HD, hemodialysis; and PD, peritoneal dialysis.

ANTIBACTERIAL AGENTS

BETA-LACTAMS

The main adverse effects are gastrointestinal (GI) disturbances, hypersensitivity reactions, and phlebitis. Hematologic disturbances, seizures, electrolyte abnormalities, liver function test (LFT) abnormalities, and interstitial nephritis may also rarely occur. Patients receiving high doses of beta-lactams should have their neurologic status monitored continuously for the presence of seizure activity. Serum creatinine (Cr) should be periodically monitored to assess dosing appropriateness and for interstitial nephritis. Complete blood counts (CBCs) should also be monitored for evidence of bone marrow suppression, as should the appearance of the skin for evidence of rash. Serum electrolytes should also be periodically monitored, as electrolyte disturbances may occur.

PENICILLINS

Amoxicillin
Amoxicillin is similar in spectrum to ampicillin but is more active than ampicillin against *Salmonella* and less active against *Shigella*.

Dosing and Administration
The usual dosage range is 250 to 500 mg PO q8h or 500 to 875 mg PO q12h.

Renal dosing:
CrCl 10 to 50 mL/min: 250 to 500 mg q8-12h
CrCl <10 mL/min: 250 to 500 mg q24h
HD: 250 to 500 mg q24h, with the daily dose administered after dialysis on dialysis days
PD: 250 mg q12h
CVVHD: 250 to 500 mg q24h

Amoxicillin/Clavulanic Acid

The addition of clavulanic acid to amoxicillin extends the spectrum of amoxicillin to include beta-lactamase-producing strains of methicillin-sensitive *Staphylococcus aureus* (MSSA), enterococci, anaerobes, *Haemophilus influenzae*, *Moraxella catarrhalis*, and some gram-negative bacilli. This agent is an oral agent of choice for bite wound infections and for step-down therapy of polymicrobial infections not involving *Pseudomonas aeruginosa*, as the agent lacks coverage of this organism.

Dosing and Administration

The usual dosage range is (a) 250 to 500 mg q8h or 500 to 875 mg PO q12h of the oral tablets; (b) 90 mg/kg/d divided q12h of the suspension; or (c) 2,000 mg PO q12h of the Augmentin XR tablet formulation.
Renal dosing:
CrCl 15 to 30 mL/min: usual dose q12h
CrCl 5 to 15 mL/min: usual dose q24h
CrCl <5 mL/min: usual dose q48h
HD: 250 to 500 mg q24-48h, with the daily dose on dialysis days administered after dialysis
PD: 250 mg q12h
CVVHD: 250 to 500 mg q24h

Key Monitoring and Safety Information

The chewable tablets and oral suspension formulations contain aspartame and should thus be used cautiously in patients with phenylketonuria.

Ampicillin

Ampicillin is considered the drug of choice for treatment of infections caused by susceptible strains of enterococci and *Listeria monocytogenes*.

Dosing and Administration

The usual dosage range for IV ampicillin is 8 to 14 g/d administered in divided doses q3-6h or as a continuous infusion. The dose of oral ampicillin is 250 to 500 mg PO q6h.
Renal dosing:
CrCl of 10 to 50 mL/min: usual dose q6-8h
CrCl <10 mL/min: usual dose q12-24h
HD: 1 to 2 g IV q12-24h, with one of the daily doses on dialysis days administered after dialysis
PD: 250 mg to 2 g q12h
CVVHD: 1 to 2 g q6-12h

Ampicillin/Sulbactam

The addition of sulbactam to ampicillin extends or restores the spectrum of ampicillin to include beta-lactamase–producing strains of MSSA, enterococci, anaerobes,

H. influenzae, *M. catarrhalis*, and some gram-negative bacilli. The sulbactam component is also active against some strains of multidrug-resistant *Acinetobacter.*

Dosing and Administration
The usual dosage is 1.5 to 3 g IV q6h.
Renal dosing:
CrCl 15 to 29 mL/min: 1.5 to 3 g q12h
CrCl 5 to 14 mL/min: 1.5 to 3 g IV q24h
HD: 1.5 to 3 g IV q24h, with the daily dose on dialysis days administered after dialysis
PD: 1.5 to 3 g IV q24h
CVVHD: 1.5 to 3 g q8h

Dicloxacillin

Dicloxacillin is a drug of choice for treating minor MSSA infections, but the agent has minimal activity against enterococci and gram-negative bacteria.

Dosing and Administration
The usual dosage range is 125 to 500 mg q6h. No dosage adjustments are required in renal failure or dialysis.

Nafcillin

Nafcillin is a drug of choice for treating MSSA infections, but the agent has minimal activity against enterococci and gram-negative bacteria.

Dosing and Administration
The usual dosage range for IV nafcillin is 4 to 12 g/d. Dose reduction should be considered in patients with significant hepatic impairment. No dosage adjustments are required in renal failure or dialysis.

Key Monitoring and Safety Information
Nafcillin may be more prone to causing neutropenia than other penicillins.

Oxacillin

Oxacillin is a drug of choice for treating MSSA infections, but the agent has minimal activity against enterococci and gram-negative bacteria.

Dosing and Administration
The usual dosage range for IV oxacillin is 4 to 12 g/d. Dose reduction should be considered in patients with significant hepatic impairment. No dosage adjustments are required in renal failure or dialysis.

Key Monitoring and Safety Information
Oxacillin may be more prone to causing drug-induced hepatitis than other penicillins. LFTs should be obtained periodically to monitor for hepatic effects, especially in patients receiving ≥12 g/d.

Penicillin G

Penicillin G remains among the drugs of choice for syphilis, *Pasteurella multocida*, *Actinomyces*, and some anaerobic infections. Penicillin is the drug of choice for group A streptococcal pharyngitis and for prophylaxis of rheumatic fever and poststreptococcal glomerular nephritis.

Dosing and Administration

The usual dosage range for IV penicillin G is 12 to 30 million U/d administered in divided doses q2-4h or as a continuous infusion. The dose of oral penicillin VK is 250 to 500 mg q6h. The usual dose of procaine penicillin is 0.6 to 1.2 million U/d. The usual dose of benzathine penicillin is 1.2 to 2.4 million U administered intermittently.

Renal dosing:

CrCl 10 to 50 mL/min: 75% of the normal daily dose

CrCl <10 mL/min: 25% to 50% of the normal daily dose

HD: 2 to 3 million U/d, with one of the daily doses administered after dialysis on dialysis days

PD: 20% to 50% of the normal daily dose

CVVHD: 75% of the normal daily dose

Key Monitoring and Safety Information

Hyperkalemia (particularly with penicillin G potassium) and hypokalemia (with penicillin G sodium) may occur. Although the potassium salt is the more commonly used penicillin G preparation, the sodium salt is available and should be given in the setting of hyperkalemia or azotemia.

Piperacillin

The extended-spectrum penicillins, including piperacillin, have improved gram-negative activity over other penicillin derivatives, including antipseudomonal activity (typically when combined with an aminoglycoside). Piperacillin also has significant activity against enterococci and anaerobes.

Dosing and Administration

The usual dosage range for piperacillin is 2 to 4 g IV q4-6h.

Renal dosing:

CrCl 10 to 50 mL/min: 3 to 4 q6-12h

CrCl <10 mL/min: 3 to 4 g q12h

HD: 2 g q8h, with one of the daily doses on dialysis days administered after dialysis

PD: 2 g q12h

CVVHD: 2 to 4 g q6-12h

Piperacillin/Tazobactam

The addition of tazobactam to piperacillin enhances the spectrum of piperacillin to include beta-lactamase-producing strains of anaerobes, gram-negative bacilli, staphylococci, and enterococci.

Dosing and Administration

The usual dosage is 3.375 to 4.5 g IV q6h.

Renal dosing:

CrCl 10 to 50 mL/min: 2.25 g q6-8h

CrCl <10 mL/min: 2.25 g IV q8h

HD: 2.25 g q8h, with one of the daily doses on dialysis days administered after dialysis

PD: 4.5 g q12h

CVVHD: 4.5 g q8h

Ticarcillin/Clavulanate

The addition of clavulanate to ticarcillin enhances the spectrum of ticarcillin to include beta-lactamase-producing strains of anaerobes, gram-negative bacilli, and staphylococci. Ticarcillin/clavulanate is not as active as piperacillin/tazobactam against enterococci.

Dosing and Administration
The usual dosage is 3.1 g IV q4-6h.
> *Renal dosing:*
> CrCl 10 to 50 mL/min: 3.1 g q8-12h
> CrCl <10 mL/min: 2 g q12h
> HD: 2 to 3.1 g q12h, with one of the daily doses administered after dialysis on dialysis days
> PD: 3.1 g q12h
> CVVHD: 3.1 g q8-12h

Key Monitoring and Safety Information
Fluid overload may occur due to the substantial sodium load in the product. Platelet aggregation defects may also be more common with ticarcillin/clavulanate than other penicillins.

CARBAPENEMS

Carbapenems have an **extremely broad spectrum of activity** against most strains of anaerobes, gram-negative bacilli, and gram-positive cocci, including strains of these organisms that produce a variety of beta-lactamases. See specific coverage notes with each medication below.

Key Monitoring and Safety Information for All Carbapenems

Seizures may occur, particularly in patients with renal failure and prior central nervous system (CNS) disorders. Patients receiving carbapenems should have their neurologic status monitored continuously for the presence of seizure activity. Serum creatinine should be closely monitored to assess dosing appropriateness in an effort to decrease seizure risk. Patients allergic to penicillin may exhibit cross-hypersensitivity reactions with carbapenems. Coadministration of carbapenems with valproic acid may cause valproic acid serum levels to decline, which increases risk of breakthrough seizures.

Doripenem

Doripenem is slightly more potent than meropenem for *P. aeruginosa*, and doripenem susceptibility testing of *P. aeruginosa* strains resistant to other carbapenems is warranted. However, doripenem does **not** provide reliable coverage against methicillin-resistant *Staphylococcus aureus* (MRSA), *Enterococcus faecium*, and *Stenotrophomonas maltophilia*.

Dosing and Administration
The usual dose is 500 mg over 1 hour every 8 hours, but the drug is also being studied for use as sustained 3-hour infusions at doses higher than 500 mg.
> *Renal dosing:*
> CrCl 30 to 49 mL/min: 250 mg over 1 hour q8h
> CrCl 11 to 29 mL/min: 250 mg over 1 hour q12h
> CrCl ≤10 mL/min: No specific recommendations are available
> HD/PD/CVVHD: No specific recommendations are available

Key Monitoring and Safety Information
See introductory section on carbapenems.

Ertapenem

Ertapenem does **not** provide reliable coverage against *P. aeruginosa, Acinetobacter, enterococci*, MRSA, and *S. maltophilia* and is thus **not suitable for empiric therapy of nosocomial infections**.

Dosing and Administration
The usual dosage is 1 g IV q24h.
    Renal dosing:
    CrCl ≤30 mL/min: 500 mg q24h
    HD: 500 mg q24h, with the daily dose on dialysis days administered after each dialysis
    PD: 500 mg q24h
    CVVHD: 1 g q24h

Key Monitoring and Safety Information
See introductory section on carbapenems.

Imipenem/Cilastatin

Imipenem does **not** provide reliable coverage against MRSA, *E. faecium*, and *S. maltophilia*. Cilastatin is microbiologically inactive but is added to imipenem to prevent renal metabolism by dehydropeptidase I, thus increasing urinary levels of imipenem.

Dosing and Administration
The usual dosage is 500 mg IV q6h or 500 to 750 mg IM q12h.
    Renal dosing:
    See Table 20-1.
    HD: 250 to 500 mg q12h
    PD: 25% of the usual dose
    CVVHD: 500 mg q6h

Key Monitoring and Safety Information
See introductory section on carbapenems. Concomitant administration of imipenem and ganciclovir may result in an increased risk of seizures.

TABLE 20-1	IMIPENEM/CILASTATIN RENAL DOSING			
Body weight (kg)	**Creatinine clearance (mL/min)**			
	≥71	**41–70**	**21–40**	**6–20**
≥70	500 mg q6h	500 mg q8h	250 mg q6h	250 mg q12h
60	500 mg q8h	250 mg q6h	250 mg q8h	250 mg q12h
50	250 mg q6h	250 mg q6h	250 mg q8h	250 mg q12h
40	250 mg q6h	250 mg q8h	250 mg q12h	250 mg q12h
30	250 mg q8h	125 mg q6h	125 mg q8h	125 mg q12h

Meropenem

Compared with imipenem, meropenem has slightly more activity against gram-negative organisms and slightly less activity against gram-positive organisms. However, meropenem does **not** provide reliable coverage against MRSA, *E. faecium*, and *S. maltophilia*.

Dosing and Administration

Meropenem may be administered as an IV bolus or infusion over 30 minutes. The usual dose is 1 g q8h or 500 mg q6h for systemic infections and 2 g q8h for meningitis.
Renal dosing:
CrCl 10 to 50 mL/min: 1 to 2 g q12h
CrCl <10 mL/min: 1 to 2 g q24h
HD: 1 to 2 g q24h, with the daily dose given after dialysis on dialysis days
PD: 1 to 2 g q24h
CVVHD: 1 to 2 g q12h

Key Monitoring and Safety Information

See introductory section on carbapenems.

MONOBACTAMS

Aztreonam

Aztreonam possesses a clinically relevant spectrum of activity that encompasses **only gram-negative bacteria**, including many strains of *P. aeruginosa*. Aztreonam does not provide reliable coverage against gram-positive or anaerobic bacteria and is also not stable to (a) AmpC chromosomal cephalosporinases produced by *Enterobacter*, *Citrobacter freundii*, or *Serratia*; or (b) extended-spectrum plasmid-mediated beta-lactamases produced by *Klebsiella*, *Escherichia coli*, and many other gram-negative bacilli. A new inhalational formulation of aztreonam is available to improve respiratory symptoms in cystic fibrosis patients with *P. aeruginosa* airway infection.

Dosing and Administration

The usual dosage is 1 to 2 g IV q8h. The dose of the inhalational formulation is 75 mg three times daily (at least 4 hours apart) for 28 days.
Renal dosing:
CrCl 10 to 50 mL/min: 50% of the usual daily dose IV
CrCl <10 mL/min: 25% of the usual daily dose IV
HD: 1 g IV q24h, with the daily dose on dialysis days administered after dialysis
PD: 25% of the usual daily dose IV
CVVHD: 1 g IV q12h

Key Monitoring and Safety Information

In contrast to cephalosporins and carbapenems, aztreonam is considered safe to use in patients with a history of beta-lactam allergy, even of a serious nature. The new inhalational formulation is only minimally absorbed systemically, but necessitates bronchodilator pretreatment to minimize the likelihood of bronchospasm.

CEPHALOSPORINS

First-generation cephalosporins have activity against streptococci, MSSA, and many community-acquired *E. coli*, *Klebsiella* spp., and *Proteus* spp. These agents have limited activity against other enteric gram-negative rods and anaerobes. **Second-generation**

cephalosporins have expanded coverage against enteric gram-negative rods and anaerobes (cefotetan and cefoxitin only). **Third-generation cephalosporins** have even broader coverage against enteric aerobic gram-negative rods, and most retain good activity against streptococci. However, these agents are not reliable for treatment of organisms producing AmpC beta-lactamases regardless of the results of susceptibility testing. The **fourth-generation cephalosporin**, cefepime, provides the broadest spectrum of the cephalosporins against aerobic gram-negative bacilli, including *P. aeruginosa* and many gram-negative bacilli resistant to third-generation cephalosporins. The **fifth-generation cephalosporin**, ceftaroline, is the first beta-lactam available for clinical use in the United States with activity against MRSA.

All cephalosporins have been associated with anaphylaxis, interstitial nephritis, anemia, and leukopenia. All patients should be asked about penicillin or cephalosporin allergies. Patients allergic to penicillins have approximately a **10% incidence of a cross-hypersensitivity reaction** to cephalosporins. These agents should not be used in a patient with a reported allergy without prior skin testing or desensitization. Prolonged therapy (>2 weeks) is typically monitored with weekly serum creatinine and CBCs.

Patients receiving cephalosporins, particularly at high doses and in the presence of renal failure, should have their neurologic status monitored continuously for the presence of seizure activity. Serum creatinine should be periodically monitored to assess dosing appropriateness. CBCs should also be monitored for evidence of bone marrow suppression, as should the appearance of the skin for evidence of rash.

FIRST-GENERATION CEPHALOSPORINS

Cefazolin

Cefazolin possesses activity against streptococci, MSSA, and many *E. coli*, *Klebsiella* spp., and *Proteus* spp. Cefazolin does **not** have activity against MRSA, enterococci, *P. aeruginosa*, and many other gram-negative organisms that produce a variety of beta-lactamases.

Dosing and Administration
The usual dosage is 1 to 2 g IV q8h.
  Renal dosing:
  CrCl 10 to 50 mL/min: 1 g q12h
  CrCl <10 mL/min: 1 g q24h
  HD: 1 g q24h, with the daily dose on dialysis days administered after dialysis
  PD: 500 mg IV q12h
  CVVHD: 1 g q12h

Cephalexin
Dosing and Administration
The usual dosage is 250 to 500 mg PO q6h.
  Renal dosing:
  CrCl 10 to 50 mL/min: 250 to 500 mg q8-12h
  CrCl <10 mL/min: 250 to 500 mg q12-24h
  HD: 250 to 500 mg q12-24h, with one of the daily doses on dialysis days administered after dialysis
  PD: 250 to 500 mg q12-24h
  CVVHD: No specific recommendations are available

SECOND-GENERATION CEPHALOSPORINS

Cefaclor

Dosing and Administration

The usual dosage is 250 to 500 mg PO q8h for the standard-release preparation or 375 mg q12h for the extended-release preparation.

> *Renal dosing:*
> CrCl 10 to 50 mL/min: 50% to 100% of the usual daily dose
> CrCl <10 mL/min: 50% to 100% of the usual daily dosage
> HD: 250 mg q8h, with one of the daily doses on dialysis days administered after dialysis
> PD: 250 to 500 mg PO q8h
> CVVHD: 250 mg PO q8h

Key Monitoring and Safety Information

Cefaclor has been associated (0.5%) with serum sickness–like reactions, most commonly in children of age <6. Symptoms of this reaction include rash, arthritis, arthralgia, and fever usually occurring 2 to 11 days into therapy. Symptoms typically resolve within a few days after discontinuation.

Cefdinir

Dosing and Administration

The usual dosage is 600 mg PO q24h or 300 mg PO q12h.

> *Renal dosing:*
> CrCl 10 to 50 mL/min: 300 mg q24h
> CrCl <10 mL/min: 300 mg q48h
> HD: 300 mg q48h, with the daily dose on dialysis days administered after dialysis
> PD: 300 mg q48h
> CVVHD: No specific recommendations are available

Cefotetan

Cefotetan is classified chemically as a **cephamycin**. A unique aspect of cefotetan is its coverage against anaerobes, including *Bacteroides fragilis*. Cefotetan is also active against most extended-spectrum beta-lactamase (ESBL)–producing gram-negative bacteria, but clinical data supporting cefotetan treatment of serious infections caused by these organisms are lacking.

Dosing and Administration

The usual dosage is 1 to 2 g IV q12h.

> *Renal dosing:*
> CrCl 10 to 50 mL/min: 1 to 2 g q24h
> CrCl <10 mL/min: 1 to 2 g IV q48h
> HD: 1 g q24h, with the daily dose on dialysis days administered after dialysis
> PD: 1 g IV q24h
> CVVHD: 1 to 2 g q24h

Key Monitoring and Safety Information

Cefotetan may cause bleeding and the disulfiram reaction (when administered concomitantly with alcohol) due to an *N*-methylthiotetrazole side chain contained on the molecule.

Cefoxitin

Cefoxitin is classified chemically as a **cephamycin**. A unique aspect of cefoxitin is its coverage against anaerobes, including *B. fragilis*. Cefoxitin is also active against most ESBL-producing gram-negative bacteria, but clinical data supporting treatment of serious infections caused by these organisms are lacking.

Dosing and Administration
The usual dosage is 1 to 2 g IV q6-8h.
   Renal failure:
   CrCl 10 to 50 mL/min: 1 to 2 g q8-12h
   CrCl <10 mL/min: 1 to 2 g q24-48h
   HD: 1 g q24-48h, with the daily dose on dialysis days administered after dialysis
   PD: 1 g IV q24h
   CVVHD: 1 to 2 g q8-12h

Cefuroxime IV

Dosing and Administration
The usual dosage is 750 mg to 1.5 g IV q8h.
   Renal dosing:
   CrCl 10 to 50 mL/min: 750 mg to 1.5 g q8-12h
   CrCl ≤10 mL/min: 750 mg to 1.5 g q24h
   HD: 750 mg to 1.5 g q24h, with the daily dose on dialysis days administered after dialysis
   PD: 750 mg to 1.5 g q24h
   CVVHD: 1 g IV q12h

Cefuroxime Axetil PO

Dosing and Administration
The usual dosage is 250 to 500 mg PO q12h.
   Renal dosing:
   CrCl 10 to 50 mL/min: 250 to 500 mg PO q12h
   CrCl ≤10 mL/min: 250 to 500 mg PO q12h
   HD: 250 to 500 mg PO q12h, with one of the daily doses on dialysis days administered after dialysis
   PD: 250 to 500 mg PO q12h
   CVVHD: No specific recommendations are available

THIRD-GENERATION CEPHALOSPORINS

Cefditoren Pivoxil

Dosing and Administration
The usual dosage is 200 to 400 mg PO q12h with food.
   Renal dosing:
   CrCl 10 to 50 mL/min: 200 mg q12-24h
   CrCl <10 mL/min: 200 mg q24h
   HD: 200 mg q24h
   PD: No specific recommendations are available
   CVVHD: No specific recommendations are available

Key Monitoring and Safety Information
Cefditoren decreases serum levels of carnitine, the clinical significance of which is unknown. However, carnitine levels normalize after 7 to 10 days. The tablets are also formulated with sodium caseinate (milk protein), and patients with a history of milk protein sensitivity should not receive cefditoren tablets.

Cefixime

Dosing and Administration
The usual dosage is 400 mg PO q24h or 200 mg PO q12h.
> *Renal dosing:*
> CrCl 21 to 60 mL/min: 300 mg q24h
> CrCl <20 mL/min: 200 mg q24h
> HD: 300 mg q24h, with the daily dose on dialysis days administered after dialysis
> PD: 200 mg PO q24h
> CVVHD: No specific recommendations are available

Key Monitoring and Safety Information
Cefiixime is 30% to 50% absorbed orally and has a diarrhea rate of up to 27%.

Cefotaxime

Cefotaxime is a drug of choice for **community-acquired pneumonia**. The drug is also established for treatment of bacterial **meningitis** and is an empiric drug of choice in this setting.

Dosing and Administration
The usual dosage is 1 g IV q6-8h for most infections and 2 g q4h for treatment of meningitis
> *Renal dosing:*
> CrCl 10 to 50 mL/min: 1 to 2 g q6-12h
> CrCl <10 mL/min: 1 to 2 g q24h
> HD: 1 g q24h, with the daily dose on dialysis days administered after dialysis
> PD: 1 g q24h
> CVVHD: 1 g q12h

Cefpodoxime Proxetil

Dosing and Administration
The usual dosage is 100 to 400 mg PO q12h.
> *Renal dosing:*
> CrCl 10 to 50 mL/min: 100 to 400 mg q24h
> CrCl <10 mL/min: 100 to 400 mg q24h
> HD: 100 to 400 mg q24-48h, with the daily dose on dialysis days administered after dialysis
> PD: 100 to 400 mg PO q24h
> CVVHD: No specific recommendations are available

Ceftazidime

Ceftazidime possesses clinically important activity against *P. aeruginosa* and is a drug of choice for infections caused by this organism. Conversely, ceftazidime may be the least active cephalosporin against gram-positive bacteria.

Dosing and Administration

The usual dosage is 1 to 2 g q8h for most infections and 2 g q8h for treatment of gram-negative meningitis.

> *Renal dosing:*
> CrCl 10 to 50 mL/min: 1 to 2 g q12-24h
> CrCl <10 mL/min: 1 to 2 g q24h
> HD: 1 g q24-48h is recommended, with the daily dose on dialysis days administered after dialysis
> PD: 500 mg q24h
> CVVHD: 1 to 2 g q12h

Ceftriaxone

Ceftriaxone is a drug of choice for **community-acquired pneumonia**. The drug is also established for treatment of bacterial **meningitis** and is an empiric drug of choice in this setting. Ceftriaxone is the drug of choice for **gonorrhea**.

Dosing and Administration

The usual dosage is 1 to 2 g IV q24h for most infections and 2 g q12h for treatment of meningitis. No dosage adjustments are recommended in renal failure or dialysis.

Key Monitoring and Safety Information

Ceftriaxone may cause biliary sludging and stones due to its high extent of biliary excretion and resultant precipitation with bile salts. Due to its biliary excretion, ceftriaxone frequently causes diarrhea. Intravenous ceftriaxone and intravenous calcium-containing products should not be coadministered in neonates due to risk of lung and/or kidney precipitation of ceftriaxone-calcium salts.

FOURTH-GENERATION CEPHALOSPORIN

Cefepime

Cefepime possesses clinically important activity against streptococci, MSSA, and gram-negative bacilli, including *P. aeruginosa* and other AmpC beta-lactamase-producing strains.

Dosing and Administration

The usual dosage is 1 to 2 g q8-12h for most infections and 2 g q8h for use in febrile neutropenia.

> *Renal dosing:*
> CrCl 10 to 50 mL/min: 1 to 2 g q24h
> CrCl <10 mL/min: 500 mg to 1 g q24h
> HD: 500 mg to 1 g q24h, with the daily dose on dialysis days administered after dialysis or 2 g after each thrice-weekly regular dialysis session
> PD: 500 mg to 1 g q24h
> CVVHD: 1 to 2 g q12h

FIFTH-GENERATION CEPHALOSPORIN

Ceftaroline

Ceftaroline is the first beta-lactam antibiotic to have clinically useful activity against MRSA, and is U.S. FDA-approved for skin and skin structure infections caused by this organism. Ceftaroline is also active against many drug-resistant pneumococci and is U.S. FDA-approved for treatment of community-acquired pneumonia. However, ceftaroline is not active against gram-negative bacteria producing ESBLs, AmpC beta-lactamase (including *P. aeruginosa*), or class A or B carbapenemases (including *Klebsiella pneumoniae* carbapenemases).

Dosing and Administration
The usual dosage is 600 mg IV q12h.
> *Renal dosing:*
> CrCl 30 to 49 mL/min: 400 mg q12h
> CrCl 15 to 29 mL/min: 300 mg q12h
> CrCl ≤14 mL/min: 200 mg q12h
> HD: 200 mg q12h, with one of the daily doses given after dialysis on dialysis days
> PD: No specific recommendations are available
> CVVHD: No specific recommendations are available

Key Monitoring and Safety Information
Ceftaroline appears to have a safety profile that is consistent with other cephalosporins. The drug was associated with more positive direct Coomb's test results than ceftriaxone in clinical trials, but no cases of hemolytic anemia occurred in these same studies.

MACROLIDES AND AZALIDES

Macrolides and azalides possess activity against many typical and atypical community respiratory tract pathogens, including *Streptococcus pneumoniae*, *Mycoplasma pneumoniae*, *Chlamydia pneumoniae*, and *Legionella pneumophila*. In addition, clarithromycin and azithromycin provide coverage against *H. influenzae* as well as *Mycobacterium avium* complex (MAC) infections. Adverse effects include GI disturbances, elevations in LFT and hepatic dysfunction, IV site reactions, rash, and, rarely, ototoxicity at high sustained doses.

Azithromycin

In addition to its activity against typical and atypical community respiratory tract pathogens, azithromycin is therapeutically useful for treatment of MAC infection and some sexually transmitted infections (STIs) including chlamydia, gonorrhea, pelvic inflammatory disease, and chancroid.

Dosing and Administration
The usual dosage is 250 to 500 mg PO q24h or 500 mg IV q24h. Dosage adjustments are not required for renal failure or dialysis.

Key Monitoring and Safety Information
See introductory paragraph in macrolide/azalide section. Unlike erythromycin and clarithromycin, **azithromycin does not inhibit cytochrome P450** hepatic enzymes and is not associated with drug interactions involving this mechanism. Azithromycin is **pregnancy category B** and has been safely used in pregnant women.

Clarithromycin

In addition to its activity against typical and atypical community respiratory tract pathogens, clarithromycin is also therapeutically useful for treatment of MAC infection and *Helicobacter pylori*–associated peptic ulcer disease.

Dosing and Administration

The usual dosage is 250 to 500 mg PO q12h or 1,000 mg PO q24h for the extended-release formulation.

> *Renal dosing:*
> CrCl 10 to 50 mL/min: 250 to 500 mg q12-24h
> CrCl <10 mL/min: 250 to 500 mg q24h
> HD: 250 to 500 mg q24h, with the daily dose on dialysis days administered after dialysis
> PD: 250 to 500 mg q12-24h
> CVVHD: 250 to 500 mg q12-24h

Key Monitoring and Safety Information

See introductory paragraph in macrolide/azalide section. Clarithromycin is **a significant inhibitor of hepatic cytochrome P450** enzymes and can increase serum levels of carbamazepine, HMG-CoA reductase inhibitors, cyclosporine, tacrolimus, theophylline, warfarin, ergotamine, dihydroergotamine, triazolam, and likely many other drugs. Clarithromycin is **pregnancy category C** and should be avoided in pregnancy.

Erythromycin

Erythromycin does **not** provide reliable coverage against *H. influenzae*, but it does possess clinically useful activity against *Chlamydia trachomatis* and *Campylobacter.*

Dosing and Administration

The usual dosage of erythromycin is 250 to 500 mg PO q6h (base, estolate, stearate), 333 mg PO q8h (base), or 400 mg PO q6h (ethylsuccinate). The usual IV dose of erythromycin lactobionate is 500 mg to 1 g IV q6h. Dosage reduction in patients with hepatic failure may be advisable. Dosage reduction is not required in renal failure or dialysis.

Key Monitoring and Safety Information

See introductory paragraph in macrolide/azalide section. Erythromycin is **a significant inhibitor of hepatic cytochrome P450** enzymes and can increase serum levels of carbamazepine, HMG-CoA reductase inhibitors, cyclosporine, tacrolimus, theophylline, warfarin, ergotamine, dihydroergotamine, triazolam, and possibly many other drugs.

AMINOGLYCOSIDES

Aminoglycosides are commonly used in severe infections caused by gram-negative aerobes as adjunctive agents and may also be used to provide synergistic activity with beta-lactams or vancomycin in the treatment of severe gram-positive infections. These agents have diminished activity in the low-pH/low-oxygen environment of abscesses and do not have activity against anaerobes. Use of these antibiotics is limited by **significant nephrotoxicity and ototoxicity**. Resistance to one aminoglycoside is not routinely associated with resistance to all members of this class.

Traditional dosing of aminoglycosides is q8h, with the upper end of the dose range reserved for life-threatening infections. **Peak and trough levels** should be obtained with the third or fourth dose and then every 3 to 4 days along with a serum creatinine. Increasing serum creatinine or peaks/troughs out of the acceptable range require immediate attention. Traditional dosing should be used for pregnant patients and in patients with endocarditis, burns covering >20% of the body, cystic fibrosis, anasarca, and CrCl <20 mL/min.

Extended-interval dosing of aminoglycosides is an alternative method of administration. A drug concentration is obtained 6 to 14 hours after the first dose, and a nomogram (Figure 20-1) is consulted to determine the subsequent dosing interval. Monitoring includes obtaining another drug concentration 6 to 14 hours after a dose every week and a serum creatinine thrice weekly. In patients who are not responding to therapy, a 12-hour level should be checked. If that 12-hour level is undetectable, extended-interval dosing should be abandoned in favor of traditional dosing. For obese patients (actual weight >20% above ideal body weight [IBW]), an obese dosing weight (ODW) should be used for determining doses in either traditional or extended-interval dosing as follows: ODW = IBW + 0.4 (actual weight – IBW). Large, infrequent dosing is not routinely recommended for use in pregnant patients, children, patients with severe renal insufficiency or renal failure, patients with cystic fibrosis, and patients with increased volume of distribution (e.g., anasarca and burn patients).

Key Monitoring and Safety Information for Aminoglycosides

Nephrotoxicity usually occurs after ≥5 days of therapy and is characterized by a reduction in glomerular filtration rate (GFR). Risk factors include hypotension, duration of therapy, associated liver disease, increased serum concentrations, advanced age, and coadministration of other nephrotoxic agents. The renal dysfunction noted is generally nonoliguric and is usually reversible with discontinuation of the agent. Serum creatinine should be monitored closely as well as serum drug levels, with the dose and frequency adjusted accordingly.

Ototoxicity associated with aminoglycosides is usually irreversible and may be vestibular or auditory. The hearing loss typically affects high-tone frequencies. Vestibular damage may manifest as nystagmus, vertigo, nausea, or vomiting. Aminoglycosides may also rarely cause neuromuscular blockade. Underlying conditions or the use of other medications that affect the neuromuscular junction enhances this effect. Hypokalemia and hypomagnesemia may also occur. Patients receiving aminoglycosides for extended periods (usually >14 days) should have baseline and regularly scheduled audiometric studies to assess for ototoxicity. Patients receiving other nephrotoxic or ototoxic agents should receive aminoglycosides with caution and be monitored closely.

Aminoglycosides can cause **fetal harm** when given to pregnant women. These agents are able to cross the placenta and may cause otologic damage. These agents should only be used during pregnancy if the potential benefits outweigh the possible risks to the fetus.

Amikacin

Amikacin has in vitro activity against a wide range of aerobic gram-negative bacilli, including some organisms resistant to other aminoglycosides. Amikacin is also useful in the treatment of infections caused by *Nocardia asteroides*, MAC, and certain species of rapid-growing mycobacteria (*Mycobacterium chelonae* and *Mycobacterium fortuitum*). As with other aminoglycosides, amikacin lacks activity against anaerobes and *S. maltophilia*.

Dosing and Administration

The usual multiple daily dose regimen is 5 to 7.5 mg/kg q8-12h. Serum peaks and troughs should be measured once the patient is at steady state. Serum **peaks** should be 20 to 30 µg/mL, with **troughs** of 5 to 10 µg/mL. Amikacin may also be given as 15 mg/kg doses administered infrequently. A random serum concentration should be checked 6 to 14 hours after the initial dose. The subsequent dosing interval should then be adjusted based on this random concentration using a nomogram (see Figure 20-1).

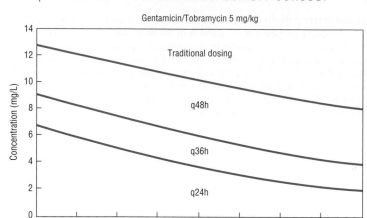

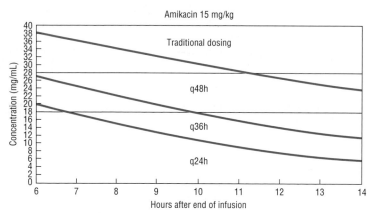

FIGURE 20-1 Nomograms for extended-interval aminoglycoside dosing.

Adapted from Reichley RM, Little JR, Bailey TC. Barnes-Jewish Hospital and Washington University School of Medicine.

Renal dosing:
CrCl 10 to 50 mL/min: 5 to 7.5 mg/kg q12-78h per levels
CrCl <10 mL/min: 5 to 7.5 mg/kg q48-72h per levels
HD: 2.5 to 7.5 mg/kg after dialysis on dialysis days only as per levels
PD: 5 to 7.5 mg/kg × 1, with serial level monitoring
CVVHD: 5 to 7.5 mg/kg q24-48h, with serial level monitoring

Key Monitoring and Safety Information
See introductory section on aminoglycosides, as well as dosing and administration section on page 441.

Gentamicin

Gentamicin is the most established and commonly used aminoglycoside for **adjunctive synergistic therapy with cell wall–active antibiotics in the treatment of serious gram-positive infections**.

Dosing and Administration

The usual multiple daily dose regimen is 1 to 1.7 mg/kg q8h. Serum peaks and troughs should be measured once the patient is at steady state. Serum **peaks** should be 3 to 5 μg/mL for gram-positive synergy and 6 to 10 μg/mL for gram-negative infections. **Troughs** should be <1 μg/mL. Gentamicin may also be given as 5 mg/kg doses administered infrequently. A random serum concentration should be checked 6 to 14 hours after the initial dose. The subsequent dosing interval should then be adjusted based on this random concentration using a nomogram (see Figure 20-1).

> *Renal dosing:*
> CrCl 10 to 50 mL/min: 1 to 1.7 mg/kg q12-48h per levels
> CrCl <10 mL/min: 1 to 1.7 mg/kg q48-72h per levels
> HD: 0.5 to 1.7 mg/kg after dialysis on dialysis days only as per levels
> PD: 1 to 1.7 mg/kg, with serial level monitoring
> CVVHD: 1 to 1.7 mg/kg q12-48h, with serial level monitoring

Key Monitoring and Safety Information

See introductory section on aminoglycosides, as well as dosing and administration section above.

Streptomycin

Streptomycin is used clinically as an alternative agent for TB, for synergistic therapy of enterococcal endocarditis in the setting of high-level gentamicin resistance, and for tularemia.

Dosing and Administration

Tuberculosis
> Daily therapy: 15 mg/kg/d (maximum, 1 g)
> Twice-weekly therapy: 25 to 30 mg/kg (maximum, 1.5 g)
> Thrice-weekly therapy: 25 to 30 mg/kg (maximum, 1.5 g)

Synergy for Endocarditis
15 mg/kg/d divided q12h in combination with cell wall–active agent (e.g., penicillin, ampicillin, and vancomycin)

Tularemia
15 mg/kg q12h
> *Renal dosing:*
> CrCl 10 to 50 mL/min: dose q24-72h per levels
> CrCl <10 mL/min: dose q72-96h per levels
> HD: 50% of the usual dose should be administered after dialysis on dialysis days only as per levels
> PD: Usual dose × 1, with serial level monitoring
> CVVHD: Usual dose q24-72h, with serial level monitoring

Key Monitoring and Safety Information

See introductory section on aminoglycosides. **Peaks** should be 20 to 35 µg/mL, and **troughs** should be <5 to 10 µg/mL. Intramuscular injections of streptomycin are often painful, and hot, tender masses may develop at sites of injection. The drug may also be administered IV.

Tobramycin

The activity of tobramycin against some strains of *Acinetobacter* spp. and *P. aeruginosa* may be greater than that of gentamicin.

Dosing and Administration

The usual multiple daily dose regimen is 1 to 1.7 mg/kg q8h. Serum peaks and troughs should be measured once the patient is at steady state. Serum **peaks** should be 6 to 10 µg/mL for gram-negative infections. **Troughs** should be <1 µg/mL. Tobramycin may also be given as 5 mg/kg doses administered infrequently. A random serum concentration should be checked 6 to 14 hours after the initial dose. The subsequent dosing interval should then be adjusted based on this random concentration using a nomogram (see Figure 20-1).

> *Renal dosing:*
> CrCl 10 to 50 mL/min: 1 to 1.7 mg/kg q24-48h per levels
> CrCl <10 mL/min: 1 to 1.7 mg/kg q48-72h per levels
> HD: 0.5 to 1.7 mg/kg after dialysis on dialysis days only as per levels
> PD: 1 to 1.7 mg/kg, with serial level monitoring
> CVVHD: 1 to 1.7 mg/kg q24-48h, with serial level monitoring

Key Monitoring and Safety Information

See introductory section on aminoglycosides, as well as dosing and administration section above.

FLUOROQUINOLONES

Fluoroquinolones are well absorbed orally, with serum levels that approach parenteral therapy. These agents are active against Enterobacteriaceae, but gram-positive activity is variable. While fluoroquinolones have activity against MSSA, they should be considered only when more traditional agents are contraindicated or inactive. Fluoroquinolones have activity against atypical community respiratory tract pathogens, but only moxifloxacin, gemifloxacin, and levofloxacin are considered reliable for pneumococcus.

Key Monitoring and Safety Information

The main adverse effects with fluoroquinolones include nausea, CNS disturbances (e.g., drowsiness, headache, restlessness, and dizziness, especially in the elderly), rashes, and phototoxicity. Patients should be counseled to use caution when performing tasks requiring alertness or coordination. Excess sunlight should also be avoided.

These agents can cause **prolongation of the QT interval** and should not be used in patients with known conduction abnormalities on ECG, patients with bradycardia, those with uncorrected hypokalemia, and those receiving class IA or

III antiarrhythmic agents. They should also be used with caution in patients receiving agents that may have an additive effect in prolonging the QT interval (e.g., erythromycin, antipsychotics, and tricyclic antidepressants [TCA]) and in patients with ongoing proarrhythmic conditions (e.g., significant bradycardia and acute myocardial ischemia). Patients at risk should be monitored closely with the use of ECGs. In patients with hepatic dysfunction or receiving other hepatotoxic drugs, LFTs should be monitored.

Fluoroquinolones should not be used routinely in patients aged <18 or in pregnant or lactating women. They can cause an age-related arthropathy and should be discontinued in patients who develop joint pain or tendinitis (most commonly the Achilles tendon), which may include the possibility of tendon rupture.

Aluminum- and magnesium-containing antacids, sucralfate, bismuth, oral iron, oral calcium, oral zinc, and enteral nutritional formulas can markedly impair absorption of oral quinolones when administered simultaneously. Staggering oral fluoroquinolone doses by at least 2 to 6 hours from these preparations is recommended.

Ciprofloxacin

Ciprofloxacin has in vitro activity against a wide range of gram-negative aerobes, including Enterobacteriaceae, *P. aeruginosa*, and other non-Enterobacteriaceae, although resistance is increasing. Ciprofloxacin is considered to be **the most clinically established oral antibiotic for treatment of *P. aeruginosa* infections**. However, it is relatively inactive against streptococci and anaerobes and therefore should not be used as monotherapy of community respiratory tract, skin, or abdominal infections.

Dosing and Administration
For most infections, an oral dose of 500 mg q12h may be used. For more severe or complicated infections, up to 750 mg q12h may be used. For uncomplicated acute cystitis, doses of 100 to 250 mg q12h or 500 mg qd of the extended-release formulation for 3 days have been used successfully. Duration of therapy depends on the type and severity of infection. The usual IV dose is 400 mg IV q12h. For more severe infections, doses of 400 mg q8h have been used.

Renal dosing:
CrCl <30 mL/min: 50% of the usual dose
HD: 200 to 250 mg q12h, with one of the daily doses administered after dialysis on dialysis days
PD: 200 to 250 mg q8h
CVVHD: 400 mg q24h

Key Monitoring and Safety Information
See introductory paragraph in fluoroquinolone section.

Gemifloxacin

Gemifloxacin's activity against *S. pneumoniae* is significantly greater than that of ciprofloxacin and levofloxacin and slightly better than that of moxifloxacin. This agent is not reliably active against *P. aeruginosa* and is only available orally, which limits inpatient usage.

Dosing and Administration

The usual dosage is 320 mg PO q24h.

  Renal dosing:
  CrCl 10 to 50 mL/min: 160 to 320 mg q24h
  CrCl <10 mL/min: 160 mg q24h
  HD: 160 mg q24h, with the daily dose given after dialysis on dialysis days
  PD: 160 mg q24h
  CVVHD: 160 to 320 mg q24h

Key Monitoring and Safety Information

See introductory paragraph in fluoroquinolone section. Skin rash occurs in 2.8% of patients, and approximately 10% of these cases are severe. The incidence of skin rash may be >15% in women under age 40 who receive 10 days of therapy. Women, patients under age 40, and postmenopausal women receiving hormone replacement therapy are at increased risk of rash.

Levofloxacin

Levofloxacin's activity against *S. pneumoniae* is greater than that of ciprofloxacin but less than that of gatifloxacin and moxifloxacin. Levofloxacin's activity against *P. aeruginosa* is inferior to that of ciprofloxacin. Levofloxacin is active against *C. trachomatis* and is an alternative treatment for this STI.

Dosing and Administration

The usual recommended dose is 500 mg IV or PO q24h. Doses of 750 mg q24h have been used for complicated skin and skin structure infections and pneumonia.

  Renal dosing:
  CrCl 20 to 49 mL/min: 500 to 750 mg × 1, then 250 to 500 mg q24h
  CrCl 10 to 19 mL/min: 500 to 750 mg × 1, then 250 to 500 mg q48h
  HD: 250 to 500 mg q48h
  PD: 250 to 500 mg q48h
  CVVHD: 500 mg q48h

Key Monitoring and Safety Information

See introductory paragraph in fluoroquinolone section.

Moxifloxacin

Moxifloxacin has activity against *S. pneumoniae*, which is greater than that of ciprofloxacin and levofloxacin. Moxifloxacin is not reliably active against *P. aeruginosa*. Moxifloxacin has clinically relevant activity against anaerobes, including *B. fragilis*, and is a monotherapy option for some abdominal infections. Moxifloxacin **should not be used for urinary tract infections** (UTIs) due to its minimal urinary excretion.

Dosing and Administration

The usual dose is 400 mg q24h. No dosage adjustments are required in renal failure or dialysis.

Key Monitoring and Safety Information

See introductory paragraph in fluoroquinolone section.

TETRACYCLINES AND GLYCYLCYCLINE

Doxycycline

Doxycycline is the treatment of choice for most rickettsial infections, including Rocky Mountain spotted fever and ehrlichiosis and can also be used to treat *Chlamydia*, *Mycoplasma*, syphilis, and outpatient community-acquired pneumonia. The drug may also be active against some multidrug-resistant gram-negative bacteria, including some *Acinetobacter* and *Klebsiella*, warranting susceptibility testing with this agent against such strains.

Dosing and Administration

The usual dose is 100 mg PO/IV q12h. No dosage adjustments are required in renal failure or dialysis.

Key Monitoring and Safety Information

GI disturbances and photosensitivity are common side effects. Esophageal ulceration, hepatic impairment, and pseudotumor cerebri may also occur. **Doxycycline should not be given to children because of its ability to discolor tooth enamel.** Doxycycline absorption may be decreased by concomitant administration with polyvalent metallic ions (e.g., magnesium, aluminum, and iron). Oral doxycycline should be administered with a full glass of water to decrease the possibility of esophageal ulceration. The drug is **pregnancy category D** and should be avoided in pregnancy. It is distributed in breast milk and should be avoided in nursing mothers.

Minocycline

Minocycline is used clinically for acne, nocardiosis, leprosy, and *Mycobacterium marinum* infections. The drug may also be active against some multidrug-resistant gram-negative bacteria, including some *Acinetobacter*, *Klebsiella*, and *Stenotrophomonas*, warranting susceptibility testing with this agent against these strains.

Dosing and Administration

The usual dose is 200 mg PO/IV × 1, then 100 mg PO/IV q12h. No dosage adjustment is required in renal failure or dialysis.

Key Monitoring and Safety Information

Vestibular disturbances occur more frequently with minocycline as compared with other tetracyclines. GI disturbances and photosensitivity are common side effects. Esophageal ulceration, hepatic impairment, and pseudotumor cerebri may also occur. Minocycline should not be given to children because of its ability to discolor tooth enamel. Minocycline absorption may be decreased by concomitant administration with polyvalent metallic ions (e.g., magnesium, aluminum, and iron). Oral minocycline should be administered with a full glass of water to decrease the possibility of esophageal ulceration. The drug is **pregnancy category D** and should be avoided in pregnancy. It is distributed in breast milk and should be avoided in nursing mothers.

Tigecycline

Tigecycline is a **glycylcycline** antibiotic that is U.S. FDA-approved for treatment of abdominal and skin/skin structure infections, as well as community-acquired pneumonia. The drug does not have activity against *P. aeruginosa* and has been shown to be **ineffective for ventilator-associated pneumonia** (VAP). The drug has also been associated with breakthrough bacteremias, which may be due to its very low blood concentrations. Tigecycline was also recently linked with **increased all-cause mortality across phase 3 and 4 clinical trials**. In vitro susceptibility to this agent should be documented as nonsusceptible strains have been reported.

Dosing and Administration
The usual dose is 100 mg × 1, then 50 mg q12h. The dose should be reduced to 100 mg × 1, then 25 mg q12h for severe hepatic failure. There are no dosage adjustments in renal failure or dialysis.

Key Monitoring and Safety Information
The most common adverse effects are nausea and vomiting, diarrhea, and headache. Hepatic dysfunction and pancreatitis may also occur. Patients allergic to tetracyclines may be cross-allergic to tigecycline. Tigecycline should not be given routinely to children because of its ability to discolor tooth enamel. The drug is **pregnancy category D** and should be avoided in pregnancy. It is likely distributed in breast milk and should be avoided in nursing mothers.

OTHER ANTIBACTERIALS

Nitrofurantoin

Nitrofurantoin is an oral antibiotic useful for uncomplicated UTIs. This drug has had a modest resurgence, as it is **frequently active against enterococci and *E. coli* that are resistant to other agents**. It has minimal activity against *P. aeruginosa*, *Serratia*, or *Proteus*. Nitrofurantoin should not be used for pyelonephritis or any other systemic infections due to its **poor systemic availability**.

Dosing and Administration
The usual dose is 50 to 100 mg qid for the macrocrystals and 100 mg q12h as the dual-release formulation. The drug should be avoided in patients with CrCl <60 mL/min, as these patients do not achieve adequate urinary concentrations and are at increased risk for toxicity.

Key Monitoring and Safety Information
Peripheral neuropathy, pulmonary reactions, hepatotoxicity, hemolytic anemia, brown urine, and rash may also occur. Probenecid and sulfinpyrazone may decrease the efficacy of nitrofurantoin by decreasing its renal elimination. Magnesium trisilicate antacids may decrease the absorption of nitrofurantoin. Although nitrofurantoin has been used for UTI suppressive therapy, this practice should be avoided because **prolonged therapy is associated with chronic pulmonary syndromes that can be fatal**. Although the drug is rated **pregnancy category B**, it should be avoided in pregnant women at term or when labor is imminent due to risk of hemolysis. It is also contraindicated in children aged <1 month due to hemolysis risk. The drug is distributed in breast milk.

Trimethoprim–Sulfamethoxazole

Trimethoprim–sulfamethoxazole (TMP-SMX) is a combination antibiotic (IV or PO) with a 1:5 ratio of TMP to SMX. This combination agent is commonly used for **uncomplicated UTIs** and is the **treatment of choice for *Pneumocystis jiroveci* pneumonia (PCP)**, ***Nocardia*, and *S. maltophilia* infections**. Many strains of MRSA are susceptible to TMP-SMX, but the drug is not reliably active against *Streptococcus pyogenes* and should, therefore, be avoided for uncomplicated cellulitis treatment.

Dosing and Administration

The usual dose is 160 mg TMP/800 mg SMX q12h. For PCP and other serious systemic infections, the dose is 15 mg/kg/d based on the TMP component.

Renal dosing:
CrCl 10 to 50 mL/min: Usual dose q12h
CrCl <10 mL/min: Usual dose q24h
HD: Dose q24h, with one of the usual daily doses on dialysis days administered after dialysis
PD: usual dose q24h
CVVHD: 2.5 to 10 mg/kg q12h

Key Monitoring and Safety Information

GI disturbances, hypersensitivity reactions, and hematologic abnormalities are common side effects. Headache, hepatitis, interstitial nephritis, hyperkalemia, and obstructive uropathy may also occur. TMP/SMX may cause a "pseudo" renal failure through **competition with serum creatinine for tubular secretion**. Isolated serum creatinine elevations in the absence of alteration in other renal function parameters should raise suspicion of this effect. TMP-SMX can increase the hypoprothrombinemic effect of warfarin. TMP-SMX can also potentiate the activity of phenytoin and oral hypoglycemic agents. Oral TMP-SMX should be administered with a full glass of water to decrease the possibility of crystalluria. The drug is **pregnancy category C** and should be avoided when possible in pregnancy, particularly during the third trimester, to minimize the possibility of kernicterus. It is distributed in breast milk and should be avoided in nursing mothers, particularly infants <2 months. If there is uncertainty with TMP/SMX dosing, serum concentrations of TMP/SMX can be monitored. Suggested serum peak concentrations of TMP and SMX are 5 to 15 and 100 to 150 µg/mL, respectively. Suggested serum trough concentrations of TMP and SMX are 2 to 8 and 75 to 120 µg/mL, respectively.

Clindamycin

Clindamycin has a predominantly gram-positive spectrum similar to that of erythromycin, with inclusion of **activity against most anaerobes**, including *B. fragilis*. Clindamycin also provides **activity against most community MRSA** isolates and is useful for treatment of minor–moderate infections caused by this organism. Clindamycin is also used for toxoplasmosis in combination with pyrimethamine and PCP in combination with primaquine, typically in sulfa-allergic patients. Metronidazole is more commonly used for intraabdominal infections due to its superior activity against *B. fragilis* relative to clindamycin.

Dosing and Administration

The usual dosage is 150 to 450 mg PO q6-8h or 300 to 900 mg IV q8h. No dosage adjustments are required in renal failure or dialysis.

Key Monitoring and Safety Information

GI disturbances (including *Clostridium difficile* **colitis**), elevations in LFTs, IV site reactions (with IV), and rash may occur. Clindamycin may enhance the activity of neuromuscular blockers and should be used cautiously in this setting.

Metronidazole

Metronidazole is more active against gram-negative versus gram-positive anaerobes, but does possess activity against *C. difficile* and *Clostridium perfringens*. **It is used as monotherapy to treat *C. difficile* colitis** and bacterial vaginosis. It is also commonly used in combination with other antibiotics to treat intraabdominal infections and brain abscesses, as well as *Giardia*, *Entamoeba histolytica*, and *Trichomonas vaginalis* infections.

Dosing and Administration

The usual dose is 250 to 500 mg PO/IV q6-12h. A single 2,000 mg dose may be used to treat trichomoniasis. Dosage reduction is suggested in severe hepatic failure. No dosage adjustments are required in renal failure or dialysis.

Key Monitoring and Safety Information

GI disturbances (e.g., nausea, vomiting, diarrhea, and dysgeusia), **disulfiram-like reactions** to alcohol, and mild CNS disturbances (headache, restlessness) may occur. Rarely, seizures and peripheral neuropathy may occur. Metronidazole can increase the procoagulant effects of warfarin. Concomitant administration of metronidazole with disulfiram may result in psychosis and confusion and should be avoided. **Alcohol ingestion should be avoided** with metronidazole and for 1 to 3 days after the last dose of the drug to prevent the disulfiram reaction.

Vancomycin

Vancomycin provides clinically useful activity against most important gram-positive pathogens, including streptococci, enterococci, MRSA, and drug-resistant pneumococci. This agent is still considered to be **a drug of choice for empiric therapy of suspected MRSA infection and remains a mainstay of therapy for treatment of gram-positive infections in beta-lactam-allergic patients**. In vitro susceptibility to this agent should be documented as nonsusceptible strains have been reported.

Dosing and Administration

The usual dose of vancomycin is 15 mg/kg of actual body weight IV q12h. Attempts should be made to limit daily doses of vancomycin to under 4 g/d, as **nephrotoxicity** risk increases beyond this limit.

> *Renal failure:*
> CrCl 10 to 50 mL/min: 15 mg/kg q24-96h per levels
> CrCl <10 mL/min: 15 mg/kg q96-168h per levels
> HD: 15 mg/kg after dialysis, with re-dosing when the concentration drops below 15 μg/mL
> PD: 15 mg/kg with re-dosing when the concentration drops below 15 μg/mL
> CVVHD: 15 mg/kg q24h with close serum level monitoring and dose titration

Key Monitoring and Safety Information

The main side effects of vancomycin are **phlebitis and rash**. **Ototoxicity and nephrotoxicity** can occur, and concurrent administration of vancomycin with other potentially nephrotoxic or ototoxic drugs may potentiate these side effects. Leukopenia and **red man syndrome** (flushing of the upper body with rapid administration of the drug) are other adverse effects.

Serum level monitoring is indicated in patients who are expected to receive ≥5 days of therapy. **Trough concentrations should be obtained one to two times weekly**. Patients with rapidly changing renal function may need more frequent serum level monitoring. Serum creatinine should also be regularly monitored to assess dosing appropriateness. Patients should also be queried about the possibility of hearing disturbances. **Doses should be adjusted to maintain the trough concentration between 10 and 20 µg/mL.** Trough concentrations <10 µg/mL are considered subtherapeutic, while trough concentrations >20 µg/mL and daily doses >4 g appear to be associated with increased nephrotoxicity.

Linezolid

Linezolid is broadly active against gram-positive bacteria, including streptococci, MSSA, MRSA, coagulase-negative staphylococci, and enterococci (including vancomycin-resistant enterococci [VRE]). The drug has emerged as a preferred agent for the treatment of hospital-acquired pneumonia (HAP) and VAP caused by MRSA. Linezolid also has unique activity against some mycobacteria and *Nocardia*. Linezolid has been associated with increased mortality in the treatment of IV line-related bacteremia and should be avoided in that setting. In vitro susceptibility to this agent should be documented as nonsusceptible strains have been reported.

Dosing and Administration

The recommended dose is 600 mg IV or PO q12h. No dosage adjustments are required in renal failure or dialysis.

Key Monitoring and Safety Information

Thrombocytopenia occurs commonly in patients receiving courses of >2 weeks. **Myelosuppression** (anemia, leukopenia, and pancytopenia) has also been reported. These hematologic parameters may return to pretreatment values following discontinuation of the drug. **Lactic acidosis** may occur, as can **peripheral and optic neuropathy** (especially with long-term use). Linezolid is a reversible, nonselective monoamine oxidase inhibitor. The consumption of large amounts of tyramine in the diet should be avoided while on linezolid to prevent possible elevations in blood pressure. Linezolid also has the **potential for interaction with adrenergic and serotonergic agents**, causing a reversible enhancement of the pressor response to agents such as dopamine or epinephrine and a risk of serotonin syndrome in patients receiving concomitant serotonergic agents, such as selective serotonin reuptake inhibitors and TCAs. CBCs should be monitored weekly in patients receiving linezolid. This is especially important in patients receiving this medication for durations >2 weeks, those with preexisting myelosuppression, and those receiving concomitant drugs that cause bone marrow suppression. Drug profiles should also be prospectively screened for potential drug interactions.

Daptomycin

Daptomycin, a **lipopeptide** antibiotic, is broadly active against gram-positive bacteria, including streptococci, MSSA, MRSA, and enterococci, including VRE. Daptomycin is a viable option for *S. aureus* bacteremia and endocarditis and has also emerged as **a preferred agent for treatment of serious VRE infections**. In vitro susceptibility to this agent should be documented as nonsusceptible strains have been reported. Daptomycin is bound by pulmonary surfactant and should not be used for the treatment of pneumonia.

Dosing and Administration

The usual dosage is 4 to 6 mg/kg IV q24h. Higher doses have been used but are not currently approved by the FDA.

Renal dosing:
CrCl <30 mL/min: 4 to 8 mg/kg q48h
HD: 4 to 8 mg/kg after each regular dialysis session
PD: 4 to 8 mg/kg q48h
CVVHD: 8 mg/kg q48h

Key Monitoring and Safety Information
Elevations in creatine phosphokinase (CPK) as well as muscle pain and weakness may occur, necessitating baseline and serial (weekly) monitoring of CPK. The drug should be discontinued in patients with unexplained myopathy and a CPK >1,000 U/L and in patients without muscle symptoms who have CPK >2,000 U/L. Daptomycin has also been recently associated with the development of eosinophilic pneumonia, and occurrence of new pulmonary symptoms during therapy should raise suspicion for the possibility of this adverse effect. Receipt of HMG-CoA reductase inhibitors in combination with daptomycin may increase the risk of myopathy and should be avoided if possible. Combined use of daptomycin and HMG-CoA reductase inhibitors necessitates more frequent CPK monitoring.

Telavancin

Telavancin is a **lipoglycopeptide** antibiotic that is **broadly active against gram-positive bacteria**, including streptococci, MSSA, MRSA, and heteroresistant vancomycin-intermediate *S. aureus*. The drug is not reliably active against VRE or vancomycin-resistant *S. aureus*. Telavancin is effective for complicated skin and skin structure infections, as well as HAP and VAP. The drug has also been anecdotally effective for bacteremia, bone and joint infections, and endocarditis.

Dosing and Administration
The usual dose is 10 mg/kg q24h.
Renal dosing:
CrCl 30 to 50 mL/min: 7.5 mg/kg q24h
CrCl 10 to 29 mL/min: 10 mg/kg q24h
CrCl <10 mL/min: No specific recommendations are available
HD: No specific recommendations are available, but a dose of 10 mg/kg after each thrice-weekly regular dialysis session has been utilized
PD/CVVHDF: No specific recommendations are available

Key Monitoring and Safety Information
The most common adverse effects are nausea and vomiting, taste disturbances, and foamy urine. Nephrotoxicity may also occur and warrants regular serum creatinine monitoring. Each dose should be administered over 1 hour to prevent red man syndrome. The drug is also associated with a minor QTc interval prolongation, which necessitates caution with combined use of other drugs that can prolong the QTc interval and avoidance of telavancin in patients with underlying cardiac conditions associated with risk of ventricular arrhythmias. Telavancin can also cause a drug-lab test interference by falsely prolonging the prothrombin time, international normalized ratio, activated partial thromboplastin time, activated clotting time, or coagulation-based factor Xa tests. These tests should be obtained immediately before or within 6 hour prior to the next dose of telavancin to minimize the possibility of this drug-lab test interference. Patients allergic to vancomycin may be cross-allergic to telavancin.

Quinupristin/Dalfopristin

Quinupristin/dalfopristin has activity against many **antibiotic-resistant gram-positive organisms**, including MRSA, *E. faecium*, and multidrug-resistant *S. pneumoniae*. The drug has minimal activity against *Enterococcus faecalis*. In vitro susceptibility to this agent should be documented as nonsusceptible strains have been reported.

Dosing and Administration

The recommended dose is 7.5 mg/kg IV q8-12h. Dosage reduction is suggested in severe hepatic failure. No dosage adjustments are required in renal failure or dialysis.

Key Monitoring and Safety Information

The main adverse effects are arthralgias and myalgias (which are frequent and often force discontinuation of therapy), IV site pain and thrombophlebitis (common when the drug is administered through the peripheral vein), and elevated LFTs. Quinupristin/dalfopristin is a significant inhibitor of CYP3A4 and can increase serum levels of drugs metabolized by that enzyme, including but not limited to carbamazepine, HMG-CoA reductase inhibitors, cyclosporine, tacrolimus, midazolam, triazolam, calcium channel blockers, and likely many other drugs.

Colistin

Colistin is a bactericidal **polypeptide** antibiotic that acts by disrupting the cell membrane of gram-negative bacteria. This drug has an **expanding role in the treatment of multiple drug-resistant gram-negative rods** (except *Proteus*, *Serratia*, *Providencia*, and *Burkholderia*). However, colistin **should only be given under guidance of an experienced clinician**, as parenteral therapy has significant CNS side effects and potential nephrotoxicity. Inhaled colistin is better tolerated with only mild upper airway irritation and has some efficacy as adjunctive therapy for *P. aeruginosa*. The drug is **not active against gram-positive bacteria**.

Dosing and Administration

The usual dose of colistin IV is 2.5 to 5 mg/kg/d divided into two to four doses, with a maximum dose of 5 mg/kg/d. The usual dose of inhaled colistin is 75 to 150 mg inhaled two to three times daily.
   Renal dosing:
   CrCl 50 to 80 mL/min: 2.5 to 3.8 mg/kg/d divided q12h
   CrCl 10 to 49 mL/min: 2.5 mg/kg/d divided q12h
   CrCl <10 mL/min: 1.5 mg/kg q36h
   HD: 2 mg/kg after each dialysis session
   PD: 0.75 to 1.5 mg/kg/d
   CVVHD: 2.5 mg/kg q48h

Key Monitoring and Safety Information

Nephrotoxicity, neurotoxicity (paresthesias, neuromuscular blockade), and **hypersensitivity reactions** are the most significant adverse effects, necessitating careful monitoring during therapy. Serum creatinine should be monitored daily early in therapy and at regular intervals for the duration of therapy. Ideally, colistin should not be coadministered with aminoglycosides, other known nephrotoxins, or neuromuscular blockers due to possible potentiation of toxicity.

Rifaximin

Rifaximin is an oral, **nonsystemic antibacterial agent** that is active against entero-toxigenic and enteroaggregative strains of *E. coli*. Rifaximin has not been shown to be effective in the treatment of GI infections due to *Campylobacter jejuni*, *Salmonella* spp., or *Shigella* spp.

Dosing and Administration
The usual dosage is 200 mg PO tid for 3 days.

Key Monitoring and Safety Information
GI disturbances and hypersensitivity reactions (i.e., rash and urticaria) may occur. Rifaximin does not have any in vivo drug interactions due to its lack of systemic absorption. Rifaximin is rated **pregnancy category C**.

ANTIMYCOBACTERIAL AGENTS

Ethambutol
Ethambutol (ETH) is used primarily for the treatment of TB and MAC infection.

Dosing and Administration
See Table 20-2.
> *Renal dosing:*
> CrCl 10 to 50 mL/min: dose q24-36h
> CrCl <10 mL/min: dose q48h
> HD: 15 to 20 mg/kg after each dialysis
> PD: 15 to 20 mg/kg q48h
> CVVHD: 15 to 20 mg/kg q24-36h

Key Monitoring and Safety Information
The primary adverse effect of ethambutol is a **dose-dependent optic neuritis**, which may manifest unilaterally or bilaterally as decreased red/green perception, decreased visual acuity, and visual field defects. At baseline, patients receiving ethambutol should have visual acuity and color perception tested. Vision should be tested monthly, with each eye tested separately. Ethambutol is not recommended in children in whom visual acuity cannot be monitored.

Isoniazid
Isoniazid (INH) is the mainstay of treatment and prevention of TB. Both MAC and *M. marinum* are resistant to isoniazid.

Dosing and Administration
For the treatment of *Mycobacterium tuberculosis*, the recommended daily dose is 5 mg/kg up to a maximum dose of 300 mg/d. For twice-weekly regimens, the recommended dose is 15 mg/kg/dose up to a maximum of 900 mg/dose. No dosage adjustments are required in renal failure or dialysis. The drug should be **avoided in severe liver disease**. Dosage reduction in milder forms of liver impairment may be warranted.

Key Monitoring and Safety Information
The incidence of **hepatitis with isoniazid increases with age and alcohol consumption**. Increases in transaminase levels may be seen, but these effects **generally do not necessitate holding the medication unless the transaminase levels are three to five**

TABLE 20-2	ETHAMBUTOL DOSING		
Dosing interval (mg/kg)	**Weight range (kg)**		
	40–55 (mg)	56–75 (mg)	76–90 (mg)
Daily mg	800	1,200	1,600[a]
3×/wk mg	1,200	2,000	2,400[a]
2×/wk mg	2,000	2,800	4,000[a]

[a]Maximum dose irrespective of body weight.

times the upper limit of normal. Baseline and monthly LFTs should be performed in patients receiving isoniazid. Patients should be monitored for signs and symptoms of liver toxicity, such as weakness, jaundice, dark urine, decrease in appetite, nausea, and vomiting. The hepatotoxicity of isoniazid may be increased by the concurrent administration of rifampin.

Peripheral and optic neuritis may also occur with isoniazid, necessitating monitoring for evidence of these effects (e.g., numbness, tingling, burning, pain in hands or feet, and blurred or loss of vision). These effects may occur more frequently in slow acetylators, patients with diabetes mellitus, and patients with poor nutrition. The concurrent administration of **pyridoxine** (vitamin B6) at doses of 25 to 50 mg PO qd may help avoid these toxicities. Other toxicities of isoniazid include hypersensitivity reactions (e.g., fever and rash), hematologic reactions (e.g., agranulocytosis, eosinophilia, thrombocytopenia, and anemia), arthritic symptoms, encephalopathy, and convulsions. Isoniazid has a direct inhibitory effect on peripheral and central dopa decarboxylase and can increase parkinsonian symptoms in patients taking levodopa. Isoniazid is distributed in breast milk. Breast-fed infants of isoniazid-treated mothers should be monitored for adverse effects.

Pyrazinamide

Pyrazinamide (PZA) is used clinically for the treatment of TB and is relied upon for its ability to shorten treatment regimens down to 6 months.

Dosing and Administration
See Table 20-3.
> *Renal dosing:*
> CrCl 10 to 50 mL/min: Usual dose q24h
> CrCl <10 mL/min: Usual dose q24-48h
> HD: 25 to 30 mg/kg three times weekly after dialysis
> PD: Usual dose q24h
> CVVHD: Usual dose q24h

Key Monitoring and Safety Information
A possible serious adverse effect of this agent is **hepatotoxicity** manifested as increases in serum aminotransferases, jaundice, hepatitis, fever, anorexia, malaise, liver tenderness, hepatomegaly, discolored urine and/or stools, or pruritus. Hepatotoxicity appears to be dose-related and may occur at any time during therapy. Patients with hepatic dysfunction or risk factors for chronic liver disease (e.g., previous hepatitis A or B infection, hepatosteatosis, alcohol or parenteral drug abuse, or other drugs associated

TABLE 20-3	PYRAZINAMIDE DOSING		
Dosing interval (g/kg)	**Weight range (kg)**		
	40–55 (g)	56–75 (g)	76–90 (g)
Daily g	1.0	1.5	2.0[a]
3×/wk g	1.5	2.5	3.0[a]
2×/wk g	2.0	3.0	4.0[a]

[a]Maximum dose irrespective of body weight.

with liver injury) may be at higher risk. Pyrazinamide also causes hyperuricemia by inhibiting the renal excretion of uric acid and should be avoided in patients with acute gout. Non-gout polyarthralgia has been reported to occur in up to 40% of patients receiving pyrazinamide. Baseline LFTs as well as uric acid concentration should be obtained before initiation of therapy. These lab tests should be repeated at periodic intervals and if clinical signs or symptoms of toxicity occur during treatment.

Rifampin

Rifampin (RIF) is active in vitro against a number of mycobacterial species, including *M. tuberculosis*, *Mycobacterium bovis*, *M. marinum*, *Mycobacterium kansasii*, and some strains of *Mycobacterium fortuitum*, *M. avium*, *Mycobacterium intracellulare*, and *Mycobacterium leprae*. The drug also has in vitro activity against many gram-positive bacteria, including *S. aureus* and *Bacillus anthracis*. In vitro activity is also seen against some gram-negative bacteria, including *Neisseria meningitidis*, *H. influenzae*, *Brucella melitensis*, and *L. pneumophila*.

Dosing and Administration
The usual dose of rifampin for the treatment of TB is 600 mg once daily IV or PO or 600 mg twice weekly as part of a multidrug therapy. A dose of 600 to 900 mg/d in divided doses is recommended for **synergistic use of rifampin for the treatment of staphylococcal prosthetic valve endocarditis**. No dosage adjustments are required in renal failure or dialysis. Dosage adjustment in severe hepatic failure should be considered.

Key Monitoring and Safety Information
The most common adverse effects of rifampin are GI disturbances. Rifampin may also cause increases in LFTs. **Hepatitis** and fatalities associated with jaundice have been reported in patients with preexisting liver disease or in those who have received concomitant hepatotoxic agents. Severe hepatic injuries have been reported in patients receiving rifampin in combination with pyrazinamide for the treatment of latent TB infections. Other hepatotoxic agents may potentiate the liver toxicity of rifampin and should be used with caution. Baseline LFTs should be performed and repeated periodically during therapy with rifampin to assess for hepatotoxicity. This may be especially important in patients receiving other agents with liver toxicity.

Thrombocytopenia, leukopenia, hemolytic anemia, hemolysis, hemoglobinuria, and decreased hemoglobin concentrations have occurred with rifampin therapy. Hypersensitivity reactions characterized by a flu-like syndrome have also occurred, as has renal failure. Edema of the face and extremities, hypotension, and shock have also been rarely reported. Red-orange discoloration of body fluids, including urine, sputum, sweat, and tears, occurs with rifampin. This may lead to permanent staining of soft contact lenses. A drug-induced lupus-like syndrome characterized by malaise, myalgias, arthritis, and peripheral edema has been reported in a few patients. Patients should be advised to take rifampin on an empty stomach either 1 hour before or 2 hours after a meal or antacids. However, if GI disturbances do occur, rifampin may be taken with a small amount of food.

Rifampin is **a potent inducer of cytochrome P4503A4** as well as 1A2, 2C9, 2C18, 2C19, and 2D6. Decreases in plasma concentrations are seen with some calcium channel blockers, methadone, digitalis, cyclosporine, corticosteroids, oral anticoagulants, haloperidol, theophylline, barbiturates, chloramphenicol, azole antifungal agents, oral or systemic hormonal contraceptive agents, various benzodiazepines, enalapril, some beta-blockers, doxycycline, levothyroxine, nortriptyline, tacrolimus, protease inhibitors, and nonnucleoside reverse transcriptase inhibitors. The patient's medication profile should be screened for potential drug interactions before rifampin is initiated.

ANTIFUNGAL AGENTS

AMPHOTERICIN B PREPARATIONS

Amphotericin B is active against a wide range of fungi, including yeasts and molds. In vitro activity is seen against *Aspergillus* spp., *Blastomyces dermatitidis*, *Coccidioides immitis*, *Cryptococcus neoformans*, *Histoplasma capsulatum*, *Paracoccidioides brasiliensis*, and most species of *Candida*. High minimal inhibitory concentration values and clinical resistance have been seen with *Pseudallescheria boydii*, *Fusarium* spp., *Candida lusitaniae*, *Trichosporon* spp., and, occasionally, with some isolates of *Candida krusei*, *Candida glabrata*, and *Aspergillus* spp. The drug is available as a conventional deoxycholate formulation and as three different lipid formulations, which have been designed to minimize toxicity while preserving the therapeutic efficacy of amphotericin B.

Infusion-related adverse effects may occur and include fever, chills, rigors, malaise, generalized aches, nausea, vomiting, and headache. Premedication with aspirin, ibuprofen, and acetaminophen may blunt response. Meperidine may be used to treat rigors but is ineffective as prophylaxis and should be used with caution in patients with decreased renal function. Antihistamines may also be useful due to the sedating effect. Other infusion-related adverse effects include hypotension, hypothermia, and bradycardia. Thrombophlebitis may also be seen at the site of infusion.

Decreases in GFR occur early during therapy and may occur in up to 80% of patients. Renal function may return to normal but may take months in some patients. This form of nephrotoxicity may be prevented with sodium loading. Pre- and posthydration with normal saline (500 to 1,000 mL) has been used. Tubular toxicity may also occur and is manifest as **hypokalemia, hypomagnesemia, and renal tubular acidosis**. Nephrotoxic agents (e.g., aminoglycosides, cyclosporine, tacrolimus, and pentamidine) may result in acute deterioration of renal function when given in combination with amphotericin B preparations. Agents causing electrolyte disturbances, such as hypokalemia seen with loop diuretics, should be used cautiously in patients being treated with amphotericin B. Electrolytes (especially potassium and magnesium) should be closely monitored during therapy. Hypokalemia induced by this antifungal agent may potentiate digitalis toxicity.

A normocytic, normochromic anemia may occur, which may not be seen until well after initiation of therapy. Ventricular arrhythmias have been seen in patients with hypokalemia, those receiving rapid infusions, and patients with renal failure. Neurotoxic effects include confusion, incoherence, delirium, depression, psychotic behavior, convulsions, tremors, blurred vision, and loss of hearing. Administration during pregnancy has resulted in increased serum creatinine levels in infants. Renal function should be closely monitored in neonates born to mothers who have received amphotericin B.

Amphotericin B Colloidal Dispersion

Amphotericin B colloidal dispersion (ABCD) is a complex of amphotericin B and cholesteryl sulfate in disc-like structures. In general, this drug is not as well-studied as other amphotericin B formulations.

Dosing and Administration

The usual recommended dose is 5 mg/kg IV once daily infused over ≥4 hours. No dosage adjustments are required in renal failure or dialysis.

Key Monitoring and Safety Information

See introductory paragraphs in amphotericin B preparations section. ABCD may be more prone to causing infusion-related reactions as compared with other lipid-based amphotericin B formulations. Hypoxia has also been associated with infusions of ABCD. Other toxicities that have been reported with ABCD include abnormalities in hepatic function, as manifested by elevations in alkaline phosphatase, conjugated bilirubin, and transaminases.

Amphotericin B Deoxycholate

Due to its increased toxicities relative to the lipid-based formulations of amphotericin B, **conventional amphotericin B use has been largely supplanted by lipid formulations** of the drug. However, conventional amphotericin B is still reasonably used for local administration, including continuous bladder irrigation or intravitreal injection.

Dosing and Administration

Usual daily doses are 0.5 to 1.0 mg/kg, with escalation from lower doses to higher doses at the start of therapy. Infusions should be over a period of ≥4 to 6 hours. No dosage adjustments are required in renal failure or dialysis.

Key Monitoring and Safety Information

See introductory paragraphs in amphotericin B preparations section. Conventional amphotericin B is the most toxic formulation of amphotericin B.

Amphotericin B Lipid Complex

Amphotericin B lipid complex (ABLC) consists of amphotericin B complexed to lipid bilayers that results in a ribbon structure.

Dosing and Administration

The recommended dose is 5 mg/kg/d IV at a rate of 2.5 mg/kg/h. No dosage adjustments are required in renal failure or dialysis.

Key Monitoring and Safety Information

See introductory paragraphs in amphotericin B preparations section. Other toxicities that have been reported with ABLC include abnormalities in hepatic function, as manifested by elevations in alkaline phosphatase, conjugated bilirubin, and transaminases.

Liposomal Amphotericin B

Liposomal amphotericin B (LAmB) is **the only true "liposomal" preparation** of the three lipid preparations available.

Dosing and Administration
The recommended dose of LAmB is 3 to 5 mg/kg/d for the treatment of systemic fungal infections. Infusions may be given over 1 hour. Doses of 3 mg/kg/d have been used for empiric therapy of suspected fungal infections in febrile neutropenia. No dosage adjustments are required in renal failure or dialysis.

Key Monitoring and Safety Information
See introductory paragraphs in amphotericin B preparations section. LAmB may be associated with **less frequent nephrotoxicity and infusion-related reactions** versus other amphotericin B formulations. Other toxicities that have been reported with LAmB include abnormalities in hepatic function, as manifested by elevations in alkaline phosphatase, conjugated bilirubin, and transaminases.

AZOLES

Fluconazole

Fluconazole is a triazole antifungal generally considered to be fungistatic, with its principal activity against *Candida* spp. and *Cryptococcus* spp. However, *C. krusei* is intrinsically resistant to fluconazole, and *C. glabrata* is considered to have dose-dependent sensitivity. Fluconazole does have activity against *C. immitis*, but it has limited activity against *H. capsulatum*, *B. dermatitidis*, and *Sporothrix schenckii* and no activity against *Aspergillus* spp. or other molds.

Dosing and Administration
The usual dosage is 100 to 400 mg/d. A single 150-mg oral dose is effective for vaginal candidiasis.
   Renal dosing:
   CrCl ≤50 mL/min: 50% of the usual daily dose q24h
   HD: 100% of the usual daily dose after each dialysis session or 50% of the usual daily dose administered daily (after dialysis session on dialysis days)
   PD: 50% of the usual daily dose q24h
   CVVHD: 100% of the usual daily dose q24h

Key Monitoring and Safety Information
Hepatitis, cholestasis, and fulminant hepatic failure have been reported to occur rarely in patients receiving fluconazole. Mild increases in LFTs have been reported to occur and are generally reversible. However, elevations to more than eight times the upper limit of normal also have been reported, as have rare fatalities. LFTs should be performed at baseline and monitored during prolonged courses of fluconazole.
   Fluconazole is a substrate of CYP3A4 isoenzyme and may also inhibit metabolism of other medications going through this isoenzyme. Rifampin has been shown to decrease the area under the curve (AUC) and half-life of fluconazole (25% and 20%, respectively). Use of these agents together may also increase the risk of hepatotoxicity. Fluconazole may also decrease the metabolism of TCAs, carbamazepine, certain benzodiazepines, warfarin, cyclosporine, tacrolimus, phenytoin, and oral sulfonylurea agents.
   According to the manufacturer, fluconazole is **pregnancy category C** and should only be used during pregnancy if the potential benefits outweigh the possible risks. Fluconazole is distributed into breast milk, with concentrations approaching those achieved in plasma. Because of this, it is recommended that fluconazole not be used in nursing women.

Itraconazole

Itraconazole is a triazole antifungal agent activity against clinically important *Aspergillus* spp. Itraconazole also has in vitro activity against *B. dermatitidis, H. capsulatum, C. immitis, S. schenckii,* and *C. neoformans.*

Dosing and Administration

The usual dose is 200 to 400 mg/d. During acute illness, loading doses of (a) 200 mg twice daily for four doses with the IV formulation or (b) 200 mg three times daily for the first 4 days with the PO formulation may be used. No dosage adjustments are required in renal failure or dialysis.

Key Monitoring and Safety Information

Serious **hepatotoxicity**, including liver failure, has been reported rarely in patients receiving triazole antifungal agents with or without preexisting liver disease. Congestive heart failure, peripheral edema, and pulmonary edema have been reported secondary to a dose-related negative inotropic effect. Hypokalemia ranging from mild to severe has also been reported in patients receiving IV and PO itraconazole for systemic fungal infections. Itraconazole **inhibits the metabolism of other drugs metabolized by the CYP3A4** isoenzyme. Concomitant use of itraconazole with quinidine or dofetilide is contraindicated due to potential increases in plasma concentrations of these agents leading to arrhythmias. Itraconazole is also contraindicated in patients receiving atorvastatin, lovastatin, and simvastatin due to the potential for rhabdomyolysis and in patients receiving certain benzodiazepines due to the potential for prolonged sedative and hypnotic effects. Itraconazole should be used with caution with other agents that are metabolized by CYP3A4 or with medications that may induce or inhibit the metabolism of itraconazole through effects on this isoenzyme. The medication profiles of patients receiving itraconazole should be carefully reviewed for potential drug interactions.

Itraconazole is rated **pregnancy category C** and should be used for the treatment of systemic fungal infections in pregnancy only when the benefits outweigh the risks to the fetus. Itraconazole is distributed into breast milk. Patients receiving oral itraconazole should have LFTs performed at baseline and at regular intervals throughout the course of therapy. Potassium levels should also be monitored due to the risk of hypokalemia. Monitoring of signs and symptoms of congestive heart failure should also occur in patients receiving prolonged courses of therapy or in those patients with predisposing risk factors.

Serum itraconazole **trough concentration monitoring is advised** to verify absorption and therapeutic levels. Desired trough concentrations are at least 0.5 to 1 µg/mL.

Posaconazole

Posaconazole is a triazole antifungal active against *Aspergillus* spp., including *Aspergillus flavus, Aspergillus fumigatus, Aspergillus niger,* and *Aspergillus terreus.* Posaconazole is also active against *Candida* spp., *C. neoformans, B. dermatitidis, C. immitis,* and *H. capsulatum.* Amongst the azole antifungals, **posaconazole is uniquely active against zygomycetes** and is the only oral antifungal with clinically relevant activity against this group of pathogens. Posaconazole is also effective for prophylaxis of invasive fungal infections in hematopoietic stem cell transplant recipients with graft-versus-host disease and in patients with hematologic malignancies experiencing prolonged neutropenia following chemotherapy.

Dosing and Administration

The usual dose for fungal infection prophylaxis is 200 mg three times daily. For treatment of serious fungal infections, the usual dose is 400 mg q12h or 200 mg q6h. No dosage adjustments are required in renal failure, dialysis, or hepatic failure.

Key Monitoring and Safety Information

Posaconazole is available as a suspension formulation. Each dose must be taken within 20 minutes of either a full meal or dose of a liquid nutritional supplement or an acidic carbonated beverage (e.g., ginger ale). Patients unable to ingest posaconazole with these concomitant meals/liquids should receive an alternate antifungal agent. Patients receiving posaconazole should have LFTs performed at baseline and at regular intervals, especially if a long course of therapy is undertaken, as **hepatotoxicity** may occur.

Despite the fact that posaconazole is **not metabolized by CYP450** enzymes, numerous drug interactions still exist due to its **effects on UDP-glucuronidation and p-glycoprotein efflux**. Rifabutin, phenytoin, cimetidine, and efavirenz significantly reduce posaconazole exposure and should not be coadministered unless benefit clearly outweighs risk. **Sirolimus is contraindicated** with posaconazole due to dramatically increased sirolimus exposure. **Cyclosporine and tacrolimus dose reduction to 75% and 33% of normal, respectively**, is recommended if these drugs are used with posaconazole. Posaconazole is also likely to interact with many other drugs, including ergot alkaloids, vinca alkaloids, certain HMG-CoA reductase inhibitors, certain calcium channel blockers, and digoxin. Monitoring for adverse effects of midazolam and protease inhibitors is required with concomitant posaconazole.

Posaconazole is **pregnancy category C** and should only be used during pregnancy if the potential benefits outweigh the possible risks.

Serum posaconazole **trough concentration monitoring** is advised to verify absorption and therapeutic levels. Desired trough concentrations are at least 0.5 to 1.5 µg/mL.

Voriconazole

Voriconazole is a triazole antifungal active against *Aspergillus* spp., including *A. flavus*, *A. fumigatus*, *A. niger*, and *A. terreus*. Voriconazole is also active against *Candida* spp., including *C. krusei*. In vitro activity is also seen against *C. neoformans*, *B. dermatitidis*, *C. immitis*, and *H. capsulatum*.

Dosing and Administration

For invasive aspergillosis and infections caused by *Fusarium* spp. and *Scedosporium apiospermum*, a loading dose of 6 mg/kg IV every 12 hours for two doses followed by 4 mg/kg IV every 12 hours is recommended by the manufacturer. Oral doses of 200 to 300 mg every 12 hours may be given once the patient is able to tolerate oral medications. Moderate renal impairment (CrCl of 30 to 50 mL/min) does not affect the pharmacokinetics of voriconazole. Accumulation of the IV excipient sulfobutyl ether beta-cyclodextrin sodium may occur in patients with moderate to severe renal failure. As a result, the IV formulation should not be used in patients with CrCl <50 mL/min unless the benefits outweigh the risks. In these circumstances, the oral formulation may be used instead. No pharmacokinetic-based dosage adjustments are required in renal failure or dialysis.

Key Monitoring and Safety Information

Transient visual disturbances, including blurred vision, changes in light perception, photophobia, and visual hallucinations, have been reported to occur in clinical trials. These may be dose-related and occur with the first few doses. Patients should be warned of the possible visual disturbances associated with the use of this agent. Other adverse events, as with other azoles, include **elevations in LFTs**, skin rash, and GI disturbances. Patients receiving voriconazole should have LFTs performed at baseline and at regular intervals, especially if a long course of therapy is undertaken, as hepatotoxicity may occur.

Voriconazole is both a **substrate and inhibitor of CYP2C9, 2C19, and 3A4** isoenzymes. Caution should be used when administering voriconazole with agents that are metabolized or inhibited/induced by the same pathways. Rifampin, rifabutin, and phenytoin have been shown to induce the metabolism of voriconazole. The metabolisms of cyclosporine, sirolimus, tacrolimus, warfarin, and omeprazole are inhibited by voriconazole. Monitoring for potential drug interactions should also be performed prospectively.

Voriconazole is rated **pregnancy category D** and can cause fetal harm if administered during pregnancy. Women becoming pregnant while receiving voriconazole should be informed of potential fetal risk.

Serum voriconazole **concentration monitoring** is advised to verify absorption and therapeutic levels. Desired trough concentrations are 0.5 to 2 µg/mL, and desired peak concentrations are 2 to 6 µg/mL.

ECHINOCANDINS

Anidulafungin

Anidulafungin is an echinocandin antifungal with in vitro activity against *Aspergillus* spp. as well as most *Candida* spp., although potency against *Candida parapsilosis* is less than for other *Candida* spp. Anidulafungin does **not** have clinically meaningful activity against *C. neoformans*, *Histoplasma*, *Blastomyces*, *Coccidioides*, and zygomycetes.

Dosing and Administration

The usual dose is 200 mg once, followed by 100 mg q24h. No dosage adjustments are recommended in renal failure or dialysis or in the setting of even severe hepatic failure.

Key Monitoring and Safety Information

To minimize risk of infusion-related reactions (e.g., rash, urticaria, flushing, dyspnea, and hypotension), the drug should be administered no quicker than 1.1 mg/min. Patients should be monitored for clinical evidence of hepatic dysfunction, including with periodic LFTs. Anidulafungin is not a significant substrate, inhibitor, or inducer of cytochrome P450 enzymes and is not expected to be associated with clinically relevant drug interactions occurring via this mechanism. Anidulafungin is **pregnancy category C**.

Caspofungin

Caspofungin is an echinocandin antifungal with in vitro activity against *Aspergillus* spp. as well as most *Candida* spp., although potency against *C. parapsilosis* is less than for other *Candida* spp. Caspofungin does **not** have clinically meaningful activity against *C. neoformans*, *Histoplasma*, *Blastomyces*, *Coccidioides*, and zygomycetes.

Dosing and Administration

Caspofungin is administered as a loading dose of 70 mg IV on day 1, followed by 50 mg IV daily thereafter. Infusions should be given over approximately 1 hour. No dosage adjustments are required in renal failure or dialysis. Patients with moderate hepatic insufficiency (Child-Pugh score 7 to 9) should receive the initial loading dose of 70 mg and then 35 mg IV daily thereafter.

Key Monitoring and Safety Information

Infusion-related reactions (i.e., pruritus, erythema, induration, and pain) and head-ache may occur. **Increases in LFTs** are the most commonly reported lab adverse effects. When administered concurrently with cyclosporine, the AUC of caspofungin has been reported to increase 35%. Due to elevations in LFTs observed with concurrent administration of cyclosporine, the manufacturer does not recommend coadministration. Reduced caspofungin levels have been observed with concomitant administration of enzyme inducers or mixed enzyme inducers/inhibitors. Reduced concentrations have been observed with efavirenz, nelfinavir, nevirapine, phenytoin, rifampin, dexamethasone, or carbamazepine. Caspofungin is **pregnancy category C**, and it is recommended to avoid its use in the first trimester. Patients should be monitored initially for allergic reactions as well as infusion-related toxicities. Patients should be monitored for clinical evidence of hepatic dysfunction, including with periodic LFTs.

Micafungin

Micafungin is an echinocandin antifungal with in vitro activity against *Aspergillus* spp. as well as most *Candida* spp., although potency against *C. parapsilosis* is less than for other *Candida* spp. Micafungin lacks clinically meaningful activity against *C. neoformans*, *Histoplasma*, *Blastomyces*, *Coccidioides*, and zygomycetes.

Dosing and Administration

The usual dose is 100 mg q24h. No dosage adjustments are recommended in renal failure or dialysis or in the setting of even severe hepatic failure.

Key Monitoring and Safety Information

To minimize risk of **infusion-related reactions** (e.g., rash, pruritis, and facial swelling), the drug should be administered over 1 hour. Patients should be monitored for clinical evidence of **hepatic dysfunction**, including with periodic LFTs. Micafungin is not a significant substrate, inhibitor, or inducer of most cytochrome P450 enzymes. But, it is a substrate for and weak inhibitor of cytochrome P4503A4. Clinically relevant drug interactions occurring as a result of this profile are unlikely. Micafungin is **pregnancy category C**.

OTHER ANTIFUNGALS

Flucytosine

Flucytosine is a fluorinated pyrimidine antifungal that is primarily used as **adjunctive therapy for cryptococcal meningitis**. The drug is also active in vitro against some strains of *C. albicans*, *C. glabrata*, *C. parapsilosis*, *C. tropicalis*, and *C. neoformans*, whereas *C. krusei* and *C. lusitaniae* are usually resistant. This agent is an **alternative treatment for candiduria**.

Dosing and Administration

The recommended dose is 100 mg/kg/d divided q6h.
> *Renal dosing:*
> CrCl 10 to 50 mL/min: 25 mg/kg q12-24h
> CrCl <10 mL/min: 25 mg/kg q24-48h
> HD: 25 mg/kg after each dialysis session
> PD: 0.5 to 1 g q24h
> CVVHD: 25 mg/kg q12-24h

Key Monitoring and Safety Information

Bone marrow suppression, including leukopenia and thrombocytopenia, is the main serious complication of flucytosine. This may occur more frequently in patients with peak concentrations >100 μg/mL. It may also occur more commonly in patients with underlying hematologic disorders, those with concurrent myelosuppression, or those receiving nephrotoxic agents that may decrease the clearance of flucytosine. Because of its effects on rapidly proliferating tissues, flucytosine may also cause **GI adverse effects**. Severe nausea, vomiting, diarrhea, and anorexia may occur. Elevations in LFTs may occur but appear to be dose-related and are generally reversible.

Nephrotoxic agents may decrease the renal clearance of flucytosine, leading to accumulation and toxicity. When given in combination with such agents, flucytosine **peak serum levels** should be monitored along with renal function, and dosage adjustments should be made accordingly. Peak serum levels should be obtained after the fifth dose. Concentrations of 25 to 100 μg/mL should be maintained. Peak serum levels should be monitored throughout therapy, especially in patients with signs of toxicity or a change in renal function or those with myelosuppression.

Flucytosine is rated **pregnancy category C** and should only be used in pregnancy when the potential benefits outweigh the possible risks. It is not known whether flucytosine is distributed into breast milk. Hematologic tests, renal function tests, and LFTs should be performed before and at frequent intervals during therapy.

ANTIVIRAL AGENTS

Antiretroviral agents used in the treatment of HIV disease are discussed in detail in Chapter 12.

GENERAL ANTIVIRALS

Acyclovir

Acyclovir's antiviral activity is limited to herpesviruses. Its greatest activity is against herpes simplex virus (HSV)-1, HSV-2, and varicella zoster virus (VZV).

Dosing and Administration

The usual dose is 200 to 800 mg three to five times daily or 5 to 10 mg/kg IV q8h.
   Renal dosing:
   CrCl 10 to 50 mL/min: Usual dose q12-24h
   CrCl <10 mL/min: 50% dose q24h
   HD: 50% dose q24h, with the daily dose administered after dialysis on dialysis days
   PD: 50% dose q24h
   CVVHD: 5 to 10 mg/kg q24h

Key Monitoring and Safety Information

Reversible **nephropathy** due to crystallization of the drug in the renal tubules is an uncommon adverse effect seen after IV administration. Preexisting renal insufficiency, dehydration, and bolus dosing may increase the risk of nephrotoxicity. This may be avoided by appropriately adjusting for renal dysfunction. **CNS toxicity** has been reported in the form of tremors, delirium, and seizures. This may be seen with high doses, in patients with impaired renal function, and in the elderly. **Phlebitis** has been associated with IV infusions. **GI disturbances** may be seen with valacyclovir and PO acyclovir. Acyclovir is distributed into breast milk, and concentrations may be higher than concurrent maternal plasma levels. Acyclovir should be used with caution in nursing mothers and only when clearly indicated. Renal function should be monitored at baseline and during therapy. Patients should also be monitored for seizure activity, especially those undergoing high-dose therapy, those with renal dysfunction, or those with a history of seizures.

Cidofovir

Cidofovir has in vitro and in vivo inhibitory activity against a broad spectrum of herpesviruses, including HSV-1, HSV-2, VZV, cytomegalovirus (CMV), Epstein-Barr virus (EBV), papillomaviruses, polyomaviruses, and adenoviruses.

Dosing and Administration

The induction dose of cidofovir is 5 mg/kg infused over 1 hour once weekly for 2 consecutive weeks. This is followed by a maintenance dose of 5 mg/kg infused over 1 hour once every other week. To reduce the risk of **nephrotoxicity, probenecid must be used concomitantly.** The recommended dose is 2 g 3 hours before the cidofovir dose, followed by 1-g doses administered at 2 and 8 hours after the completion of the infusion for a total dose of 4 g. Patients should also receive 1 L 0.9% sodium chloride over 1 to 2 hours immediately before each cidofovir infusion. For patients who can tolerate it, a second infusion of 1 L 0.9% sodium chloride should be initiated concomitantly with or immediately after the cidofovir dose and should be infused over 1 to 3 hours. **Cidofovir is contraindicated in patients with a serum creatinine of >1.5 mg/dL**, a CrCl of ≤55 mL/min, or a urine protein concentration ≥100 mg/dL. If renal function changes during therapy, the dose should be reduced to 3 mg/kg for an increase in serum creatinine of 0.3 to 0.4 mg/dL above baseline.

Key Monitoring and Safety Information

Dose-related **nephrotoxicity** is the principal side effect of IV cidofovir and is characterized by proteinuria, azotemia, glycosuria, and metabolic acidosis. Fanconi syndrome may also occur. Proteinuria may occur in up to 50% of patients receiving maintenance doses of 5 mg/kg every other week; elevated serum creatinine may occur in 15%. **Neutropenia** may occur in 20% of patients. Other adverse effects when combined with probenecid include fever, nausea, emesis, diarrhea, headache, rash, asthenia, anterior uveitis, and ocular hypotony. Topical application is associated with burning, pain, pruritus, and occasionally ulceration. Concurrent use of nephrotoxic agents increases the risk of nephrotoxicity. Cidofovir has mutagenic, gonadotoxic, embryotoxic, and teratogenic effects and is considered **a potential human carcinogen**. It may cause **infertility** in humans. It is unknown whether cidofovir is excreted in breast milk.

Serum creatinine concentration and urine protein should be determined within 48 hours before each dose. Proteinuria may be an early sign of nephrotoxicity. Due to neutropenia associated with cidofovir, it is recommended that leukocyte counts with differentials be monitored during therapy. It is also recommended that signs and symptoms of uveitis be monitored along with intraocular pressure and visual acuity.

Famciclovir

Famciclovir is converted to the active triphosphate form of penciclovir, which has activity against HSV-1, HSV-2, and VZV.

Dosing and Administration
The usual dose for treatment of HSV or VZV infection is 500 mg q8-12h. Chronic suppressive therapy doses are 125 to 250 mg q12h.

> *Renal dosing:*
> CrCl 10 to 50 mL/min: Usual dose q12-24h
> CrCl <10 mL/min: 50% dose q24h
> HD: 50% dose q24h, with the daily dose administered after dialysis on dialysis days
> PD: No specific recommendations are available
> CVVHD: No specific recommendations are available

Key Monitoring and Safety Information
Famciclovir appears to be well tolerated in both immunocompetent and immuno-compromised patients. The most common adverse effects reported include headache, nausea, and diarrhea, which are generally mild to moderate in severity.

Foscarnet

Foscarnet is active against HSV-1, HSV-2, VZV, and CMV. Because it does not require phosphorylation by thymidine kinase, **foscarnet remains active against many resistant strains of HSV and CMV.**

Dosing and Administration

CMV Retinitis
The recommended dose is 60 mg/kg infused over 1 hour q8h or 90 mg/kg infused over 1.5 to 2 hours q12h for 14 to 21 days. This induction regimen is followed by a maintenance regimen of 90 to 120 mg/kg/d infused over 2 hours.

Acyclovir-Resistant Mucocutaneous Herpes Simplex Virus
The recommended dose is 40 mg/kg q8-12h for 14 to 21 days.

Herpes Zoster in Immunocompromised Patients
The recommended dose is 40 mg/kg q8h for 10 to 21 days or until complete healing occurs. Higher doses of 60 mg/kg q8h have also been used.

> *Renal dosing:*
> See Tables 20-4 and 20-5.
> HD: 45 to 65 mg/kg/dose postdialysis (three times/wk)
> PD: 45 mg/kg q24h
> CVVHD: 60 mg/kg q24-48h

Key Monitoring and Safety Information
The major dose-limiting side effect of foscarnet is **nephrotoxicit**y with azotemia, mild proteinuria, and sometimes acute tubular necrosis. Renal function should be meticu-lously monitored during therapy and converted to creatinine clearance in mL/min/kg body weight to allow dosage adjustments to be made according to specific manufac-turer guidelines. Renal impairment usually begins during the second week of therapy and is reversible within 2 to 4 weeks after cessation of the medication in most patients. Concurrent administration with other nephrotoxic drugs (e.g., amphotericin B, cido-fovir, aminoglycosides, and IV pentamidine) may result in additive nephrotoxicity.

Metabolic abnormalities may include hypocalcemia or hypercalcemia, hypophos-phatemia or hyperphosphatemia, hypomagnesemia, and hypokalemia. Concurrent use with IV pentamidine also may increase the risk of hypocalcemia. Potential CNS side effects include headache, tremor, irritability, seizures, and hallucinations. Other side effects may include fever, rash, diarrhea, nausea, vomiting, abnormal LFTs,

TABLE 20-4	INDUCTION DOSING OF FOSCARNET IN PATIENTS WITH ABNORMAL RENAL FUNCTION			
	Herpes simplex virus		**Cytomegalovirus**	
CrCl in mL/min/kg	Equivalent mg/kg to 40 mg/kg q12h	Equivalent mg/kg to 40 mg/kg q8h	Equivalent mg/kg to 60 mg/kg q8h	Equivalent mg/kg to 90 mg/kg q12h
>1.4	40 q12h	40 q8h	60 q8h	90 q12h
>1–1.4	30 q12h	30 q8h	45 q8h	70 q12h
>0.8–1	20 q12h	35 q12h	50 q12h	50 q12h
>0.6–0.8	35 q24h	25 q12h	40 q12h	80 q24h
>0.5–0.6	25 q24h	40 q24h	60 q24h	60 q24h
≥0.4–0.5	20 q24h	35 q24h	50 q24h	50 q24h
<0.4	NR	NR	NR	NR

NR, not recommended.

anxiety, fatigue, and genital ulcerations. There are case reports of seizure activity with concomitant administration of foscarnet and ciprofloxacin.

Foscarnet should be administered by an infusion pump **at a rate not exceeding 1 mg/kg/min**. Patients should be **adequately hydrated** before and during administration to minimize the risk of nephrotoxicity. A total of 750 to 1,000 mL normal saline or 5% dextrose should be administered before the first dose. With additional doses of 90 to 120 mg/kg, 750 to 1,000 mL of fluid should be administered concurrently with each dose; 500 mL of fluid should be administered with each dose of 40 to 60 mg/kg. Renal function, electrolytes, and CBCs should be monitored at least two to three times a week during induction therapy and at least once every 1 to 2 weeks during maintenance therapy.

There are no adequate and well-controlled studies in pregnant women, and the drug should only be used when the potential benefits outweigh the potential risks. It is not known whether foscarnet is distributed in breast milk.

TABLE 20-5	MAINTENANCE DOSING OF FOSCARNET IN PATIENTS WITH ABNORMAL RENAL FUNCTION	
CrCl in mL/min/kg	**Equivalent mg/kg to 90 mg/kg once daily**	**Equivalent mg/kg to 120 mg/kg once daily**
>1.4	90 q24h	120 q24h
>1–1.4	70 q24h	90 q24h
>0.8–1	50 q24h	65 q24h
>0.6–0.8	80 q48h	105 q48h
>0.5–0.6	60 q48h	80 q48h
≥0.4–0.5	50 q48h	65 q48h
<0.4	NR	NR

NR, not recommended.

Ganciclovir

Ganciclovir is a **potent inhibitor of CMV replication**, with inhibitory concentrations 10- to >50-fold lower than acyclovir for CMV strains. Ganciclovir also has inhibitory activity against HSV-1, HSV-2, EBV, and VZV.

Dosing and Administration

For the treatment of CMV disease, the induction dose is 5 mg/kg q12h for 2 to 3 weeks, followed by a maintenance dose of 5 mg/kg/d IV; 6 mg/kg IV 5 d/wk; or 1,000 mg three times daily PO with food. **Ganciclovir implants** may also be used for the treatment of CMV retinitis. Each implant contains 4.5 mg of ganciclovir and is designed to release the drug over a 5- to 8-month period.

> *Renal dosing:*
> CrCl 10 to 50 mL/min: 25% to 50% dose q24h
> CrCl <10 mL/min: 25% dose three times weekly
> HD: 25% dose after each regular dialysis session (three times weekly)
> PD: 25% dose three times weekly
> CVVHD: 1.25 to 2.5 mg/kg q12-24h

Key Monitoring and Safety Information

Myelosuppression is the principal dose-limiting toxicity, with neutropenia occurring in 15% to 40% of patients and thrombocytopenia in 5% to 20%. These effects are usually reversible with drug cessation. Concomitant use with zidovudine may increase the risk of hematologic toxicity. Neutrophil counts and platelet counts should be monitored every 2 days during twice-daily dosing of ganciclovir and at least weekly thereafter. Neutrophil counts should be monitored daily in patients who have previously experienced leukopenia. Ganciclovir should not be administered if the absolute neutrophil count falls below 500 cells/mm^3 or if the platelet count falls below 25,000/mm^3.

Potential **CNS side effects** (e.g., headache, behavioral changes, convulsions, and coma) may occur in 5% to 15% of patients. Other side effects include infusion-related phlebitis, azotemia, anemia, rash, fever, LFT abnormalities, nausea, vomiting, and eosinophilia.

Ganciclovir is rated **pregnancy category C** and should be used only when potential benefit outweighs risk. It is not known whether ganciclovir is distributed in breast milk. Because of the potential for serious adverse reactions in breast-fed infants, it is recommended that nursing mothers discontinue nursing while they are receiving the drug and that they do not resume nursing until ≥72 hours after the last dose.

Valacyclovir

Valacyclovir is an acyclovir prodrug with antiviral activity limited to herpesviruses. Its greatest activity is against HSV-1, HSV-2, and VSV.

Dosing and Administration

The dose for treatment of herpes zoster infection is 1,000 mg PO q8h for 7 days. The dose for treatment of genital HSV infection is 1,000 mg PO q12h for 10 days for initial episodes and 500 mg PO qd for 5 days for recurrent episodes.

> *Renal dosing:*
> CrCl 10 to 50 mL/min: Usual dose q12-24h
> CrCl <10 mL/min: 500 mg q24h
> HD: 500 mg q24h, with the daily dose after dialysis on dialysis days
> PD: 500 mg q24h
> CVVHD: 500 mg q24h

TABLE 20-6	VALGANCICLOVIR RENAL DOSING	
CrCl (mL/min)	Induction dose	Maintenance dose
≥60	900 mg bid	900 mg qd
40–59	450 mg bid	450 mg qd
25–39	450 mg qd	450 mg q2d
10–24	450 mg q2d	450 mg twice weekly

Key Monitoring and Safety Information

Adverse effects are **similar to those noted with acyclovir**. Thrombotic thrombocytopenic purpura with hemolytic uremic syndrome has occurred in immunocompromised patients receiving high doses of valacyclovir. Renal function should be monitored at baseline and during therapy. Patients should also be monitored for seizure activity, especially those undergoing high-dose therapy, those with renal dysfunction, and those with a history of seizures.

Valganciclovir

Valganciclovir is a ganciclovir prodrug that is a potent inhibitor of CMV replication. Ganciclovir also has inhibitory activity against HSV-1, HSV-2, and VZV.

Dosing and Administration

For the treatment of active CMV retinitis in patients with normal renal function, the induction dose is 900 mg (two 450-mg tablets) twice daily for 21 days with food. After the induction dose, or in patients with inactive CMV retinitis, the recommended maintenance dosage is 900 mg once daily with food.

Renal dosing:

See Table 20-6.

HD/PD/CVVHD: It is recommended to avoid valganciclovir in these situations

Key Monitoring and Safety Information

Adverse effects are **similar to those noted with ganciclovir**. Other adverse effects associated with valganciclovir include diarrhea, nausea, vomiting, abdominal pain, headache, and pyrexia. Because valganciclovir is considered a **potential teratogen and carcinogen** in humans, caution should be observed in handling broken tablets. Tablets should not be broken or crushed, and direct contact of broken or crushed tablets should be avoided.

ANTI-INFLUENZA AGENTS

Oseltamivir

Oseltamivir is a **neuraminidase inhibitor that is active against both influenza A and B virus**.

Dosing and Administration

The recommended treatment dose of oseltamivir is 75 mg PO q12h for a total of 5 days. It should be **initiated within 48 hours of symptom onset**.

Renal dosing:
CrCl <30 mL/min: 75 mg q48h
HD: 30 mg three to four times weekly
PD: 30 mg one to two times weekly
CVVHD: 75 mg q12h

Key Monitoring and Safety Information

The main side effects are nausea and vomiting. These GI side effects usually occur after the first dose and resolve after 1 to 2 days with continued dosing. They may be reduced by taking oseltamivir with food. Oseltamivir should only be used in pregnancy when the potential benefits outweigh the possible risks. In animal studies, both the prodrug and active drug have been found distributed in breast milk. Caution is recommended if used in nursing mothers.

Zanamivir

Zanamivir is an inhalational **neuraminidase inhibitor active against both influenza A and B virus**.

Dosing and Administration

Zanamivir is given via two inhalations of dry powder (5 mg/inhalation for a total of 10 mg) q12h for the treatment of influenza A and B infection. A Rotadisk is loaded into the supplied plastic breath-activated Diskhaler inhalation device. One blister is pierced, and zanamivir is dispersed into the airstream created by inhalation of the patient. Each Rotadisk contains four blister packets of 5 mg and supplies enough medication for 1 day. Optimal response to therapy is seen when zanamivir is initiated **within 2 days of symptom onset**. No dosage adjustments are required in renal failure or dialysis.

Key Monitoring and Safety Information

In patients with underlying airway disease, **bronchospasm and allergic-like reactions** have been reported. As a result, caution should be used when zanamivir is used in patients with underlying airway diseases, such as asthma and chronic obstructive pulmonary disease. Patients with airway diseases should be instructed to have a fast-acting bronchodilator available when inhaling zanamivir and to discontinue use and contact their physician if they experience worsening respiratory symptoms.

REFERENCES

1. McEvoy GK, ed. *AHFS Drug Information, 2012.* Bethesda, MD: American Society of Health-System Pharmacists, Inc.; 2012.
2. PDR Network. Physicians' Desk Reference. 66th ed. Montvale, NJ: PDR Network; 2011.
3. Lexi-Drugs. Lexi-Comp, Inc. http://www.lexi.com/. Accessed May 22, 2012.
4. Brunton LL, Chabner BA, Knollmann, eds. *Goodman and Gilman's The Pharmacological Basis of Therapeutics.* 12th ed. New York, NY: McGraw-Hill; 2011.
5. Aronoff GR, Bennet WM, Berns JS, et al., eds. *Drug Prescribing in Renal Failure: Dosing Guidelines for Adults and Children.* 5th ed. Philadelphia, PA: American College of Physicians; 2007.
6. Treatment Guidelines from The Medical Letter. The Medical Letter, Inc. http://medicalletter.org/. Accessed May 22, 2012.

Index

Note: Locators following 'f' and 't' refer to figures and tables respectively.

CCS1012